ENDOCRINE
AND NONENDOCRINE
HORMONE-PRODUCING
TUMORS

Proceedings of the Annual Clinical Conferences on Cancer
sponsored by The University of Texas at Houston
M. D. Anderson Hospital and Tumor Institute,
and published by Year Book Medical Publishers, Inc.

TUMORS OF THE SKIN
TUMORS OF BONE AND SOFT TISSUE
RECENT ADVANCES IN THE DIAGNOSIS OF CANCER
CANCER OF THE GASTROINTESTINAL TRACT
CANCER OF THE UTERUS AND OVARY
NEOPLASIA IN CHILDHOOD
BREAST CANCER: EARLY AND LATE
LEUKEMIA-LYMPHOMA
REHABILITATION OF THE CANCER PATIENT
ENDOCRINE AND NONENDOCRINE HORMONE-PRODUCING
TUMORS

ENDOCRINE AND NONENDOCRINE HORMONE-PRODUCING TUMORS

A Collection of Papers Presented at the
Sixteenth Annual Clinical Conference on Cancer, 1971,
at The University of Texas at Houston
M. D. Anderson Hospital and Tumor Institute,
Houston, Texas

YEAR BOOK MEDICAL PUBLISHERS, INC.
35 East Wacker Drive, Chicago

Reprinted from

ENDOCRINE AND NONENDOCRINE
HORMONE-PRODUCING TUMORS

Copyright © 1973 by Year Book Medical Publishers, Inc.

Library of Congress Catalog Card Number: 73-77494
International Standard Book Number: 0-8151-0209-7

Acknowledgments

FOR THEIR SUPPORT in making possible both the Sixteenth Annual Clinical Conference and the publication of this monograph, the staff of The University of Texas at Houston M. D. Anderson Hospital and Tumor Institute gratefully acknowledges the assistance of the Texas Division of the American Cancer Society, the Division of Continuing Education of The University of Texas Graduate School of Biomedical Sciences at Houston, and the Regional Medical Program of the United States Public Health Service.

The program was arranged and organized by a committee composed of the following staff members of M. D. Anderson Hospital: Naguib A. Samaan, chairman; C. Stratton Hill, Jr., co-chairman; and members Raymond Alexanian, Emil Frei, III, Robert C. Hickey, Michael L. Ibanez, William V. Leary, Robert D. Lindberg, Felix N. Rutledge, Sidney Wallace, and Darrell N. Ward.

This volume was prepared for publication by the following members of the M. D. Anderson Hospital Department of Publications: R. W. Cumley, Joan E. McCay, Dorothy M. Beane, Susan Birkel Freitag, Carol Baxter, Susan Jane Baily, Elizabeth A. Klomp, Walter J. Pagel, Deborah D. Rylander, and Bonnie S. Somyak.

Many of the illustrations in this volume were prepared by members of the M. D. Anderson Hospital Department of Medical Communications.

Contents

ENDOCRINE
AND NONENDOCRINE
HORMONE-PRODUCING
TUMORS

Introduction

R. LEE CLARK, M.D., M.Sc., D.Sc. (Hon.)

*President, The University of Texas at Houston M. D. Anderson
Hospital and Tumor Institute, Houston, Texas*

DESIGNED AS A FORUM for the exchange of ideas and information about the
various clinical aspects of cancer diagnosis and treatment, the Annual
Clinical Conference on Cancer sponsored by The University of Texas at
Houston M. D. Anderson Hospital and Tumor Institute is open to Texas
physicians and all others who are interested in the most current developments on these specific topics.

Through the exchange of experiences and findings between staff members at M. D. Anderson Hospital and the distinguished guest lecturers
from cancer research and treatment centers throughout the country, the
interested clinician can continue broadening his education and enlarging
the scope of his knowledge. Although such an exchange of knowledge is
in itself highly rewarding to the physician, it is ultimately the cancer patient who benefits most from such a Conference. And that, after all, is the
true purpose of such a meeting.

Beginning in 1956, previous Clinical Conferences have dealt with many
subjects, including breast cancer, melanoma, childhood cancer, cancer of
the head and neck, rehabilitation of cancer patients, tumors of skin, cancer
chemotherapy, and others. This, the Sixteenth Annual Clinical Conference, is concerned with a subject which should be of great interest to the
cancer-oriented physician: endocrine and nonendocrine hormone-producing tumors.

Our thanks are extended to the Texas Division of the American Cancer
Society and to the United States Public Health Service for their assistance
in making this Clinical Conference possible.

The Heath Memorial Award

R. LEE CLARK, M.D., M.Sc., D.Sc. (Hon.)

*President, The University of Texas at Houston M. D. Anderson
Hospital and Tumor Institute, Houston, Texas*

ON THIS OCCASION, my University of Texas colleagues and I have mixed feelings of sadness and pride, a sense of loss and also of gain.

The feelings of sadness and loss result from the untimely death, in June 1971, of William Womack Heath. Mr. Heath and his wife, Mavis Barnett Heath, established this memorial award in remembrance of three of Mr. Heath's brothers.

William Heath was an exceptional individual. His life was dedicated to the service of his fellow man, and he chose many outlets for this dedication. His wife, Mavis, was a steady source of encouragement and support for his many activities throughout their 44-year marriage.

Mr. Heath interspersed his university education, acquired at Lon Morris Junior College, Texas Christian University, and The University of Texas Law School, with teaching in a one-room county school and as principal of a high school in Grimes County, Texas.

In 1924, at the age of 20, and before completion of law school, he was elected County Attorney and served two terms. In order to take the bar examination, it was necessary for him to appear in District Court following the election to have his disabilities as a minor removed. He served one term as County Judge, and then in 1933, at age 29, he was appointed Secretary of State by Governor Miriam Ferguson. Two years later, he became Assistant Attorney General in charge of state affairs and the insurance division. In 1937, he resigned to enter the private practice of law.

In 1957, he was appointed a member of the State Board of Hospitals and Special Schools to fill an unexpired term; during that time he was elected chairman of that board.

In 1959, he was appointed by the Governor to The University of Texas Board of Regents. From 1962 to 1967, he served two terms as Chairman of the Board. Mr. Heath responded to his extensive experiences with other individuals with personal growth and a broadened scope of understanding.

3

Over the years, he developed an almost limitless capacity for human sympathy.

Upon his resignation from The University of Texas Board of Regents, he was appointed United States Ambassador to Sweden by President Johnson. During this service, in 1968, he was named Distinguished University of Texas Alumnus.

Mr. Heath was a close personal friend of former President Johnson and was instrumental in having The University of Texas designated as the home of the Lyndon Baines Johnson Library. The State of Texas and the nation have lost a valuable citizen.

Mr. and Mrs. Heath originally established this memorial award six years ago to acknowledge an individual who has made "outstanding contributions to the better care of the cancer patient by the clinical application of basic cancer knowledge." The privilege of presenting this award occasions pride and appreciation for the significant medical gains contributed by the recipient, Dr. Jerome W. Conn, who will be introduced by Dr. Hickey.

Introduction of Heath Memorial Award Recipient

ROBERT C. HICKEY, M.D.

Director, The University of Texas at Houston M. D. Anderson
Hospital and Tumor Institute, Houston, Texas

DOCTOR JEROME W. CONN is a true academician who has served well his alma mater, the University of Michigan. He graduated as a Doctor of Medicine from the University of Michigan, and it is there that he performed his monumental works; this association spans 43 years.

Dr. Conn epitomizes the triad of purposes (namely service, research, and education) to which our own institution is dedicated. His life has been dedicated to excellence in laboratory science and to its practical application in two equally vital areas, at the patient's bedside and in teaching.

His outstanding abilities in all of these challenging areas are reflected in the many and varied awards he has received. He has been awarded both the Banting Medal and, in 1963, the Banting Memorial Award, presented by the American Diabetes Association for his contributions to better management of the diabetic patient. Such awards as the Claude Bernard Medal, the Phillips Memorial Award of the American College of Physicians, honorary fellowship in the American College of Surgeons, and the Career Research Award of the United States Public Health Service are all testimonies of deserved admiration from the nation's scientific community. He presently is a member of many national committees and boards for the U. S. Government, and serves on the World Health Organization Panel of Experts on Degenerative Diseases.

At home in Ann Arbor, a true test, Dr. Conn was chosen "the outstanding faculty member" of the entire University of Michigan faculty in 1961 and awarded the Henry Russel Lectureship. Again, in 1968, the University Board of Regents awarded him a Distinguished University Professorship in the name of Louis Harry Newburgh. Dr. Newburgh was the school's first Professor of Clinical Investigation, and it was in his laboratory, in 1935, that Dr. Conn began his lifelong venture of studying the human endocrine system.

Although Dr. Newburgh's laboratory was then concentrating on the causes and control of obesity and of fluid and electrolyte balance, Dr. Conn developed an early intense interest in the search for diabetogenic substances in patients with insulinomas and for the etiologies of hypoglycemia.

Dr. Conn has made major contributions in the detection and management of pancreatic, adrenal, and pituitary tumors and also has developed a method for early detection of diabetes. His work on diabetes mellitus and its relation to cancer opened new pathways for cancer research.

The two major areas of Dr. Conn's investigations are: (1) adrenal cortical function and its relation to electrolyte metabolism and to the physiology of the renin-angiotensin-aldosterone system and of hypertension (referred to as "The Big Discovery" by his colleagues) and (2) carbohydrate metabolism in the prediabetic state, especially in the clinical states producing hypoglycemia and the conditions resulting in loss of carbohydrate tolerance.

The description of a new clinical syndrome, primary aldosteronism (Conn's syndrome), was published by Dr. Conn in 1955, but the preliminary work that led to this delineation was begun in 1943. At this time, Dr. Conn organized and was made Chief of the Section of Endocrinology and Metabolism at the University of Michigan Medical School, one of the first sections of its kind in the United States. This same year, Dr. Conn and his co-workers participated in a study to determine why American troops could not acclimate rapidly to jungle temperatures. Their findings revealed a substance (later identified as aldosterone in 1953) secreted by the adrenal glands that lowered the sodium content of sweat and urine. The kidneys eventually were able to "escape" from the intense salt-saving activity of this hormone, allowing for sodium homeostasis and shielding of the soldier from excessive loss of salt in his sweat. The salt pills routinely given to the American troops were slowing down this adaptive process. The problem was solved by withholding salt tablets on board ships en route to the tropics and acclimatizing the soldiers with mild exercise.

In 1954, Dr. Conn saw a hypertensive patient with low sodium content in her sweat and hypothesized that the patient was secreting excessive amounts of aldosterone and, therefore, might have an adrenal tumor. After eight months of exhaustive balance studies, surgical removal of the adrenal gland containing the tumor confirmed the hypothesis and eliminated the hypertension in this patient.

Much work has since been done on primary aldosteronism, which is almost always caused by adrenal cortical adenoma. Because the current tests for the screening of hypertensive individuals are very complex, Dr. Conn and his colleagues have been searching for simpler methods of tumor detection. The exact prevalence of adenoma- or tumor-induced hypertension is not yet known, but it is thought to be about seven to eight per cent of the total number of hypertensive cases. Occasionally, primary aldosteronism is secondary to adrenal carcinoma or hyperplasia; on rare occasions, it occurs in the absence of any adrenal histologic changes detectable by light microscopy.

Until now, the two most successful approaches to detection of primary aldosteronism have been adrenal venography, which has been about 80 per cent effective, and direct adrenal venous plasma analysis, which can detect a twofold increase of aldosterone secretion on the involved side.

Dr. Conn's accomplishments are reflected in the long list of his awards and honors, in approximately 350 published articles, in contributions to 17 books on hypertension, metabolism, and endocrinology, and in his reputation as a superior teacher and lecturer. Regarding these latter talents, I quote from a 1968 issue of the *University of Michigan Medical Center Journal:* Dr. Conn's "subjects are usually complicated. Yet he speaks with such clarity, in beautifully constructed sentences . . . that the listener is carried along with his topic, through the labyrinth of the subject to the completion of the lecture." And, in his role "as frequent honorary lecturer to learned gatherings around the world, the splendid impression he leaves as a diplomat and representative of the best in medicine . . . is a force for goodwill in these troubled times."

Dr. Conn honors us by his presence, and certainly we are truly proud to join the ranks of those around the world who have honored Dr. Conn and who have had the opportunity to learn from him.

THE HEATH MEMORIAL LECTURE

Visualization of Adrenal Abnormalities by Photoscanning after Administration of Radiocholesterol

J. W. CONN, M.D., W. H. BEIERWALTES, M.D.,
E. L. COHEN, M.D., R. MORITA, M.D.,
A. N. ANSARI, M.D., AND K. R. HERWIG, M.D.

Departments of Internal Medicine and Surgery,
University of Michigan Medical School, Ann Arbor Michigan

THE MATERIAL that I have chosen to present is new and largely unknown, although recent reports have appeared (Conn *et al.,* 1971a and b; Lieberman *et al.,* 1971; Morita *et al.,* 1972). It, of course, has been known for many years that the adrenal gland not only is very high in its content of cholesterol but that it uses this compound as a precursor in its biosynthesis of steroidal hormones. It is capable of synthesizing cholesterol *de novo* from acetate, but it also uses preformed cholesterol from the blood stream. For these reasons, a number of investigators in the recent past have worked on the possibility that a radioactive form of cholesterol might be sufficiently concentrated in the adrenal cortex to make photoscanning of that organ possible.

The first practical approach to this goal was realized when Dr. Raymond E. Counsell (1970), at the University of Michigan, synthesized a stable cholesterol compound with a stable iodine molecule substituted at the 19 position. Various degrees of radioactivity of the compound could then be achieved by isotope exchange with either ^{125}I or [131]I. It was then quickly shown in dogs (Counsell *et al.,* 1970) and in man (Beierwaltes *et al.,* 1971) with the use of [131]I-19-iodocholesterol (1) that there occurred sufficient concentration of radioactivity in the adrenal glands for photoscanning, (2) that soon after injection, the adrenal cortex to liver and the

9

adrenal cortex to kidney concentration ratios were 30, and (3) that by eight days after injection, the ratios exceeded 100.

Since then, my Endocrinology group, in collaboration with our Division of Nuclear Medicine, headed by Dr. William Beierwaltes, has been exploring a number of clinical states associated with abnormalities of the adrenal cortex. I shall present some of the exciting findings that we have observed to date.

Briefly, the technique that has been employed so far is as follows: A tracer dose of ^{131}I-19-iodocholesterol in 1 to 20 mg. of synthetic 19-iodocholesterol is injected intravenously, the thyroid gland being protected by administration of five drops of Lugol's solution twice daily. Total radioactivity injected has been between 0.6 and 2 mc. Scanning by means of a computer-assisted Anger gamma camera is done four to six days, and again eight to ten days, after administration of the radioactive material. In addition, however, we (Morita *et al.*, 1972) have described a method for estimating the percentage uptake of administered radioactivity by each adrenal gland. Thus, we have not only a visual image but a confirmatory numerical expression as well.

Results

Figure 1 shows the chemical configuration of ^{131}I-19-iodocholesterol. For purposes of orientation, Figure 2 shows the Anger camera image of both adrenal glands as they appear normally. The two light spots in the center are images of the left and right adrenal glands. Because these are all posterior view photographs, the left center spot is the left adrenal gland. The increased radioactivity observed at the periphery on the right side is from liver, and the lower peripheral activity is from bowel.

It is well established that the two steroids of major physiological importance released from the adrenal glands are cortisol and aldosterone. The adrenal cortex can also make androgenic and estrogenic compounds. Under pathological conditions, this can result in feminizing and masculinizing syndromes. Time has not yet permitted us to evaluate these rarer conditions by radiocholesterol scanning; we have, however, looked carefully at cortisolism and aldosteronism.

Cushing's Syndrome

Excessive production of cortisol produces characteristic physical changes which the experienced clinician can recognize even in the early stages. Eighty-five per cent of the cases are caused by excessive and inappropriate

^{131} I-19-IODOCHOLESTEROL

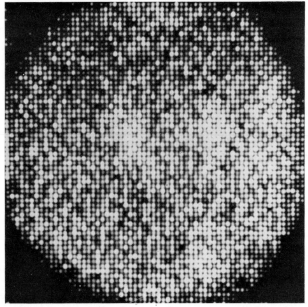

(19-iodocholest-5-ene-3β-ol-^{131}I)

FIG. 1 (*top*).—See text.
FIG. 2 (*bottom*).—Anger camera scan of normal adrenals (posterior view) (see text).

secretion of adrenocorticotropin (ACTH) from the anterior pituitary gland, which induces bilateral adrenal hyperplasia. The remaining cases are the result of adrenal cortical tumor (adenoma or carcinoma), and a few result from the production of an ACTH-like compound produced by tumors of nonendocrine origin. This also induces bilateral adrenal hyperplasia. The distinction between adrenal tumor and hyperplasia has rested upon the relative suppressibility of cortisol production with large doses of dexamethasone, since tumors are not suppressible and bilateral adrenal hyperplasia is partially suppressible. Photoscanning after radiocholesterol gives a rapid visual solution to many of these problems.

Figure 3, the scan of an 18-year-old girl with nonsuppressible Cushing's syndrome, shows a large right adrenal shadow with heavy uptake of radioactivity and no uptake on the contralateral side. This, of course, represents atrophy of the contralateral gland because of suppression of ACTH by the tumor.

Figure 4 shows the 3½-cm. adenoma removed from this patient. In this connection, it is of interest that in the two patients with adrenal carcinoma scanned to date, uptake of radioactivity did not occur. Thus, while our experience is small, it suggests that a patient with Cushing's syndrome who shows little or no uptake of radioactivity by either gland may have a carcinoma in one of them.

Conversely, a scan of the usual variety of Cushing's syndrome, which is caused by excessive ACTH stimulation of both adrenal glands, shows (Fig. 5) two large adrenal glands that stand out like headlights. The scan on the left is before dexamethasone, and that on the right is after three days of dexamethasone, 8 mg. per day. With this amount of dexamethasone, this patient did suppress 17-hydroxycorticosteroid excretion to below 50 per cent of base line values, which usually means bilateral hyperplasia. It is evident, however, that this amount of suppression did not decrease adrenal uptake of radiocholesterol. Thus, in a patient with Cushing's syndrome, the visualization of two headlamps means hyperplasia. One headlamp with contralateral suppression means adenoma, and lack of bilateral uptake of radioactivity probably means carcinoma.

There is another place where the radiocholesterol test can play a unique function. In these days of total bilateral adrenalectomy for Cushing's syndrome, it is not unusual to observe regression of the disease for a year or two, followed by its recrudescence. This means either that a small fragment of adrenal tissue was inadvertently left in the patient, or that an accessory adrenal has blown up in response to heavy ACTH stimulation. We believe that the former explanation is more likely because we have now scanned four patients of this kind, and in all four, the remnant was

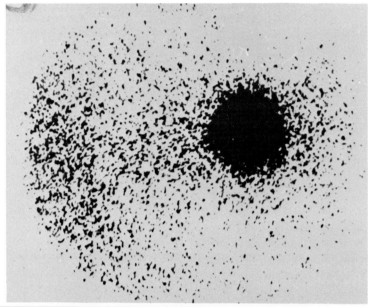

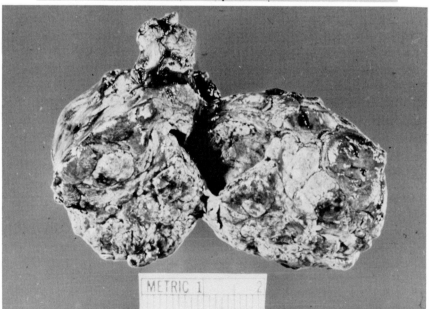

FIG. 3 (*top*).—Right adrenal tumors as shown by radiocholesterol scan of patient with Cushing's syndrome (posterior views).

FIG. 4 (*bottom*).—Adrenal tumor which was excised from patient whose scan is shown in Figure 3.

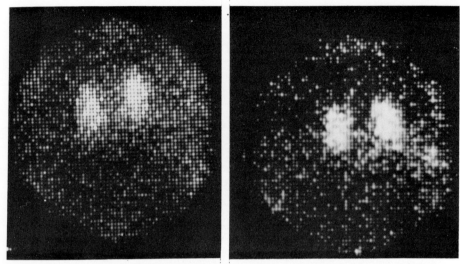

FIG. 5.—Scan from patient with Cushing's syndrome caused by bilateral hyperplasia before and after dexamethasone (see text).

FIG. 6.—Scan from patient with recurrent Cushing's syndrome 10 years after "total" bilateral adrenalectomy. Radioactivity shows the position of the hyperplastic remnant.

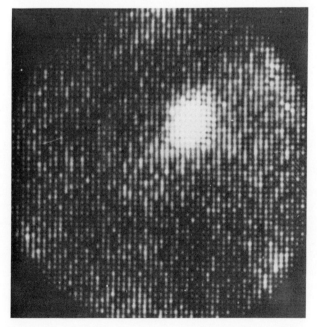

localized in the right side. This is the more difficult side for the surgeon, since he must peel off the last remnant of adrenal tissue close to the inferior vena cava.

Figure 6 shows an example of this. "Total" bilateral adrenalectomy took place in our hospital 10 years ago. Recurrence of Cushing's syndrome was obvious three years later. Reoperation disclosed much scar tissue but no adrenal remnant, and Cushing's syndrome persisted. Treatment for the next seven years has been with ortho-p'-DDD and aminoglutethimide with only moderate success. The scan on this patient indicates where the surgeon must look for the remnant.

Primary Aldosteronism

In primary aldosteronism, we have a different set of facts with which to contend. The clinical diagnosis is much less evident. In another paper (see pages 213 to 223, this volume), I shall discuss the clinical and biochemical manifestations of primary aldosteronism in detail. It is sufficient to say now that the basic diagnostic criteria consist of overproduction of aldosterone, subnormal plasma renin activity, and normal cortisol production. In contrast to Cushing's syndrome, where tumor is a minor cause, 85 per cent of patients satisfying the criteria for primary aldosteronism have tumors, while only 15 per cent have bilateral hyperplasia; the mechanism by which this form of hyperplasia is produced is unknown. There are at present no testing procedures by which a preoperative distinction can be made between tumor and hyperplasia. A computerized system, called Quadric Analysis, has been devised by Ferris and his colleagues (1970) for predicting preoperatively which will be found at operation, but there has been insufficient experience with this method to date.

The second fact to be considered is that aldosterone-producing tumors are characteristically small, 75 per cent measuring 8 to 20 mm. in diameter. Because of their small size and relative avascularity, conventional methods such as nephrotomography, retroperitoneal pneumography, and arteriography rarely detect these tumors.

In previous communications, we (Conn et al., 1969, 1971b) have pointed out the important advantages to both the surgeon and the patient of being able, in cases of primary aldosteronism, to localize the side of the tumor preoperatively. Since more than 90 per cent of aldosterone-producing tumors are unilateral, identification of a tumor on one side (1) provides a better than 90 per cent chance that it is the only side involved, (2) allows for much less extensive surgical procedure (unilateral posterior operation), and (3) minimizes the possibility of bilateral hyperplasia. Thus, we have concentrated our efforts on methods that would give us a preoperative indication of which adrenal gland contains the tumor.

Since 1968, we have been highly successful with selective adrenal venography for tumor identification and have visualized aldosterone-producing tumors in 32 (84 per cent) of 38 tumor-bearing glands. There are, however, several disadvantages inherent in the procedure of adrenal venography. First, it requires that someone be highly skilled in the techniques of adrenal vein catheterization. Second, one occasionally ruptures tiny medullary vessels in the course of the procedure and can observe extravasation of contrast material under the fluoroscope as it occurs. Usually, small extravasations result only in a transient episode of back pain. If, however, intra-adrenal bleeding should continue, it can result in complete loss of the involved gland, and if bilateral, it results in acute, followed by chronic, adrenal cortical insufficiency. Let us assume, however, that in the course of diagnostic adrenal venography which turns out to be negative, extravasation of contrast material is observed in one side only. How would we ever know the ultimate outcome of that single gland? If it had been destroyed, the contralateral gland would take over its function, and apart from a pain in the back for two or three days, the patient would apparently recover completely. I called back for the radioactivity test just such a patient who had had severe left back pain after venography two years previously. Figure 7 shows the computer-assisted Anger camera picture which gives an image of the right adrenal gland but shows complete absence of the left adrenal gland.

The disadvantages of adrenal venography then are: (1) the need for an expert with a catheter, (2) the occasional intra-adrenal hemorrhages which are produced, (3) it may be impossible to enter one or both of the adrenal veins with a catheter, and (4) about five per cent of patients who present a good indication for adrenal venography give a history of previously having had alarming reactions to administration of contrast media, a clear contraindication to adrenal venography.

The other current technique for preoperative localization of aldosterone-producing tumors consists of determination of aldosterone concentrations in adrenal venous blood, again obtained by catheterization of the adrenal veins. We have done many such determinations and are convinced that some errors are inevitable because it is not possible to be certain that the blood draining through the catheter is wholly of adrenal origin. Melby and his associates (1967) seem to have been more successful in this respect. In any case, this approach to lateralization of the tumor requires a similar degree of expertise with the catheter and, even in the best hands, it frequently is impossible to catheterize one of the adrenal veins, particularly the right one.

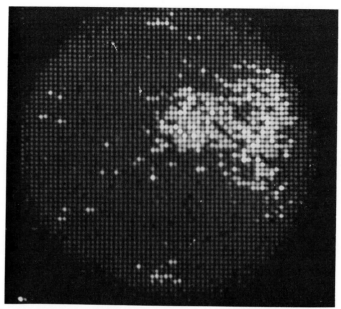

Fig. 7.—Scan from patient two years after extravasation of contrast medium in left adrenal during venography. The left gland takes up no radioactivity. The radioactivity in the right peripheral field is in liver.

I should like to present two typical examples of what we have found with the use of radiocholesterol in four consecutive cases of primary aldosteronism with tumor. I shall also present the findings in one case of "idiopathic" aldosteronism (bilateral hyperplasia), which was unique in that one adrenal was twice as large as the other, although both showed definite hyperplasia of the zona glomerulosa.

Figure 8 shows a scan of a patient with a right-sided aldosterone-producing tumor. It is clear that there is increased concentration of radioactivity within the right adrenal area. It also shows the right-sided tumor as depicted in the right venogram (the venograms are anterior views). Figure 9 shows the tumor itself, which is about 20 mm. in its longest dimension.

Figure 10 is the scan of a patient with a left-sided aldosterone-producing tumor. It shows concentration of radioactivity in the left adrenal gland; the left-sided venogram shows the tumor as well. Figure 11 shows the 20-mm. tumor removed at the time of operation.

Figure 12 shows the scan of a patient with bilateral hyperplasia. The right adrenal gland was almost twice as large as the left. It is of interest that the concentration of radioactivity in the larger adrenal gland is evenly

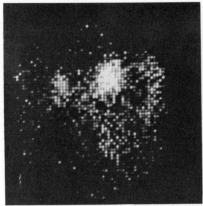
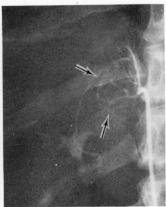
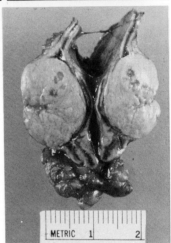

FIG. 8 (*top*).—Primary aldosteronism with right adrenal tumor. Comparison of scan and venogram.

FIG. 9 (*right*).—Tumor removed from patient shown in Figure 8.

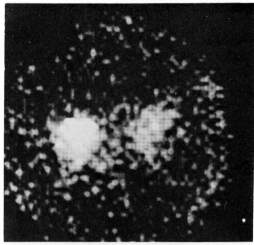
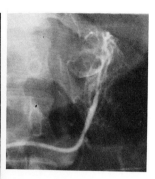

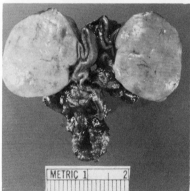

FIG. 10 (*top*).—Primary aldosteronism with left adrenal tumor. Comparison of scan and venogram.

FIG. 11 (*left*).—Tumor removed from patient shown in Figure 10.

dispersed, rather than concentrated. It was not possible to do an adrenal venogram on this patient because she previously had collapsed and had laryngeal edema upon administration of contrast medium for pyelography. On the basis of the scan, our preoperative diagnosis was right-sided adrenal tumor.

Special Studies

Special studies were conducted on three patients to test the versatility of the radiocholesterol testing procedure. The first of these was to repeat the whole scanning procedure after the tumor had been removed. The left side of Figure 13 was taken preoperatively and shows the tumor in the

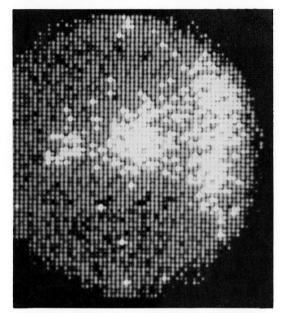

Fig. 12.—"Idiopathic" aldosteronism (see text).

Fig. 13.—Special study. Comparison of scans before and after removal of right adrenal tumor in primary aldosteronism.

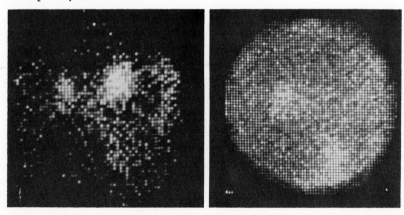

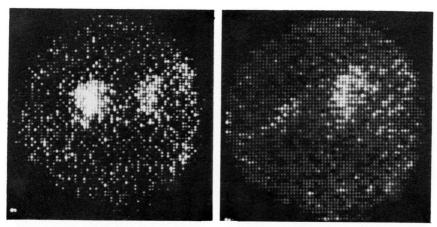

FIG. 14.—Special study. Comparison of scans before and after removal of left adrenal tumor in primary aldosteronism.

FIG. 15.—Special study. Preoperative comparison of Anger camera image before (*left panel*) and after dexamethasone administration (*right panel*) in primary aldosteronism (tumor). Note (*right panel*) that the tumor image persists while the left gland no longer takes up radioactivity.

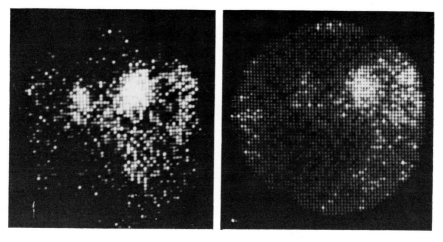

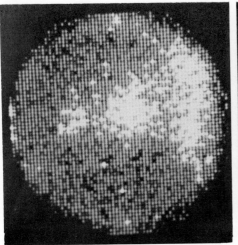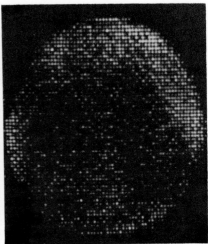

FIG. 16.—Special study. Preoperative comparison of Anger camera image before (*left panel*) and after dexamethasone administration (*right panel*) in "idiopathic" aldosteronism (bilateral hyperplasia). Note (*right panel*) complete suppression of uptake of radioactivity by both adrenal glands.

right adrenal gland; the scan on the right was taken three days after operation. It shows no radioactivity on the side from which the tumor was removed, but one does see the remaining left adrenal gland.

Similarly, Figure 14 compares the preoperative scan (left) showing the left-sided adrenal tumor with the repeated scan 83 days after removal of the left-sided tumor. The tumor is gone and there is small residual activity in the one third of the gland that was allowed to remain in the patient when the tumor was removed. The right side has increased its radioactivity slightly, probably in compensation for the small remnant on the left. Thus, after seeing the postoperative scans, one's confidence in the procedure increases rapidly.

Preoperatively, we chose for special study two cases (Figs. 8 and 12). We administered dexamethasone, 2 mg. per day, for three days before repeating the radiocholesterol test. The idea was that we might suppress the uptake of radioactivity by normal adrenal tissue and make the tumor stand out in bold relief.

Figure 15 compares the scans of the tumor patient before and after dexamethasone, both in the preoperative period. On the right, after dexamethasone, the image of the normal left adrenal has essentially disappeared, but the tumorous right gland has taken up a large amount of cholesterol.

Conversely (Fig. 16), in the patient who proved at operation to have "idiopathic" aldosteronism and two large hyperplastic adrenals, the images of both glands have disappeared, despite the fact that the right gland had originally taken up twice as much radioactivity as the left.

Summary

It is clear from what you have seen that in the case of Cushing's syndrome, the technique of photoscanning after administration of radiocholesterol can easily aid one in distinguishing between adenoma and bilateral hyperplasia and, with further experience, may aid in distinguishing adenoma from carcinoma. The technique also delineates the absence of a functioning adrenal gland, either functionally suppressed, destroyed, or removed.

The ability to visualize the characteristically small aldosterone-producing tumor, following a simple intravenous injection of a tracer dose of radiocholesterol, eliminates the important disadvantages inherent in adrenal vein catheterization. The results, while encompassing only a total of four consecutive cases of aldosterone-producing tumor, indicate that so far radiocholesterol has been just as effective as adrenal venography in lateralizing the tumor. While venography provides better circumscription of the tumor, the major objective is to determine the side of the lesion, and this can be accomplished by the simpler technique.

The dramatic postoperative disappearance from the Anger camera picture of the image of the tumorous gland, together with the precipitous decrease of uptake of radioactivity on that side, provides clear evidence that this new technique will acquire many functions.

In addition, it now seems possible that a positive distinction can be made preoperatively between primary aldosteronism (tumor) and "idiopathic" aldosteronism (bilateral hyperplasia), although we have studied this in only one patient with each type of syndrome. By combining dexamethasone suppression with adrenal photoscanning, uptake of radioactivity was inhibited bilaterally in "idiopathic" aldosteronism, while in primary aldosteronism it was inhibited only in the gland contralateral to the tumor. These results with dexamethasone suppression must be viewed with caution because the data are sparse, but they provide the possibility of preoperative determination of the anatomical diagnosis. Of particular interest are the contrasting results obtained in the two forms of bilateral adrenal hyperplasia. In the ACTH-dependent hyperplasia of Cushing's syndrome, no decrease of adrenal uptake of radioactivity was observed after large doses of dexamethasone, while small doses completely eradicated uptake of radioactivity in the bilateral hyperplasia of "idiopathic" aldosteronism. This technique may thus provide a new approach to the study of the pathophysiology of some adrenal disorders.

Acknowledgments

Supported in part by U. S. Public Health Service Grant AM10257; U. S. Public Health Service Training Grant AM05001; 5MO1-FR-4204, Division of Research Facilities and Resources; U. S. Public Health Service Training Grant CA-05134-09; and Atomic Energy Commission Contract AT (11-2) 2031.

REFERENCES

Beierwaltes, W. H., Lieberman, L. M., Ansari, A. N., and Nishiyama, H.: Visualization of human adrenal glands in vivo by scintillation scanning. *Journal of the American Medical Association*, 216:275-277, April 12, 1971.

Conn, J. W., Beierwaltes, W. H., Lieberman, L. M., Ansari, A. N., Cohen, E. L., Bookstein, J. J., and Herwig, K. R.: Primary aldosteronism: Preoperative tumor visualization by scintillation scanning. *Journal of Clinical Endocrinology and Metabolism*, 33:713-716, October, 1971a.

Conn, J. W., Morita, R., Cohen, E. L., Beierwaltes, W. H., McDonald, W. J., and Herwig, K. R.: Primary aldosteronism: Photoscanning of tumors after [131]I-19-iodocholesterol. *Archives of Internal Medicine*, 129:417-425, March, 1971b.

Conn, J. W., Rovner, D. R., Cohen, E. L., Bookstein, J. J., Cerny, J. C., and Lucas, C. P.: Preoperative diagnosis of primary aldosteronism. *Archives of Internal Medicine*, 123:113-123, February 1969.

Counsell, R. E., Ranade, V. V., Blair, R. J., Beierwaltes, W. H., and Weinhold, P. A.: Tumor localizing agents. IX. Radioiodinated cholesterol. *Steroids*, 16: 317-328, September 1970.

Ferris, J. B., Brown, J. J., Fraser, R., Kay, A. W., Neville, A. M., O'Muircheartaigh, I. G., Robertson, J. I. S., Symington, T., and Lever, A. F.: Hypertension with aldosterone excess and low plasma-renin: Preoperative distinction between patients with and without adrenocortical tumor. *The Lancet*, 2:995-1000, November 14, 1970.

Lieberman, L. M., Beierwaltes, W. H., Conn, J. W., Ansari, A. N., and Nishiyama, H.: Diagnosis of adrenal disease by visualization of human adrenal glands with [131]I-19-iodocholesterol. *The New England Journal of Medicine*, 285:1387-1393, December 16, 1971.

Melby, J. C., Spark, R. F., Dale, S. L., Egdahl, R. H., and Kahn, P. C.: Diagnosis and localization of aldosterone-producing adenomas by adrenal-vein catheterization. *The New England Journal of Medicine*, 277:1050-1056, 1967.

Morita, R., Leiberman, L. M., Beierwaltes, W. H., Conn, J. W., Ansari, A. N., and Nishiyama, H.: Percent uptake ^{131}I radioactivity in the adrenal from radioiodinated cholesterol. *Journal of Clinical Endocrinology and Metabolism*, 34: 36-43, January 1972.

Clinical Investigation Program of the American Cancer Society

A. HAMBLIN LETTON, M.D., F.A.C.S.*

Georgia Baptist Hospital, Atlanta, Georgia

To UNDERSTAND the present Clinical Investigation Program of the American Cancer Society, that portion of the research program which is clinically oriented, it is necessary to review the development of the Society's research program.

The Society has been interested in research since its inception. Shortly after the Society was founded in 1913 (then called the American Society for the Control of Cancer), a Committee on Statistics was established to conduct epidemiological research. This committee collected convincing evidence that some cancer patients could be cured if treated early enough— a revolutionary concept at the time. This disclosure was influential in changing the then prevailing attitude of hopelessness about cancer.

The Society recognized that the future control of cancer requires answers that only research could provide. Since they believed that this research would be of such a magnitude that the finances of the Society could not support it, they brought influence to bear on the Congress and the Administration to support this research. It was through the continued efforts of the American Cancer Society that the National Cancer Institute (the first of the Institutes of Health) was established by President Roosevelt in 1935.

Later, the Society established a section on Epidemiology and Statistics. Epidemiology is the only area, even today, in which the Society conducts scientific research. It was this section that conducted the Hammond-Horn studies of 1952-1955 which established a definite causal relationship between cigarette smoking and lung cancer. This section was also responsible for developing the Cancer Prevention Study, an investigation of environmental, demographic, and medical factors significant to the onset of cancer.

---

*President, American Cancer Society, Inc.

Initiated in 1960, this investigation has obtained information from more than 1,000,000 participants. The analysis and collection of these data are continuing.

In 1945, the Society decided to expand the scope of its work, and added research support to its programs of education and service. This decision was based on a growing recognition of the cancer problem, a problem which created the need for a driving force that would stimulate and encourage the development of cancer research and help to raise money to finance it. It was clear that in addition to governmental involvement, voluntary effort was essential and that the American Cancer Society, by assuming this responsibility, could complement the government's activities and join with it to provide a broad and balanced program of cancer research support. So in 1945, the Society asked the National Research Council to act, under contract, as its advisory agent on research. The Council, by establishing a Committee on Growth within its Division of Medical Sciences, served the Society by reviewing applications for research and personnel grants and by keeping it informed of significant developments in cancer research.

In 1947, the Society broadened its research support activities, adding Institutional Research Grants to help provide urgently needed facilities for cancer research in the medical schools and other research institutions. These institutional grants were administered within the Society's National Office rather than by the National Research Council. The Society's program continued to expand, and by 1955, it had grown so much in size and complexity that the Society's Board of Directors decided to dissolve the arrangement with the National Research Council and to consolidate all of its research activities within the National Office. This had taken effect by early 1957.

Between 1957 and 1966, two important changes were made. First, the range of personnel grants, limited originally to postdoctoral fellowships, was expanded to include other categories of training and research. Second, the Institutional Research Grant Program, designed originally to stimulate the development of cancer research facilities in the large universities and institutes, was expanded to include a broader range of educational and research centers. In 1966, the Research Program of the Society was examined again and a Council on Projection and Analysis was added. This was in response to an analysis of the Research Program by a group of experts, including Dr. Richard Shope of the Rockefeller Institute, who concluded his recommendations with the plea, "The time has now arrived when intelligent direction and leadership will have to be introduced into cancer research to assure that we hew to the line of fixing our objectives of solving human cancer problems more closely than in the past."

Since its inception, the Research Program of the Society has responded to changing times and new requirements and has been under constant review. It has broadened its programs, reorganized its scientific advisory committees, and developed new ones to meet new needs. It is not difficult, therefore, to understand the action of the Board of Directors, under the leadership of its president, Dr. Sidney Farber, in establishing a Clinical Investigation Program in 1969. This was done to accomplish the goal of speeding to the patient the benefits of current research. The Society was not alone in recognizing that much of the research it was supporting was allowing the discovery of more and more about cancer in mice but not enough about cancer in man. This is the same kind of frustration that comes from the expectation of "breakthroughs" following the striking advances of the 1940's and 1950's in chemotherapy and hormone therapy which failed to develop into curative therapy. Following each lead took the researchers deeper and deeper into the cell and further and further away from the bedside.

To emphasize the new direction sought and to stimulate research using the patient as the experimental model, the Society announced its Clinical Investigation Program. The principal purpose of the program was to speed the application of information derived from research to the patient with cancer and to add to our knowledge of cancer by studying the patient. This program added a new dimension to the Research Program of the Society in seeking, stimulating, and supporting applicatory and developmental projects in the prevention, diagnosis and management of cancer in man. This active role was a natural progression toward development of projection functions coming from the Council on Projection and Analysis, formed in 1966.

To add to its identity as a patient-oriented program, it was originally placed in the Medical Affairs Department rather than the Research Department and was administered by a staff officer who was clinically skilled and oriented toward the management of cancer in the patient. A separate Scientific Advisory Committee, consisting entirely of specialists in the major disciplines related to cancer in human beings, was established.

Under the Clinical Investigation Program, $643,500 was awarded to 18 grantees in fiscal year 1969; $1,554,797 was awarded to 32 grantees in fiscal year 1970. In addition to supporting clinical studies through this mechanism, it is emphasized that the American Cancer Society provided considerable support for clinically oriented studies through grants administered by the Research Department. For example, in fiscal year 1970, of the $19.1 million awarded through the Research Department, $2.9 million supported studies concerned partially or wholly with "cancer chemotherapy." This included fundamental and applied work such as basic pharma-cology, toxicology, and animal and human studies. In the same year, ap-proximately $2 million was granted for the support of fundamental and applied studies in radiobiology and radiotherapy, and another $1.6 million was awarded for the support of surgical, other therapeutic and diagnostic studies.

It was recognized from the first that clinical investigation is in fact re-search. So, in November 1970, the Clinical Investigation Program was in-corporated into the general research program. However, the identity of this clinical research program has been maintained to give it emphasis, and grant requests for the support of clinical studies are referred to the Clinical Investigation Scientific Advisory Committee for review and evaluation. Other proposals concerned with preclinical aspects are reviewed by addi-tional committees such as Immunology and Chemotherapy, Epidemiology, Diagnosis and Therapy, *etc.* For example, in fiscal year 1971, 69 grant appli-cations were reviewed by the Clinical Investigation Committee, and an additional 34 clinically oriented studies were reviewed by other commit-tees. Since clinical research very often necessitates a team approach involv-ing basic science and clinical disciplines simultaneously, our Scientific Advisory Committee for Clinical Investigation has suggested that their re-views would be more effective if these disciplines were represented on the Committee. We have acted on this suggestion by appointing a clinical in-vestigator with extensive experience in basic immunology.

At this time, we have no plans to change our support of research if and when the Conquest of Cancer legislation comes into being. In fact, we be-lieve that we will be called upon even more heavily in the future when this program develops. I do, however, expect to see an increase in our emphasis on the patient, his family, and their problems. I am hoping there will be an increase in public and professional education activities, as well as in service and rehabilitation. We must utilize the information from the research lab-oratory when it is of greatest benefit to the patient. This means education of the public to seek such information and education of the professional to apply it. We must help the victims of cancer to overcome their disabilities. You will remember from St. Matthew, Our Master is quoted as having said, "For what is a man profited if he shall gain the whole world and lose his own soul?" We might paraphrase that: "What is a man profited if we cure him of cancer and he loses his ability to live?" We must, through our service and rehabilitation activities assure quality of survival. I repeat to you. that we have no plans at the present time to change our support of the research portion of the American Cancer Society.

As a volunteer health organization, we plan to carry out the role that the

National Institutes of Health delineated so clearly: "Their concern (that is, the volunteer health agencies) will lead them into new areas of research. both clinical and basic; their desire to enlist the best scientific minds in the fight against disease will lead them to support the work of young scientists at the beginning of their careers, as well as the work of the seasoned investigators; and the flexibility of their organizations will enable them to blaze new trails with the minimum of delay. It may also be expected that continued, active involvement with research will further strengthen the role that the American Cancer Society is uniquely suited to play, that of preparing the way for the fullest utilization of the new knowledge that research will yield."

Pituitary Syndromes

O. H. PEARSON, M.D.

*Department of Medicine, Case Western Reserve University
School of Medicine, Cleveland, Ohio*

Six anterior pituitary hormones have been isolated and identified, and methods for the precise measurement of these hormone levels in blood have been developed. Clinical evidence of hypersecretion of four pituitary hormones has been recognized in association with pituitary neoplasms. As yet, no instance of a pituitary neoplasm associated with hypersecretion of gonadotrophins—follicle stimulating hormone (FSH) and luteinizing hormone (LH)—has been reported. Some of the clinical features of the hormone-producing pituitary tumors will be reviewed.

Hypersecretion of Growth Hormone (HGH)

HGH hypersecretion produces gigantism (proportionate growth) in children and acromegaly (disproportionate growth) in adults and usually is associated with an acidophilic or chromophobe adenoma of the pituitary. In adults, there is enlargement of the skeleton, especially of the skull, of the hands and feet, and also thickening of the skin, subcutaneous tissue, and viscera. Initially, growth of the head, hands, and feet may call attention to the disorder because of increasing size of hat, gloves, or shoes. The progressive facial and acral changes are often so gradual that the patient, family, or friends may not recognize the changes until they are well advanced. The fully developed condition produces a grotesque appearance of the face which is readily recognized.

The face appears massive and coarse, and the lips and the nose are large and thick. The supraorbital ridges bulge, the lower jaw protrudes, the teeth may become separated, and malocclusion frequently occurs. The skin and subcutaneous tissues become thick and spongy. The larynx and sinuses enlarge, and the voice develops a peculiar resonance and cavernous quality. The tongue is enlarged, and the speech may be thick. The hair tends to be

31

coarse. Hirsutism of the face, body, and extremities is frequently seen in women. The hands and feet become thick and broad.

Associated disturbances commonly seen in acromegaly are hypermetabolism (not hyperthyroidism), hyperhidrosis, impaired glucose tolerance or clinical diabetes mellitus, hypogonadism, arthritic complaints, and paresthesias of the hands (carpel-tunnel syndrome). Manifestations associated with the presence of a pituitary tumor are headache, visual impairment, and enlargement of the sella turcica. The course of the disease often is insidiously progressive, and late manifestations consist of progressive muscular weakness, degenerative bone disease, hypertension, coronary artery disease, and cerebral arteriosclerosis.

Diagnosis is usually suspected from the appearance of the patient and is confirmed by measurement of plasma HGH levels. Elevated plasma HGH levels which are not suppressed after administration of glucose are pathognomonic of acromegaly. Provocative tests usually demonstrate autonomous secretion of HGH, although paradoxical responses frequently are seen after glucose, arginine, or insulin administration, suggesting that some hypothalamic control over HGH secretion by the tumor is maintained.

Treatment for acromegaly remains a problem for a number of patients with this disorder. When plasma HGH measurements became available, it was apparent that conventional radiation therapy of the pituitary failed to restore HGH levels to normal in many patients. Roth, Gorden, and Brace (1970) restudied the use of conventional radiation therapy and found that 4,000 R of cobalt therapy directed to the pituitary produces significant lowering of serum HGH levels but that even after several years most patients continue to have hypersecretion of HGH. With high energy radiation in patients with acromegaly (see Lawrence, pages 39 to 61, this volume), the results are better. However, several years are required to restore HGH secretion to normal, and in many patients this is never accomplished. In the past, surgical treatment of acromegaly was confined to those patients who had evidence of extrasellar extension of their tumors. In these patients, it was often impossible to remove all of the tumor, and active acromegaly persisted despite surgical and radiation therapy. With improvement in the surgical hypophysectomy techniques, surgical removal of the tumor has resulted in prompt correction of the disorder. When the tumor is not excessively enlarged and is confined to the sella turcica, removal often results in the restoration of HGH levels to normal or below. Medical treatment for acromegaly with large doses of estrogen or progestational agents is usually ineffective.

Illustrative Cases

CASE 1.—A 14-year-old boy complained of headache. He was noted to be very tall for his age. X-ray examination revealed an enlarged sella turcica; serum HGH levels were notably elevated and were not suppressed during a glucose tolerance test. Proton beam irradiation of the pituitary utilizing the Bragg peak failed to alleviate the incapacitating headaches, and although serum HGH levels declined about 50 per cent, at one and a half years posttreatment they still were elevated. The patient grew 5 in. in height during this period. Transphenoidal microsurgical removal of the tumor resulted in immediate relief of the headache and a reduction of HGH levels to near normal.

CASE 2.—A 40-year-old Negro male developed polydipsia and polyuria and was found to have diabetes mellitus which responded to insulin therapy (80 units daily). Three years later, he was suspected of having acromegaly because of his need for enlarging sizes of shoes and gloves. This was confirmed by HGH measurements, and X-ray studies showed an enlarged sella turcica. ^{90}Yttrium rods were implanted within the sella turcica. There was prompt remission of the diabetes mellitus postoperatively and glucose tolerance returned to normal. Serum HGH became undetectable, and there was striking regression of the soft tissue swelling of the face, hands, and feet.

CASE 3.—A 35-year-old woman noted enlargement of the hands and feet, coarsening of facial features, and increasing hirsutism. A diagnosis of acromegaly was confirmed by serum HGH assays and X-ray evidence of an enlarged sella turcica. ^{90}Yttrium rods were implanted into the sella turcica, and postoperatively there was striking regression of the soft tissue swellings. HGH and insulin secretions declined to normal postoperatively without significant change in the normal glucose tolerance curves.

Hypersecretion of ACTH

Cushing's disease is a pituitary disorder characterized by hypersecretion of adrenocorticotrophic hormone (ACTH), which in turn produces hypersecretion of cortisol. Hypersecretion of cortisol produces Cushing's syndrome. An occult pituitary tumor may be present at the time of diagnosis, but most often the sella turcica is not enlarged and the pituitary gland may not show a recognizable histological abnormality. Small basophilic tumors of the anterior pituitary are seen at autopsy in about 25 per cent of patients with Cushing's syndrome.

Diagnosis of Cushing's disease is confirmed by the finding of elevated urinary excretion of 17-hydroxycorticosteroids (17-OHCS), elevated plasma cortisol levels, and lack of diurnal variation in plasma cortisol levels. Plasma ACTH levels are elevated or at least inappropriate for the elevated plasma cortisol levels. This is in contrast to the low levels of ACTH seen in patients with Cushing's syndrome caused by adrenal neoplasm. Dexamethasone suppression tests are also useful in distinguishing Cushing's disease from Cushing's syndrome resulting from adrenal neoplasm or the ectopic ACTH syndrome. Large doses of dexamethasone (*e.g.*, 2 mg. every six hours) will induce a significant suppression of urinary 17-OHCS secretion below control levels in most patients with Cushing's disease, whereas no suppression occurs in patients with adrenal neoplasm or ectopic ACTH syndrome. This indicates that ACTH secretion is abnormal in Cushing's disease but not autonomous.

Treatment for Cushing's disease in patients with occult tumors of the pituitary is usually accomplished by surgical hypophysectomy. In most patients who have normal-sized sella turcicas, conventional radiation therapy to the pituitary (cobalt—5,000 R) or heavy particle radiation (7,500 rads) will induce lasting remissions after three to six months in about 30 per cent of cases. In younger patients in whom preservation of gonadal function is desirable, bilateral total adrenalectomy is the treatment of choice when radiation therapy fails or when a more rapid reversal of adrenal hyperfunction is needed. With older patients in whom maintenance of fertility is not a problem, surgical hypophysectomy may afford optimum results. Medical therapy of hypercorticism may be useful in patients with advanced disease who may be poor risks for surgical procedures. O,p' DDD (1,1-dichloro-2-[o-chlorophenyl]-2-[p-chlorophenyl] ethane) or a combination of aminoglutethimide and metyrapone are effective agents in suppressing adrenocortical hyperfunction.

ILLUSTRATIVE CASES

CASE 1.—A 10-year-old girl was found to have Cushing's syndrome. She was treated by a right total and left subtotal adrenalectomy and radiation therapy (4,000 R) to the pituitary gland. Remission of the Cushing's syndrome lasted one and a half years, followed by recurrence. The remaining adrenal tissue on the left was removed surgically but no improvement occurred. Laboratory studies at this time revealed elevated plasma and urinary 17-OHCS levels, and plasma ACTH was elevated (1.2 mU/100 ml.). A [90]Yttrium rod was inserted into the pituitary gland via a transnasal, transphenoidal approach. Prompt remission of the Cushing's disease followed and has been maintained for eight years.

Although pituitary tumors may be present when Cushing's disease is diagnosed, they are more commonly observed after treatment by bilateral total adrenalectomy. In one series, 10 per cent of patients who underwent adrenalectomy for Cushing's disease developed pituitary tumors. The development of the pituitary tumor is usually heralded by intense pigmentation of the skin (similar to that seen in Addison's disease). This condition is referred to as Nelson's syndrome. The pituitary tumors are chromophobe adenomas but in several instances these tumors have shown unusual invasive properties, with the development of cranial nerve palsies and distant metastases in one case. Preferred treatment appears to be surgical hypophysectomy.

CASE 2.—A 39-year-old woman underwent bilateral total adrenalectomy for treatment for Cushing's disease which was followed by remission of the Cushing's syndrome. One year later, she noted such increasing pigmentation of the skin over the entire body that she appeared negroid. She otherwise remained asymptomatic for 11 years at which time persistent headache developed and enlargement of the sella turcica was noted. Plasma ACTH levels were notably elevated (1,000 mU/100 ml.). 90Yttrium pituitary implantation relieved the headache and lowered the plasma ACTH levels but did not influence the pigmentation. Subsequent surgical hypophysectomy failed to eliminate the elevated plasma ACTH levels, suggesting that the pituitary tumor had extended beyond the sella turcica.

Hypersecretion of Prolactin (HPr)

Nonpuerperal galactorrhea and amenorrhea have been observed in women in association with chromophobe adenomas of the pituitary gland. This condition is referred to as the Forbes-Albright syndrome (Forbes, Henneman, Griswold, and Albright, 1954), following their report of 15 patients, eight of whom had enlarged sella turcicas; three patients were shown to have chromophobe adenomas at operation. Recently, sensitive and specific assays for human prolactin have been developed which are capable of measuring normal serum prolactin levels. Studies of patients with Forbes-Albright syndrome associated with pituitary tumors have demonstrated elevated serum prolactin levels which were restored to normal or below after surgical removal of the tumor, thus establishing that these are prolactin-secreting tumors. Diagnosis of this syndrome can now be confirmed by radioimmunoassays of serum prolactin. L-Dopa is an effective agent in suppressing normal serum prolactin levels, and preliminary studies suggest that this drug fails to suppress serum prolactin levels in patients with pituitary tumors. Surgical removal of prolactin-secreting pituitary tumors appears to be the treatment of choice. Medical treatment with L-Dopa is effective in correcting galactorrhea and amenorrhea in patients without obvious pituitary tumors (Turkington, 1971).

ILLUSTRATIVE CASES

CASE 1.—A 27-year-old woman had noted amenorrhea for seven years and galactorrhea for five years. Studies revealed notably elevated serum HPr levels (150 ng./ml.) as compared to those of normal women (less than 20 ng./ml.). Serum HPr levels were not influenced by administration of perphenazine, which usually induces a prompt rise in serum HPr levels in normal women. X-ray studies revealed an asymmetrically enlarged sella turcica. A transnasal, transsphenoidal microsurgical exploration of the sella turcica was performed. A large pituitary adenoma was found which had displaced the normal-appearing anterior pituitary gland to one side. By microsurgical dissection, it was possible to remove the adenoma without disturbing the normal-appearing gland. Postoperatively, there was disappearance of milk secretion within one week, and a spontaneous menstrual period began on the eighth postoperative day. Adrenal and thyroid gland functions remain normal postoperatively, and serum HPr was less than 10 ng./ml.

CASE 2.—A 52-year-old man noted sudden impairment of vision and examination disclosed bitemporal hemianopsia. The patient was otherwise asymptomatic except for moderate gynecomastia which had been present for several years. X-ray films and pneumoencephalogram disclosed massive enlargement of the sella turcica with suprasellar extension. A transfrontal craniotomy was performed, and a large chromophobe adenoma was found which could be only partially resected. Preoperative serum HPr levels were elevated (750 ng./ml.). Culture of pituitary tumor obtained at operation revealed that it was synthesizing HPr.

Hypersecretion of Thyrotropin (TSH)

Hyperthyroidism in association with a pituitary tumor is uncommon. Three cases have been reported in which there is good evidence that a pituitary tumor was secreting excessive amounts of TSH producing hyperthyroidism. A well-documented case has recently been reported by Hamilton, Adams, and Maloof (1970). In this patient, partial removal of a chromophobe adenoma failed to correct the hyperthyroidism and serum TSH levels remain elevated. After 4,600 R of conventional external irradiation to the pituitary area, there was remission of the hyperthyroidism and serum TSH levels returned to normal. Remission of hyperthyroidism after irradiation of a pituitary tumor has been reported in two additional patients.

Summary

Four types of hormone-secreting tumors of the anterior pituitary gland now have been well documented. With the newly available sensitive and specific assays for the anterior pituitary hormones, earlier diagnosis of these lesions should be possible. Satisfactory treatments for correction of both the endocrine disorders and the neoplasms are available if the disease is not too far advanced.

Acknowledgment

This investigation was supported by grants from the U.S.P.H.S., CA-05197-12, RR 80, and the American Cancer Society, T 461.

REFERENCES

Forbes, A. P., Henneman, P. H., Griswold, G. C., and Albright, F.: Syndrome characterized by galactorrhea, amenorrhea, and low urinary FSH: Comparison with acromegaly and normal lactation. *Journal of Clinical Endocrinology,* 14: 265-271, 1954.

Hamilton, C. R., Jr., Adams, L. C., and Maloof, F.: Hyperthyroidism due to a thyrotropic-producing pituitary chromophobe adenoma. *The New England Journal of Medicine,* 283:1077, 1970.

Roth, J., Gorden, P., and Brace, K.: Efficacy of conventional pituitary irradiation in acromegaly. *The New England Journal of Medicine,* 282:1385-1390, 1970.

Turkington, R. W.: Inhibition of prolactin secretion and successful therapy of the Forbes-Albright syndrome with L-dopa. *Proceedings of the Society for Clinical Research,* 44:44, 1971.

Heavy Particles in Acromegaly and Cushing's Disease

JOHN H. LAWRENCE, M.D.,
CLAUDE Y. CHONG, M.D., Ph.D.,
JAMES L. BORN, M.D., JOHN T. LYMAN, Ph.D.,
MICHAEL D. OKERLUND, M.D.,
JOSEPH F. GARCIA, Ph.D.,
JOHN A. LINFOOT, M.D.,
CORNELIUS A. TOBIAS, Ph.D., AND
EDWARD MANOUGIAN, M.D.

*Donner Laboratory & Donner Pavilion, University of California,
Berkeley, California*

THE RELATIVE RADIORESISTANCE of the normal pituitary gland has long been known (Lawrence, Nelson, and Wilson, 1937). The hyperplastic or adenomatous glands such as we find in acromegaly, Cushing's disease, Nelson's syndrome, and chromophobe adenoma are also relatively resistant; as a result, the treatment for pituitary disorders with externally delivered radiation poses a problem. Metabolic effects from conventional pituitary irradiation procedures are not usually seen because of the limitation placed on the pituitary dose in order to avoid possible damaging doses to surrounding vital structures such as cranial nerves, hypothalamus, and temporal lobes. Therefore, when animal studies carried out by Tobias, Anger, and Lawrence (1952) in 1948 (demonstrating that the Bragg peaks of 190-Mev deuteron and 340-Mev proton beams could be used successfully to eradicate transplanted mammary tumors in mice by passing the heavy-particle beam through the animal's body with the Bragg peak located at the tumor site) indicated that heavy particles were suitable for effective and intense irradiation of small volumes deep within the body, their use for pituitary irradiation in animals was immediately investigated (Tobias *et al.*, 1954). On finding that it is possible to suppress pituitary function with heavy particles safely in animals, our interest was again aroused regarding the possible use of heavy particles for treating human disease.

In 1954, 340-Mev protons were first used to suppress pituitary function in patients with far-advanced metastatic breast cancer (Lawrence, 1957; Tobias et al., 1958). Since 1957, higher-energy 910-Mev alpha particles have been used, and their therapeutic applications have been extended to include the treatment of patients with disorders of the pituitary gland, including acromegaly, Cushing's disease, Nelson's syndrome, and chromophobe adenoma (Lawrence et al., 1970; Lawrence, 1964; Linfoot et al., 1970; Tobias, Lyman, and Lawrence, 1971; Linfoot et al., 1971). With these high-energy heavy particles, it is possible to overcome the relative insensitivity of the pituitary gland to externally delivered radiations and to safely deliver sufficiently large doses of energy to the pituitary area to treat successfully patients with these pituitary disorders. In addition, the patient is ambulatory during the treatment period, the procedure is painless, and there is no need to enter the cranium either surgically or by needle.

Acromegaly

Acromegaly, a disorder of the pituitary gland first described by Marie in 1886, is usually caused by an eosinophilic tumor of the pituitary gland, and the resultant hypersecretion of growth hormone leads to the development of the many symptoms and signs of acromegaly. The life expectancy of these patients is known to be reduced. One study reported that in 100 patients with acromegaly, 50 per cent had died before the age of 50 years and 89 per cent by the age of 60 years (Evans, Briggs, and Dixon, 1966). Another study reported that the number of deaths in 194 patients was almost twice that expected from a matched general population (Wright, Hill, Lowy, and Fraser, 1970). In addition, both of these studies reported an increased incidence of deaths from cardiovascular and cerebrovascular causes. Surgical partial hypophysectomy or limited doses of X rays had been, until recently, the usual therapeutic methods. However, because the pituitary gland is relatively radioresistant, metabolic effects from X-ray or gamma-ray irradiation of the pituitary are rarely seen (Hamwi, Skillman, and Tufts, 1960; Roth, Gorden, and Brace, 1970; Christy, 1969) with the limited doses that can be used safely without damaging surrounding vital structures such as cranial nerves, hypothalamus, and temporal lobes. After such treatment, long periods of relief from signs and symptoms are not achieved and life expectancy remains poor. With the availability of cortisone for replacement therapy, surgical hypophysectomy has been used with considerable success (Hamberger, Hammer, Norlen, and Sjögren,

1960; Hardy and Wigser, 1965; Ray, Bronson, Horwith, and Mautelen, 1968) as have pituitary implants of [198]Au or [90]Y (Molinatti *et al.*, 1962; Kaufman *et al.*, 1966; Jadresic and Poblete, 1967; Fraser and Wright, 1968), and more recently cryosurgery (Rand *et al.*, 1966) and thermocautery (Zervas, 1969). However, using an externally delivered high-energy heavy-particle beam from a cyclotron, it is possible to safely deliver sufficiently large doses to the pituitary area to control the excessive growth-hormone secretion and thereby to treat acromegaly successfully.

Following heavy-particle therapy, relief from symptoms and signs is gradually achieved. Headache, the most frequent and troublesome symptom encountered, has either improved significantly or disappeared in most patients within one year. Lethargy and weakness, symptoms which are difficult to assess but which nevertheless adversely affect the patient's psychological outlook and ability to continue normal activities, improve following therapy. No further acral enlargement has occurred in any of the patients following treatment and had decreased in one third of the patients within four years after completion of treatment. The typical coarse, heavy, facial appearance of these patients underwent satisfying changes in 35 per cent of the group followed for at least four years. This was evident in a refinement and decrease in mass of the supraorbital ridges, the malar prominences, the jaw, and the nose. Primarily, the changes occur in the soft tissue mass, but there is also evidence of change in the bones, as demonstrated by comparative head casts, by X-ray examination of the hands and feet, and by studies of calcium metabolism.

The plasma growth hormone levels, as determined by radioimmunoassay (Garcia *et al.*, 1967), were elevated in all patients before treatment (median 21.5 mμg./ml., range 5.3 to 213). Subsequently, growth hormone levels fell in all patients (Fig. 1); values were within normal limits ($\leq$ 5 mμg./ml.) in 30 per cent of the patients within two years, in 68 per cent within six years, and in 95 per cent within eight years. Although the most striking metabolic changes are noted when values of 5 mμg./ml. or less are achieved, significant metabolic improvements are generally seen when the growth hormone level drops to 10 mμg./ml. or less. This level had been reached by 68 per cent of the patients within two years, 85 per cent within five years, and 96 per cent within seven years. In addition, abnormalities in carbohydrate metabolism, including insulin resistance, diabetic-type glucose tolerance curves, and the presence of diabetes mellitus, disappear following treatment.

The remaining normal pituitary gland continues to function, and cortisone replacement therapy has been required in only one third of those patients whom we have followed for at least two years. Onset of replace-

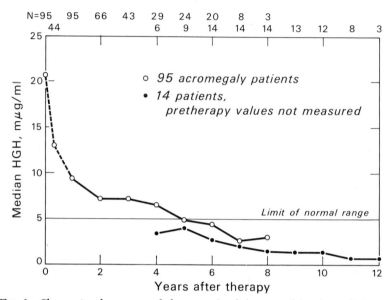

Fig. 1.—Change in plasma growth hormone level (measured by the radioimmuno-assay method) in 109 patients with acromegaly who have been re-evaluated one or more years after completion of heavy-particle pituitary irradiation. For 95 patients, growth hormone determinations were made both before therapy and from 1 to 12 years after therapy; for the remaining 14 patients, pretreatment determinations were not made by this method, but determinations were made from 4 to 12 years after treatment, and their values (closed dots) are consistent with the other group.

ment therapy was usually between two and four years after completion of heavy-particle therapy, although the range extends to 12 years. As expected, the amount of dose has an effect on this subsequent need; when patients are divided into low (3,000 to 5,900 rads), medium (6,000 to 7,800 rads), and high (8,200 to 12,000 rads, including X rays) dose groups, we find that only 18 per cent (5 of 28) of the low-dose and 32 per cent (12 of 37) of the medium-dose groups required cortisone replacement, whereas 72 per cent (10 of 14) of the high-dose group subsequently showed hypoadrenocorti-cism. About 35 per cent of the patients required thyroid replacement at some time following treatment; however, this was more difficult to assess because many of these patients had been placed on thyroid therapy before treatment without clear documentation of the need for such therapy. About 10 per cent of the men required androgen therapy, slightly more than 10 per cent of the women required estrogen therapy. Three patients have be-come pregnant since therapy, and the wives of three other patients have also become pregnant (subsequent deliveries were normal). Thus far, about one third of the patients developed some degree of hypopituitarism as a result of achieving adequate control of their disease. Hypopituitarism develops slowly in most cases, and therefore young couples are encouraged to initiate their families promptly after treatment. However, we have so far no clinical evidence of sterility in any of these patients. All patients and their attending physicians are alerted to the possible eventual need for adrenal as well as other types of hormonal replacement, and the patients carry a card indicating this need under conditions of stress such as infection, operation, or injury.

With improvement in the metabolic picture, it is reasonable to expect extension of comfortable and chronological life in these patients to normal or nearly normal for their age group and for a group of people with similar incidence of vascular disease or other independent disease processes. Only nine of the 153 patients treated during the past 13½ years have died. As seen in Figure 2, the median survival for the group is now 11 years. Comparing the 1971 curve with that calculated in 1969, one notes that as the follow-up period increases, the survival curve approaches that of a treated diabetic population.

FIG. 2.—Comparison of the 1971 and 1969 survival curves for our series of 153 patients with acromegaly who have been treated with heavy particles; the median survival for the group is now 11 years, and as the follow-up period increases, the survival curve approaches that of a treated diabetic population.

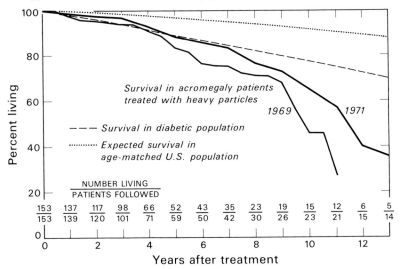

The increased incidence of deaths from cardiovascular and cerebrovascular causes which has been noted in other studies of deaths in series of acromegalic patients (Evans, Briggs, and Dixon, 1966; Wright, Hill, Lowy, and Fraser, 1970) was also apparent in our series: four of the nine deaths were the result of cardiovascular disease, and these patients all had cardiomegaly and hypertension before heavy-particle therapy. (It seems clear to us that many patients referred for treatment have been considered poor risks for other therapeutic procedures such as operation, cryosurgery, or radioactive implants.) One suffered a coronary occlusion 3½ years after treatment; there was no postmortem examination since he died in another city and we were not advised immediately. One had mild obstructive airway disease of the lungs and arteriosclerotic heart disease with some degree of failure before heavy-particle therapy. (He had been considered a poor candidate for both transsphenoidal hypophysectomy and cryohypophysectomy because of his cardiopulmonary problems.) He went into congestive heart failure with notable ventricular irritability and died 14 months after completion of heavy-particle therapy; portmortem findings revealed pulmonary embolism, cardiac hypertrophy and dilation, generalized arteriosclerosis, and eosinophilic adenoma of the pituitary gland with fibrosis and scarring. One patient who had advanced cardiovascular disease before heavy-particle therapy died from cardiac failure within six months; postmortem examination revealed a greatly enlarged heart (the head was not examined). One suffered a cerebrovascular accident and died nine years after completion of heavy-particle therapy; postmortem findings revealed a somewhat enlarged heart, generalized arteriosclerosis with ischemic degeneration and infarction of the brain, and partial radiation necrosis of the anterior lobe of the pituitary gland.

Of the remaining five patients who have died, one took his own life seven months after treatment before the maximum effect of therapy was achieved; microscopic study of the pituitary gland showed some vessel sclerosis. Another died of an accidental overdose of barbiturates five years after completion of heavy-particle therapy; postmortem findings revealed changes in the pituitary consistent with old necrosis and hemorrhage in an adenoma. One patient, whose growth hormone level remained high, was given proton-beam therapy (12,000 rads in a single dose) elsewhere three years after being treated here, and one year later died with acute myeloblastic leukemia; postmortem findings revealed absence of the pituitary, secondary to irradiation. One patient died because of severe systemic toxemia (*Histoplasma capsulatum*) approximately four years after heavy-particle therapy. Postmortem findings in the brain and pituitary revealed minimal dystrophic calcification of the optic nerve, focal acidophilic hyperplasia of the anterior pituitary, and minimal fibrosis of the pituitary; no changes were found attributable to irradiation. The other patient died because of meningioma at another medical center 11 years after completion of heavy-particle therapy (the patient and his wife refused treatment for the meningioma); postmortem examination revealed radiation atrophy of the pituitary gland with no residual tumor. The meningioma was benign and was in an area of the brain estimated to have received 300 rads; it seems unlikely that a cause-effect relationship between therapy and tumor is present.

It is of interest to note that we did find an extrapituitary intracranial tumor in a second patient in this series, but in his case, the second tumor was diagnosed before heavy-particle therapy was administered. When we first saw this 40-year-old man in April 1969, he had a five-year history of onset of acromegalic signs and symptoms with the diagnosis being made in November 1967. We found his fasting growth hormone level to be 12.9 mμg./ml.; his symptoms were mild, his visual fields normal, and the skull X-ray films within normal limits. However, the pneumoencephalogram revealed, in addition to slight sellar enlargement without evidence of a suprasellar lesion, a deformity of the left temporal horn, suggesting the presence of a mass in the left middle fossa. Cerebral ^{99m}Tc studies and bilateral internal carotid arteriograms confirmed the presence of a mass in the left temporal region, but since there were no clear-cut signs or symptoms related to this mass, it was thought to be a cyst or slowly growing tumor (possible diagnosis included meningioma, gliomatous cyst, and arachnoid cyst). The patient refused surgical exploration because of the increased risk that a general anesthetic would present (he had serious lung disease with a history of asthma, bronchitis, and bronchiectasis, and a thoracotomy done at age ten for a lung abscess). A decision concerning the temporal lobe mass was therefore postponed and the intrasellar eosinophilic tumor was treated with heavy particles in June 1969. During subsequent follow-up visits in June 1970 and June 1971, brain scans have revealed no change in the temporal lobe mass. His acromegaly has improved; the plasma growth hormone fell to normal levels within one year and remains there (3.0 mμg./ml.); his symptoms of headaches, excessive perspiration, and lethargy have all diminished.

Significant amounts of previous radiation contribute to an increased incidence of complications after heavy-particle therapy. Six of the patients treated before 1961 had already received from one to three courses of X-ray therapy, the total doses ranging from 2,000 to 5,275 rads. However, when we first saw the patients, they still had active and progressive acromegaly, and we accepted them with reluctance for heavy-particle treatment. Three of these six patients subsequently developed mild ocular complications which were not progressive; two developed transient diplopia 14 months following retreatment with heavy particles (they are both doing well 12½ years since treatment), and the third developed a quadrant cut two years following retreatment with heavy particles (this did not progress, and the patient died nine years after treatment from a cerebral vascular accident at the age of 68). These mild ocular complications were presumed to have resulted from therapy, and their occurrence further reinforces our belief that heavy-particle therapy should be limited to those patients who have not received previous X-ray or gamma-ray therapy. Since 1961, we have not accepted such patients for treatment with heavy particles. Further, we strongly believe that the presence of any significant extrasellar extension of the pituitary adenoma requires the serious consideration of surgical treatment. In several patients without field cuts, suprasellar extensions were found only after carefully conducted tomographic pneumoencephalography; this procedure is now done routinely before heavy-particle treatment. In many cases, arteriograms are also done, and in some cases, cavernous venograms are valuable. Suprasellar tumor extensions were found in eight patients; four of this group who had large tumor extensions were referred for surgical hypophysectomy, and the remaining four were treated with heavy particles after surgical removal of the suprasellar extension.

Two other patients who were treated before 1961, before pneumoencephalography and tomography were routinely performed before acceptance for heavy-particle therapy, experienced mild ocular complications. At ten months posttherapy, one developed bilateral, small, upper-field cuts which have remained stable for the past ten years. The other complained of transient diplopia at three weeks and of difficulty in focusing his eyes when driving eight weeks after therapy. He developed symptoms compatible with uncinate seizures which have not been constant at 15 months posttherapy. (Extensive psychiatric evaluation and testing indicated the possibility that these might have resulted from the patient's personality structure.) Both of these patients are currently doing well more than ten years since treatment.

With our current selection criteria (i.e., rejection of patients who have received prior X-ray or gamma-ray therapy and requirement of pneumoencephalography and tomography before treatment), the dosage delivered to the brain tissue surrounding the pituitary gland and to the cranial nerves has been limited to less than 3,500 rads. Of the 136 patients treated since 1961, 131 were treated with the plateau portion of the beam, using a biplanar rotational technique. We have experienced no neurological complications in this large group. The other five patients had very large pituitary tumors and were therefore treated with the Bragg peak, because it is not possible by the present rotation technique to give sufficient doses to the sella turcica unless the Bragg peak is employed. Two of these patients, treated with 12 portals, have had excellent responses and show no evidence of side effects. The other patients were treated with six portals; two of these developed transient diplopia, and the other developed transient unilateral scotoma immediately following treatment. The scotoma may have been unrelated to the treatment since it cleared rapidly, and the patient has no sign of ocular difficulty 18 months following treatment. Of the two who developed transient diplopia, one underwent transfrontal surgical therapy for a small suprasellar extension and has shown definite improvement since then. The other has recently developed uncinate seizures which are controlled by anticonvulsant therapy.

Our total experience using heavy particles to treat this large number of patients (153) over a 13½-year period is encouraging and indicates that good control of acromegaly can be achieved by this safe method with a very low incidence of side effects.

Chromophobe Adenoma

During the past ten years, 910-Mev alpha particles have been used to treat 17 patients with nonfunctioning or chromophobe adenomas of the pituitary gland. This series was limited because our selection criteria exclude patients with suprasellar extension or with massive enlargement of the sella turcica. The method of treatment is the same as described for acromegalic patients, with the range of heavy-particle doses being 4,000 to 8,000 rads delivered in 12 days. Four patients were panhypopituitary at the time of treatment; three of these had undergone previous transfrontal surgical decompression, and the other one had a 25-year history of hypopituitarism. Although the remaining 13 patients were not clinically hypopituitary, most of them did have diminished growth hormone responses to provocative testing. Two of this group subsequently developed hypothyroidism, and one developed secondary adrenal insufficiency. In one patient, transnasal surgical decompression was successfully performed following further intrasphenoidal tumor extension. Three patients in the group have died, two from unrelated cardiovascular complications and one from complications following a transnasal hypophysectomy which was performed at another institution in an attempt to relieve intractable headaches.

Cushing's Disease and Nelson's Syndrome

The clinical syndrome we now call Cushing's disease was formerly called the pluriglandular syndrome and was first described by Cushing in 1932. He believed this disorder to be caused by a basophilic adenoma of the anterior lobe of the pituitary gland (Cushing, 1932). Similar clinical pictures were noted later, however, with benign or malignant adrenal tumors (usually unilateral) and adrenocortical hyperplasia (always bilateral), leading many investigators during the ensuing years to believe that the condition was usually caused by primary adrenal hyperfunction. Surgical adrenalectomy, made possible by the availability of adrenocorticosteroid therapy as a substitution therapy for these patients, was successful for some. However, when the very sensitive radioimmunoassay method for measuring plasma hormones became available, it was demonstrated that small amounts of adrenocorticosteroids (ACTH) are released by these patients in spite of their high circulating levels of hydrocortisone. In addition, roentgenologically detectable pituitary tumors were found in 15 to 25 per cent of the patients, and it was further noted that many of these tumors were not detectable until after bilateral surgical removal of the adrenal glands. It also was observed that the incidence of Nelson's syndrome (Nelson, Meakin, and Thorn, 1960), which develops following total adrenalectomy, was lower in those patients who had received pituitary irradiation before adrenalectomy. As a result of these findings, and in line with Cushing's earlier concept, it more recently has been proposed that this syndrome is the result of an altered hypothalamic-pituitary-adrenal axis associated with hypothalamic pituitary overactivity. Thus, there has been a renewed interest in the pituitary gland as the initial site for therapy of this disorder. Since 1959, we have used this approach to treat 25 patients. Nineteen were treated to control adrenal hypersecretion through the administration of heavy particles to the pituitary gland; the remaining six had previously been treated elsewhere for Cushing's syndrome by bilateral adrenalectomy and then, after developing Nelson's syndrome, were referred to us for heavy-particle treatment of the pituitary gland.

Three additional patients with Cushing's syndrome, who were referred to us for pituitary heavy-particle therapy, were found to have adrenal tumors and were referred back for adrenal surgery. One of these had an adrenal carcinoma and subsequently died of metastatic carcinoma. The other two responded well to surgical removal of adrenal adenomas. Most of the 19 patients treated with heavy particles for primary adrenal hyperplasia received from 9,000 to 15,000 rads in 12 days (one patient received only 6,000 rads in 12 days). Four had previously undergone unsuccessful adrenal surgery. One had bilateral adrenalectomy and subsequently developed Cushing's syndrome, presumably from accessory adrenal tissue; three had undergone subtotal adrenalectomies, with further removal of the remnant considered surgically too difficult. With the exception of some of the tests in these patients with prior adrenal surgery, all patients could be characterized as having elevated urinary 17-ketosteroids. In most patients, the plasma cortisol level was modestly to definitely elevated and in all patients, the circadian or nyctohemeral rhythm was abnormal. All patients showed an exaggerated steroid response to ACTH and to the oral or intravenous administration of metyrapone. The patients with adrenal remnants or accessory adrenal tissue were maximally ACTH stimulated; as expected, their responses to suppression and stimulation tests were more like those observed in patients with adrenal adenomas. Dexamethasone suppression was determined in eight patients, of whom two showed normal suppression with a low dose (2 mg./day) of dexamethasone and six suppression of at least 50 per cent with the high dose (8 mg./day). The ACTH values, available only in the recent patients, were not found to be notably elevated, the expected finding in bilateral adrenal hyperplasia.

Seventeen of the 19 patients have been followed long enough for analysis of results (Fig. 3). Following treatment, there was a significant fall in the urinary base line 17-hydroxycorticosteroids (17-OHCS). The exaggerated response to metyrapone, seen in all patients who had not undergone prior adrenal surgery, was also dramatically obliterated by heavy-particle pituitary therapy. In two patients who had transient remissions and then suffered relapse, the metyrapone response diminished and then returned to or exceeded the pretreatment levels. Of the successfully treated patients, four developed normal nyctohemeral or circadian rhythms following treatment. Eleven who were tested showed suppression of plasma cortisol during an overnight dexamethasone (2 mg./day) suppression test, but only five suppressed to less than 5 μg./ml.

Sixteen patients have undergone partial or complete remissions. One patient who had had a unilateral adrenalectomy did not return for follow-up evaluation, but studies elsewhere demonstrated failure to respond and without our being consulted, he subsequently had a total adrenalectomy there, nine months after our treatment (if a longer waiting period had been allowed, this might not have been necessary). Two patients who had shown earlier remissions later suffered relapse and underwent total adrenalectomy at 7 and 38 months posttreatment. Two patients remained in partial remission two years after treatment. Two of the patients had been treated too recently to be evaluated, but preliminary data from the referring physicians indicate some clinical improvement in all. No patient with Cushing's disease receiving heavy particles to the pituitary has developed Nelson's syndrome.

The response rate in the 17 patients for whom we have follow-up information appears to be significantly better than that obtained in patients treated with conventional radiation: no more than 25 to 30 per cent of pa-

CUSHING'S DISEASE

Patient	Adrenal Surgery	Years Duration, Post Heavy-Particle Pituitary Irradiation	Urinary 17-OHCS				Plasma 17-OHCS Circadian Rhythm Pre/Post
			Baseline Pre/Post	Metyrapone Pre/Post	ACTH Pre/Post	Dexamethasone (8 mg/day) Pre	
1 KLE F 37	Unilateral + 3 mon	12.4	↑/N	↑/N	↑/N	S	A/N
2 SCT F 45	Total + 38 mon	8.5	↑/N/↑++	↑/N/↑++	↑/↓/↑++	S	A/A
3 CX M 17		7.8	↑/N	↑/N	↑/N	S	A/A*
4 MCC F 35		6.3°	↑/N	↑/N	↑/↓	S	A/N*
5 VEG F 56	Subtotal Pre-Rx	6.3	↗/N	→/→	→/→	NS	A/N*
6 ASH M 24	Total+ Pre-Rx	5.8	↑/N	↗/↗	→/→	S	A/A
7 DIX F 38		5.7	↗/N	↑/N	↑/	S	A/N*
8 ODN F 34		5.4	↑/N	↑/N	↑/	S	A/A**
9 P DN F 19		5.0	↑/↓	↗/N	↑/	S	A/A*
10 DAM M 46	Unilateral Pre-Rx Total + 9 mon	4.7	↑/?/↑++	↑/?/↑++	↑/	S	A/
11 DOR M 42	Total + 7 mon	4.5	↑/N/↑++	↑/↓/↑++	↑/↓/↑++	S	A/A
12 DNS F 43		3.1	↑/↓	↑/↓	↑/	S	A/A**
13 K.DN F 23		2.6	↑/↓	↑/N	↑/	S	A/A**
14 HNT M 39		1.3	↑/↓°°	↑/ °°	↑/↓°°	S	A/A°°
15 JON F 39		1.0	↑/N	↑/N		S	A/A**
16 SLT F 26	Subtotal Pre-Rx	1.0	↑/N	↗/↓		S	A/A**
17 MOE F 31		0.6	↗/↗	↑/↓		S	A/A*

° Patient died 76 mos. after heavy-particle therapy
°° Developed secondary adrenal insufficiency 3 mos. after treatment
+ Accessory adrenal still present
++ Values during initial response and relapse given; cortisone replacement post adrenalectomy.

* Overnight dexamethasone suppression test (2 mg at 11:00 p.m.) was > 5 µg/100 ml.
** Overnight dexamethasone suppression test (2 mg at 11:00 p.m.) was normal (<5 µg/100 ml).

N = Normal
A = Abnormal
S = Adequately suppressed
NS = Not adequately suppressed

↑ = Increased
↗ = Slightly Increased
→ = No change
↓ = Decreased from Pre-Rx value, but not yet normal

FIG. 3.—Changes in urinary and plasma steroids in patients with Cushing's disease treated with heavy-particle pituitary irradiation.

tients show permanent response to such radiation therapy (Liddle, 1967). The further advantage of this form of treatment seems to be that it is a direct approach to the pathological secretion of ACTH. Furthermore, this approach prevents the subsequent development of pituitary tumors in the rare patient who may require adrenalectomy later. A disadvantage is that other trophic hormones are at risk, and the problem of infertility must be considered. Only one patient thus far has developed hypoadrenalism, and a few have developed hypogonadism or hypothyroidism (follow-up intervals range from several months to 12 years). None of the patients has developed any signs of other radiation side effects, although one developed an incomplete third-nerve palsy seven years after treatment. This cleared, coincidentally, following a cavernous sinus venogram. Since most of the patients who received less than 10,000 rads have suffered relapse, it would appear that higher doses are required. Such doses will probably produce the desired results in a much higher percentage of patients, and we are currently conducting such a program.

As indicated previously, six patients had undergone total adrenalectomies elsewhere and were subsequently referred to us for heavy-particle pituitary therapy when Nelson's syndrome developed. Four of these six patients had enlarged sella turcicas; the enlargement had developed after bilateral adrenalectomy (Table 1). In one patient, a suprasellar extension was removed before heavy-particle treatment. The heavy-particle doses given this group of patients ranged from 5,000 to 10,000 rads delivered in 12 days. All patients had elevated plasma ACTH levels before treatment. A fall in serum ACTH levels was observed in the two cases in which we had both pretreatment and posttreatment radioimmunoassay ACTH determinations. A stabilization or decrease in pigmentation was observed in all six patients.

One patient with Nelson's syndrome had an invasive pituitary tumor and died four years after treatment, following a difficult operation to relieve a large suprasellar extension. This patient had shown dramatic loss of pigmentation when she moved from the mountains, and this was interpreted to be a sign of clinical improvement. Her plasma ACTH levels were significantly elevated before treatment (bioassay ACTH determination, 100 mU./100 ml.). Subsequent ACTH determinations were done by radioimmunoassay method, and the plasma level of 1,000 pg./ml. at seven months following treatment had fallen to 600 pg./ml. at 20 months. However, the ACTH level again increased and was notably elevated (greater than 2,500 pg./ml.) just before brain surgery. Postmortem examination revealed a malignant pituitary adenoma which had extended superiorly to involve the optic chiasm, left optic nerve and tract, and inferior portion of the internal capsule. The intrasellar portion of the pituitary adenoma showed radiation fibrosis, but there were areas of well-preserved tumor tissue invading bone laterally. Although the tumor had the appearance of the chromophobe tumors which are often associated with patients with Cushing's disease treated by bilateral adrenalectomy (except for pleomorphism of some of the cells), no distant metastases were found. Infarction of the cerebral cortex followed the difficult decompression. This case suggests the tendency to invasiveness and malignancy of these tumors and emphasizes the need for aggressive management of these patients. It also indicates the importance of the serious consideration of attacking the pituitary gland first, and not the adrenals, in patients with Cushing's disease when ectopic ACTH-producing tumors and adrenal adenoma or carcinoma can be ruled out.

TABLE 1.—PITUITARY TUMORS IN PATIENTS WITH NELSON'S SYNDROME TREATED WITH HEAVY PARTICLES

Patient			At Time of Adrenalectomy			At Time Pigmentation Noted and Subsequent Changes		At Time of Heavy-Particle Pituitary Irradiation	
			Date	Adrenal surgery	Sella size	Date	Sella size	Date	Sella size
1. RIC	F	32	7/54	Subtotal	Normal (9 × 11 mm)	1959	No report	11/61	Enlarged
			11/57	Total	"Deeper" (12 × 13 mm)	9/61	Enlarged (15 × 16 mm)		
2. PHL	F	30	3/59	Total	Normal	6/64	Progressively enlarged	11/64	Enlarged (died 9/69 following surgery for invasive pituitary tumor)
3. GRY	F	38	7/54	Total	Normal	1960	Normal	11/64	Normal
4. BRU	M	18	2/62	Total	Normal	1962	Normal	10/66	Normal
5. WYK	F	28	11/63	Total	No report	5/65	Normal (asymmetry)	1/68	Enlarged
						9/67	Subtle interval change; expanding lesion of pituitary		
6. BER	M	17	7/65	Total	Normal	6/66	Normal	5/69	Enlarged
						1/69	Enlarged; suprasellar extension excised 3/69		

It is apparent from the literature that Cushing's disease is a serious illness (Liddle, 1967; Plotz, Knowlton, and Ragan, 1952; Rovit and Duane, 1969; Fraser *et al.*, 1971; Welbourn, Montgomery, and Kennedy, 1971) with 50 per cent of the patients dying within five years, and that treatment is urgent. Nelson's syndrome, in the opinion of many endocrinologists, is also a very serious disease. There may be the complication of invasiveness of the tumor—a tumor which may or may not be evident by sellar enlargement (Fraser *et al.*, 1971). Invasiveness of pituitary tumors in Cushing's disease, with or without previous adrenalectomy or pituitary irradiation, has been reported by many investigators (Fraser *et al.*, 1971; Welbourn, Montgomery, and Kennedy, 1971; Cohen and Dible, 1936; Thompson and Eisenhardt, 1943; Forbes, 1947; Feiring, Davidoff, and Zimmerman, 1953; Sheldon, Golden, and Bondy, 1954; Kernohan and Sayre, 1956; Montgomery, Welbourn, McGaughey, and Gleadhill, 1959; Salassa *et al.*, 1959; Shrank and Turner, 1960; Haugen and Loken, 1960; Scholz, Gastineau, and Harrison, 1962; Simkin, Panish, Palmer, and Cohen, 1962; Ray, 1964; Rovit and Berry, 1965; Hartog *et al.*, 1965; Minagi and Steinback, 1968; Clinicopathologic Conference, 1969). It has also been pointed out that the invasiveness of pituitary tumors associated with Cushing's syndrome seems to be much more common than in chromophobe adenomas unassociated with Cushing's syndrome or in eosinophilic adenomas, although invasive tumors do occur in all these syndromes (Jefferson, 1954; Bailey and Cutler, 1940; Weinberger, Adler, and Grant, 1940; Spark and Biller, 1943; Kraus, 1945; Walsh, 1949; Richmond, 1958; Newton, Burhenne, and Palubinskas, 1962; Martins, Hayes, and Kempe, 1965). Of the verified pituitary tumors in Cushing's series, 3 per cent were classified as adenocarcinomatous (11 of 338 tumors in patients treated by Cushing between 1913 and 1932 and followed by Henderson in 1939 and by German and Flanigan in 1962).

It seems to be increasingly believed by more and more investigators that when disorders such as primary adrenal tumors and ACTH-producing cancers can be ruled out, Cushing's disease is caused by hyperactivity of the hypothalamic-pituitary-adrenal axis. Therefore, in most cases, the pituitary gland, and not the adrenal, should be the target for its treatment. When a sufficient radiation dose is delivered to the pituitary gland, such as can be done using heavy particles, then a much higher percentage of patients with Cushing's disease will respond to pituitary therapy. Furthermore, if the pituitary gland does receive heavy-particle radiation initially, and if adrenalectomy is later required (and in our experience, this is uncommon), there will probably not be the subsequent development of Nelson's syndrome; thus, a serious problem can be avoided. None of our patients whose initial treatment for Cushing's disease was heavy-particle pituitary irradiation has thus far developed hyperpigmentation or evidence of pituitary tumor following radiation. In summary, because of the demonstrated efficacy, the capability of administering higher doses with heavy particles, and the possible role of pituitary irradiation in the prevention of later development of postadrenalectomy hyperpigmentation, heavy-particle pituitary irradiation is an effective treatment for Cushing's disease and can now be considered an established method of treatment.

Radiation Necrosis

Irradiation of large volumes of brain tissue and shortening of the fractionation intervals are known generally to increase the likelihood of late radionecrosis in radiation therapy. It is known that a radiation dose of 3,200 rads delivered to a relatively large field over a 10-day fractionation period may produce radiation necrosis in some cases, while larger doses delivered through smaller fields may produce little or no radiation changes (Lindgren, 1958; Berg and Lindgren, 1958). Cases of necrosis of brain tissue following treatment for acromegaly with electromagnetic radiation such as X rays and gamma rays have been reported in the literature. Recently, Peck and McGovern (1966) cited three such cases in addition to one case following X-ray therapy for chromophobe adenoma. The brain and cranial nerves can only tolerate doses up to the range of 3,000 to 5,000 rads. In our own series of patients, we have avoided giving such doses to the surrounding tissues—the dosimetry is such that most of the administered heavy-particle dose goes to the pituitary gland and relatively little goes to the surrounding area, and with the Bragg peak the dosimetry is even better (Fig. 4). Use of the Bragg peak is desirable in treating conditions such as Cushing's disease, Nelson's syndrome, and other neoplasms where higher doses are required. However, because accurate localization of the Bragg peak is extremely difficult by current methods, Bragg-peak therapy must be employed cautiously in cases where there is marked tumor asymmetry or difficulty in discerning the lateral margin of the tumor. Problems also occur in correcting for air gap and for bone absorption. However, once technical difficulties are overcome, the Bragg peak with multiaxial rotation will provide optimum treatment for lesions requiring large doses of irradiation and those with vulnerable normal tissue in the vicinity. For the treatment of acromegaly, however, the dose needed is relatively low (usually 5,000 to 6,000 rads in 11 days, corresponding to perhaps 6,000 to 7,000 rads of conventional radiation in 30 days), so that the rotation technique using the plateau is usually quite adequate. Although in theory it should be possible by the use of careful alignment and multiple fields or rotations to deliver safely an adequate dose to the acro-

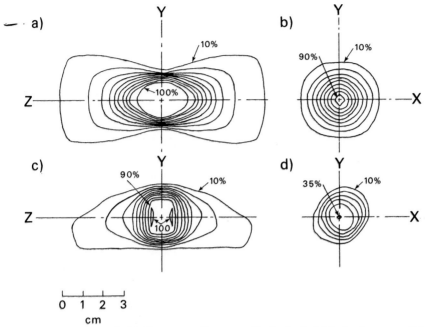

Fig. 4.—Comparison of isodose curves for two methods of administering heavy-particle pituitary irradiation: upper diagrams (*A, B*) show the dose distribution for the plateau-rotation method; lower diagrams (*C, D*) show the dose distribution for the Bragg-peak, multiple-field method. In each case, the aperture is a circle, ⅜ inch in diameter. The coronal sections (left diagrams, *A* and *C*) are through the center of the pituitary; the sagittal sections (right diagrams, *B* and *D*) are 15 mm. from the midline of the pituitary, showing the dose differential between the two methods at a point which represents the medial surface of the temporal lobe in an average patient.

megalic pituitary with high-voltage X rays and gamma rays (Lawrence *et al.*, 1962; Benbow *et al.*, 1966), convincing evidence on any fairly large series of patients awaits further clinical evaluation.

Another consideration is the question of possible relationship between malignant transformation in pituitary tumors and radiation therapy, and several authors have reported the development of pituitary sarcomas in patients who had received radiation therapy for pituitary tumors. In 1959, Terry, Hyams, and Davidoff reported three cases of pituitary sarcoma occurring from three to 12 years after administration of X-ray therapy for chromophobe adenoma. In 1963, Goldberg, Sheline, and Malamud reported two cases of pituitary sarcoma which occurred 10 years and 20 years after pituitary irradiation for acromegaly. In 1964, Greenhouse reported one case of pituitary sarcoma which occurred nine years after X-ray therapy for acromegaly, and at a Cancer Seminar on Intracranial Tumors in 1962, Wheelock reported one case of pituitary sarcoma occurring 12 years after initial X-ray therapy for acromegaly. At that seminar, Taveras mentioned two cases of pituitary sarcoma which occurred 10 or more years after irradiation therapy, and Zimmerman commented on his observation of three pituitary sarcomas which had received previous irradiation. However, the literature does not clearly answer the question of causal relationships one way or the other. A definitely increased incidence of intracranial tumors in patients treated with radiation compared to those not receiving radiation has not been absolutely established. Pituitary sarcomas are rare; furthermore, it would be difficult to find a large control group for comparison because so many patients with pituitary adenomas eventually receive radiation therapy. There is also the problem of establishing malignancy in these cases. It is generally believed, however, that even if a causal relationship were to be proved, it would not negate the value of radiotherapy in the management of pituitary adenomas. Thus far, only one patient in this series has developed an intracranial tumor following treatment. This patient refused surgical procedures and died from a meningioma (benign) 10 years after pituitary irradiation for acromegaly; as previously noted, the dose to the area involved was in the region of only 300 rads.

Summary

Heavy-particle therapy provides a form of treatment with no mortality and extremely low morbidity and results in dramatic and definite improvement in the signs and symptoms of patients with acromegaly and Cushing's syndrome (adrenal hyperplasia). In general, patients with Cushing's disease require larger amounts of radiation than do those with acromegaly. Heavy-particle treatment in Nelson's syndrome appears less favorable, a finding which emphasizes the need for aggressive prevention or treatment of this disorder. In the case of patients with chromophobe adenoma, heavy-particle treatment appears to compare favorably with conventional methods of treatment, but the selection criteria interfere with a satisfactory evaluation of our limited series. However, in a larger series, the higher doses that can be delivered with heavy particles should result in better results and longer average survival.

Acknowledgments

These studies were made possible by the generous assistance of many individuals. The authors would especially like to thank Mr. James Vale and his crew for their skillful operation of the cyclotron, Mr. Jerry Howard for his efficient operation of the Medical Control Room, Mr. Robert Walton for his valuable help in the Medical Cave, and Miss Janice DeMoor for her preparation of material for this manuscript (without her talents this lecture and paper would not have been possible)—J. H. L. This paper was submitted for publication in November 1971.

REFERENCES

Bailey, O. T., and Cutler, E. C.: Malignant adenomas of the chromophobe cells of the pituitary body. *Archives of Pathology,* 29:368-399, 1940.

Benbow, R. M., von Essen, C. F., Rowe, J. W., and Stedeford, J. B.: Treatment design for pituitary suppression utilizing 6-Mev photons. *Radiology,* 87:64-67, 1966.

Berg, N. O., and Lindgren, M.: Time-dose relationship and morphology of delayed radiation lesions of the brain in rabbits. *Acta Radiologica* (Supplement), 167:1-118, 1958.

Christy, N. P.: When to hospitalize in acromegaly. *Hospital Practice,* 4:54-57, February 1969.

Clinicopathological Conference: The case of the persistent pituitary. Presented at the Royal Postgraduate Medical School. *British Medical Journal,* 2:557-560, 1969.

Cohen, H., and Dible, J. H.: Pituitary basophilism associated with a basophil carcinoma of the anterior lobe of the pituitary gland. *Brain,* 59:395-407, 1936.

Cushing, H.: The basophil adenomas of the pituitary body and their clinical manifestations (pituitary basophilism). *Bulletin of the Johns Hopkins Hospital,* 50:137-195, 1932.

Evans, H. M., Briggs, J. H., and Dixon, J. S.: The physiology and chemistry of growth hormone. In Harris, G. W., and Donnovan, B. T., Eds.: *The Pituitary Gland.* University of California Press, 1966, Vol. 1, pp. 439-491.

Feiring, E. H., Davidoff, L. M., and Zimmerman, H. M.: Primary carcinoma of the pituitary. *Journal of Neuropathology and Experimental Neurology,* 12:205-223, 1953.

Forbes, W.: Carcinoma of the pituitary gland with metastases to the liver in a case of Cushing's syndrome. *Journal of Pathology and Bacteriology,* 59:137-144, 1947.

Fraser, R., Doyle, F. H., Joplin, G. F., Burke, C. W., and Arnot, R.: The treatment of Cushing's disease by pituitary implant of Y-90 or Au-198. (In press, 1971.)

Fraser, T. R., and Wright, A. D.: Treatment of acromegaly and Cushing's disease by ^{90}Y implant for partial ablation of the pituitary. In Astwood, E. B., and Cassidy, C. B., Eds.: *Clinical Endocrinology II.* New York, New York, Grune and Stratton, 1968, pp. 78-92.

Garcia, J. F., Linfoot, J. A., Manougian, E., Born, J. L., and Lawrence, J. H.: Plasma growth hormone studies in normal individuals and acromegalic patients. *Journal of Clinical Endocrinology and Metabolism,* 27:1395-1402, 1967.

German, W. J., and Flanigan, S.: Pituitary adenomas: A follow-up study of the Cushing series. In *Clinical Neurosurgery*, Baltimore, Maryland, The Williams and Wilkins Co., 1964, Vol. X, pp. 72-81.

Goldberg, M. D., Sheline, G. E., and Malamud, N.: Malignant intracranial neoplasms following radiation therapy for acromegaly. *Radiology*, 80:465-470, 1963.

Greenhouse, A. H.: Pituitary sarcoma. A possible consequence of radiation. *Journal of the American Medical Association*, 190:269-273, 1964.

Hamberger, C. A., Hammer, G., Norlen, G., and Sjögren, B.: Surgical treatment of acromegaly. *Acta Oto-Laryngologica (Stockholm)*, Supplement 158:168-172, 1960.

Hamwi, G. J., Skillman, T. G., and Tufts, K. C., Jr.: Acromegaly. *American Journal of Medicine*, 29:690-699, 1960.

Hardy, J., and Wigser, S. M.: Trans-sphenoidal surgery of pituitary fossa tumors with televised radiofluoroscopic control. *Journal of Neurosurgery*, 23:612-619, 1965.

Hartog, M., Doyle, F., Fotherby, K., Fraser, R., and Joplin, G. F.: Partial pituitary ablation with implants of gold-198 and yttrium-90 for Cushing's syndrome with associated adrenal hyperplasia. *British Medical Journal*, 2:393-395, 1965.

Haugen, H. N., and Loken, A. C.: Carcinoma of the hypophysis associated with Cushing's syndrome and Addisonian pigmentation. *Journal of Clinical Endocrinology*, 20:173-179, 1960.

Henderson, W. R.: Pituitary adenomata: Follow-up study of surgical results in 338 cases (Dr. Harvey Cushing's series). *British Journal of Surgery*, 26:811-921, April 1939.

Jadresic, A., and Poblete, M.: Stereotaxic pituitary implantation of yttrium-90 and iridium-192 for acromegaly. *Journal of Clinical Endocrinology and Metabolism*, 27:1502-1507. 1967.

Jefferson, G.: The invasive adenomas of the anterior pituitary. *Sherrington Lecture No. III*. Liverpool, England, University Press, 1954.

Kaufman, B., Pearson, O. H., Shealy, C. N., Chernak, E. S., Samaan, N., and Storaasli, J. P.: Transnasal-transsphenoidal yttrium-90 pituitary implantation in the therapy of acromegaly. *Radiology*, 86:915-920, 1966.

Kernohan, J. W., and Sayre, G. P.: Tumors of the pituitary gland and infundibulum. Section 10, Fascicle 36, In *Atlas of Tumor Pathology*. Washington, D. C., Armed Forces Institute of Pathology, 1956, 81 pp.

Kraus, J. E.: Neoplastic diseases of the human hypophysis. *Archives of Pathology*, 39:343-349, 1945.

Lawrence, J. H.: Particules lourdes en thérapie. *La Presse Medicale*, 72:1349-1352, 1964.

Lawrence, J. H.: Proton irradiation of the pituitary. *Cancer*, 10:795-798, 1957.

Lawrence, J. H., Nelson, W. O., and Wilson, H.: Roentgen irradiation of the hypophysis. *Radiology*, 29:446-454, 1937.

Lawrence, J. H., Tobias, C. A., Born, J. L., Sangalli, F., Carlson, R. A., and Linfoot, J. H.: Heavy particle therapy in acromegaly. *Acta Radiologica*, 58:337-347, 1962.

Lawrence, J. H., Tobias, C. A., Linfoot, J. A., Born, J. L., Lyman, J. T., Chong, C. Y., Manougian, E., and Wei, W. C.: Successful treatment of acromegaly:

Metabolic and clinical studies in 145 patients. *Journal of Clinical Endocrinology and Metabolism*, 31:180-198, 1970.

Liddle, G. T.: Cushing's syndrome. In Eisenstein, A. B., Ed.: *The Adrenal Cortex*. Boston, Massachusetts, Little, Brown and Co., 1967, pp. 523-551.

Lindgren, M.: On tolerance of brain tissue and sensitivity of brain tumours to irradiation. *Acta Radiologica*, Supplement 170:1-73, 1958.

Linfoot, J. A., Chong, C. Y., Garcia, J. F., Cleveland, A. S., Connell, G. M., Manougian, E., Okerlund, M. D., Born, J. L., and Lawrence, J. H.: Heavy-particle therapy for acromegaly, Cushing's disease, Nelson's syndrome, and non-functioning pituitary adenomas. In Lawrence, J. H., Ed.: *Progress in Atomic Medicine: Recent Advances in Nuclear Medicine*. New York, New York, Grune and Stratton, 1971, Vol. III, pp. 219-238.

Linfoot, J. A., Lawrence, J. H., Tobias, C. A., Born, J. L., Chong, C. Y., Lyman, J. T., and Manougian, E.: Progress report on the treatment of Cushing's disease. *Transactions of the American Clinical and Climatological Association*, 81:196-212, 1970.

Marie, P.: Sur deux cas d'acromégalie. Hypertrophie singulière non-congénitale, des extrémites supérieures, inférieures, et céphalique. *Review de Medicine (Paris)*, 6:297-333, April 1886.

Martins, A. N., Hayes, G. J., and Kempe, L. G.: Invasive pituitary adenomas. *Journal of Neurosurgery*, 22:268-276, 1965.

Minagi, H., and Steinbach, H. L.: Roentgen aspects of pituitary tumors manifested after bilateral adrenalectomy for Cushing's syndrome. *Radiology*, 90:276-280, 1968.

Molinatti, G. M., Camanni, F., Massara, F., Olivetti, M., Pizzini, A., and Guiliani, G.: Implantation of yttrium-[90] in sella turcica in sixteen cases of acromegaly. *Journal of Clinical Endocrinology and Metabolism*, 22:599-611, 1962.

Montgomery, D. A. D., Welbourn, R. B., McGaughey, W. T. E., and Gleadhill, C. A.: Pituitary tumours manifested after adrenalectomy for Cushing's syndrome. *The Lancet*, 2:707-710, 1959.

Nelson, P. H., Meakin, J. W., and Thorn, G. W.: ACTH-producing pituitary tumors following adrenalectomy for Cushing's syndrome. *Annals of Internal Medicine*, 52:560-569, March 1960.

Newton, T. H., Burhenne, H. J., and Palubinskas, J.: Primary carcinoma of the pituitary. *American Journal of Roentgenology, Radium Therapy and Nuclear Medicine*, 87:110-120, 1962.

Peck, F. C., Jr., and McGovern, E. R.: Radiation necrosis of the brain in acromegaly. *Journal of Neurosurgery*, 25:536-542, 1966.

Plotz, C. M., Knowlton, A. I., and Ragan, C.: The natural history of Cushing's syndrome. *The American Journal of Medicine*, 13:597-614, 1952.

Rand, R. W., Solomon, D. H., Dashe, A. M., and Heuser, G.: Cryohypophysectomy in acromegaly. *Transactions of the American Neurological Association*, 91:324-325, 1966.

Ray, B. S.: Surgery of recurrent intracranial tumors. In *Clinical Neurosurgery*. Baltimore, Maryland, The Williams and Wilkins Co., 1964, Vol. X, pp. 1-30.

Ray, B. S., Horwith, M., and Mautalen, C.: Surgical hypophysectomy as a treatment for acromegaly. In Astwood, C. B., and Cassidy, C. E., Eds.: *Clinical Endocrinology II*. New York, New York, Grune and Stratton, 1968, pp. 93-102.

Richmond, J. J.: Pituitary tumors: The role of radiotherapy. *Proceedings of the Royal Society of Medicine*, 51:911-914, 1958.

Roth, J., Gorden, P., and Brace, K.: Efficacy of conventional pituitary irradiation in acromegaly. *The New England Journal of Medicine*, 282:1385-1391, 1970.

Rovit, R. L., and Berry, R.: Cushing's syndrome and the hypophysis: A re-evaluation of pituitary tumors and hyperadrenalism. *Journal of Neurosurgery*, 23: 270-295, 1965.

Rovit, R. L., and Duane, T. D.: Cushing's syndrome and the pituitary tumors: Pathophysiology and ocular manifestations of ACTH-secreting pituitary adenomas. *American Journal of Medicine*, 46:416-427, March 1969.

Salassa, R. M., Kearns, T. P., Kernohan, J. W., Sprague, R. G., and MacCarty, C. S.: Pituitary tumors in patients with Cushing's syndrome. *Journal of Clinical Endocrinology and Metabolism*, 19:1523-1539, 1959.

Scholz, D. A., Gastineau, C. F., and Harrison, E. G., Jr.: Cushing's syndrome with malignant chromophobe tumor of the pituitary and extracranial metastasis: Report of a case. *Proceedings of the Staff Meetings of the Mayo Clinic*, 37:31-42, 1962.

Sheldon, W. H., Golden, A., and Bondy, P. K.: Cushing's syndrome produced by a pituitary basophil carcinoma with hepatic metastases. *American Journal of Medicine*, 17:134-142, 1954.

Shrank, A. B., and Turner, P.: Pituitary adenoma with Cushing's syndrome, *British Medical Journal*, 1:849-852, 1960.

Simkin, B., Panish, J. F., Palmer, W. S., and Cohen, S.: Cushing's syndrome associated with a basophilic carcinoma of the pituitary. *Annals of Internal Medicine*, 56:495-503, March 1962.

Spark, C., and Biller, S. B.: Acromegaly with long-standing tumor infiltration of cavernous sinuses. *A.M.A. Archives of Pathology*, 35:93-111, 1943.

Terry, R. D., Hyams, V. J., and Davidoff, L. M.: Combined nonmetastasizing fibrosarcoma and chromophobe tumor of the pituitary. *Cancer*, 12:791-798, 1959.

Thompson, K. W., and Eisenhardt, L.: Cushing's syndrome. *Journal of Clinical Endocrinology*, 3:445-452, 1943.

Tobias, C. A., Anger, H. O., and Lawrence, J. H.: Radiological use of high energy deuterons and alpha particles. *American Journal of Roentgenology, Radium Therapy and Nuclear Medicine*, 67:1-27, 1952.

Tobias, C. A., Lawrence, J. H., Born, J. L., McCombs, R. K., Roberts, J. E., Anger, H. O., Low-Beer, B. V. A., and Huggins, C.: Pituitary irradiation with high-energy proton beams. A preliminary report. *Cancer Research*, 18:121-134, 1958.

Tobias, C. A., Lyman, J. T., and Lawrence, J. H.: Some considerations of physical and biological factors in radiotherapy with high-LET radiations including heavy particle, pi mesons, and fast neutrons. In Lawrence, J. H., Ed.: *Progress in Atomic Medicine: Recent Advances in Nuclear Medicine*. New York, New York, Grune and Stratton, 1971, Vol. III, pp. 167-218.

Tobias, C. A., Van Dyke, D. C., Simpson, M. E., Anger, H. O., Huff, R. L., and Koneff, A. A.: Irradiation of the pituitary of the rat with high energy deuterons. *American Journal of Roentgenology, Radium Therapy and Nuclear Medicine*, 72:1-21, 1954.

Walsh, F. C.: Bilateral total ophthalmoplegia with adenoma of the pituitary

gland. Report of two cases; an anatomic study. *Archives of Ophthalmology,* 42:646-654, 1949.
Weinberger, L. M., Adler, F. H., and Grant, F. C.: Primary pituitary adenomas and the syndrome of the cavernous sinus. *Archives of Ophthalmology,* 24: 1197-1236, 1940.
Welbourn, R. B., Montgomery, D. A. D., and Kennedy, T. L.: The natural history of treated Cushing's syndrome. *British Journal of Surgery,* 58:1-16, January 1971.
Wheelock, M. C.: Eosinophilic adenoma of the pituitary with sarcomatous changes. In del Regato, J. A., Ed.: *Cancer Seminar.* Colorado Springs, Colorado, Penrose Cancer Hospital, 1963, Vol. III, pp. 77-79.
Wright, A. D., Hill, D. M., Lowy, C., and Fraser, T. R.: Mortality in acromegaly. *Quarterly Journal of Medicine,* 39:1-16, 1970.
Zervas, N. T.: Stereotaxic radiofrequency surgery of the normal and abnormal pituitary gland. *The New England Journal of Medicine,* 280:429-437, 1969.

The Radiologic Changes in Pituitary Lesions

SIDNEY WALLACE, M.D.

Department of Diagnostic Radiology, The University of Texas at Houston M. D. Anderson Hospital and Tumor Institute, Houston, Texas

ENDOCRINOLOGICAL MANIFESTATIONS of sellar and parasellar lesions are the result of pituitary hyper- or hypofunction or of hypothalamic impairment. The radiologic changes are dependent upon the size and localization of the lesion. Tumor localization and the possible etiologic agents may be categorized as follows:

Intrasellar—pituitary adenomas and adenocarcinomas, craniopharyngiomas, myoblastomas, adamantinomas, arachnoidal cysts, pituitary cysts, "empty" sella, dilated third ventricle extending into the sella, pseudotumor cerebri, and apparent sellar enlargement associated with increased intracranial pressure.

Suprasellar—pituitary adenomas with suprasellar extension, craniopharyngiomas, optic and hypothalamic gliomas, meningiomas, teratoid tumors, ectopic pinealomas, aneurysms, and a dilated third ventricle.

Retrosellar—pituitary lesions with retrosellar extension, meningiomas, chordomas, osteochondromas, chondrosarcomas, osteosarcomas, basilar artery aneurysms, and brain stem gliomas extending anteriorly.

Parasellar—pituitary tumors with parasellar extension, meningiomas, aneurysms of the cavernous portion of the carotid artery, and neuromas of the trigeminal nerve.

Infrasellar—pituitary tumors with inferior extension, nasopharyngeal carcinomas, and sphenoid sinus carcinomas.

Intra-axial—colloid cysts of the third ventricle, tuberous sclerosis, hypothalamic gliomas, and inflammatory lesions, *e.g.*, sarcoidosis, *etc.* Metastases can be found in any of the above-listed sites.

There is no constant relationship between the volume of the sella turcica

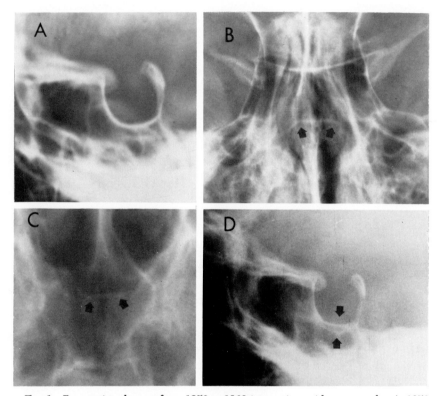

Fig. 1.—Progressive changes from 1953 to 1969 in a patient with acromegaly: *A*, 1953 —sella turcica, lateral projection; *B*, 1953—sella turcica, PA projection (→ : floor of the sella); *C*, 1953—sella turcica, base view (→ : anterior portion of the sella turcica); *D*, 1963—sella turcica, lateral projection (→ : double floor).

and the size of the pituitary gland. On the average, 80 per cent of the volume of the sella turcica is occupied by the pituitary gland, allowing significant enlargement before any obvious radiographic changes can be appreciated. The pituitary gland may increase in size at the expense of the venous sinuses and as much as double in size, *e.g.*, during pregnancy, without altering the bony cavity. In addition, the sella turcica has a fairly wide range of normal volumetric measurement, 282 cu. mm. to 1,096 cu. mm., as calculated by Di Chiro and Nelson (1962) utilizing the formula:

$$V = \tfrac{1}{2}DLW,$$

a modification of the determination of the volume of an ellipsoid:

$$V = 4/3 \, \pi \, D/2 \times L/2 \times W/2,$$

where D = maximum depth, L = maximum length, and W = maximum

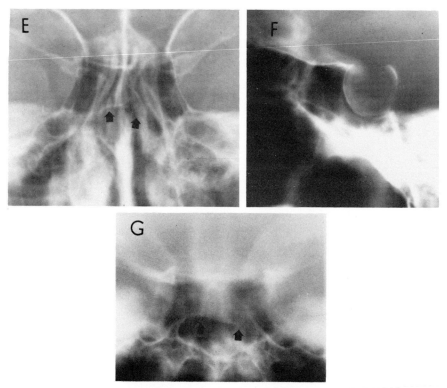

Fig. 1 (*continued*).—*E*, 1963—sella turcica, PA projection (→: depression of the floor on the left); *F*, 1969—sella turcica, tomogram of the lateral view demonstrating thinning and bowing of the dorsum sella and more acute angulation of the tuberculum resulting from enlargement by the expanding eosinophilic adenoma; *G*, 1969—sella turcica, AP tomogram (→ : demonstrating depression of the floor and enlargement of the sella).

width. The pituitary may exceed the volume of the bony sella by 10 to 20 per cent without being observed roentgenographically. These possibilities may explain the normal radiologic findings reported in 8 to 13 per cent of pituitary tumors (Lombardi, 1967).

Alterations in the contour of the sella turcica as the result of erosion and destruction of the bony confines by an expanding intrasellar process precede the radiologic recognition of obvious volumetric changes. These findings include: (1) sharpening of the inferior aspect of the clinoids, (2) alteration of the angle between the tuberculum sellae and the anterior wall of the sella turcica resulting in a balloon-shaped or cup-shaped sella, (3) thinning and depression of the sellar floor which when asymmetric results in the appearance of a "double floor" in the lateral projection, and (4) straightening and thinning the dorsum sellae. Tomography in the antero-posterior, lateral, and base projections may assist in the delineation of these changes in contour.

The gradual alteration of the contour of the sella is illustrated by a patient (Fig. 1), examined radiographically over a period from 1953 to 1969. Headache was her only complaint in 1963, at which time the roentgenogram of the sella turcica demonstrated a depression of the sellar floor. Clinical evidence of acromegaly was obvious in 1969 when an eosinophilic adenoma was managed surgically.

Another patient (Fig. 2) presented with notable progressive increase in skin pigmentation after bilateral adrenalectomy for Cushing's disease. This complex, Nelson's syndrome (Nelson and Meakin, 1959), is believed to be the result of an increase in the amount of melanocyte-stimulating hormone (MSH) released from the pituitary. Her sella turcica was within normal volumetric measurements. However, the contour of the sella was altered, as manifested by an angulation and sharpening of the tuberculum sellae. There was unilateral erosion of the sellar floor.

An increase in the volume of the sella turcica is a definite indication for

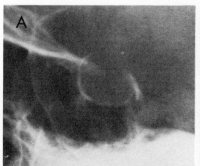
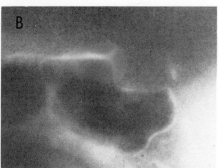
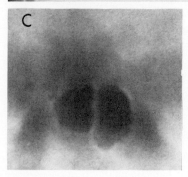

Fig. 2.—Alterations in the contour of the sella turcica produced by a pituitary adenoma: Nelson's syndrome; A and B, sella turcica, lateral projection and tomogram. The tuberculum sellae is sharpened and angulated. There is some thinning of the dorsum sella; C, sella turcica, tomograms in the AP projection. There is depression of the floor of the sella on the right.

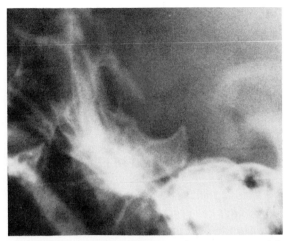

Fig. 3.—A J-shaped sella in an optic glioma is producing this type of destruction of the sella. In Figure 5A, the J shape is caused by a craniopharyngioma.

further clinical and radiological examinations and hormonal assays. With a sella which is borderline in size and which has normal, sharply defined contours and a lack of clinical signs and symptoms, further radiologic examination is rarely rewarding.

Enlargement of the sella may be associated with a "characteristic" change in contour, such as the "balloon-shaped" sella which is frequently seen with the slowly growing eosinophilic adenoma, the "cup-shaped" sella in chromophobe adenoma, and the "J-shaped" sella attributed to optic glioma (Fig. 3). These are not specific in that the balloon and cup shapes may be seen in any type of pituitary tumor, while a J shape may be normal or seen in Hurler's disease, craniopharyngioma, aneurysm, or with any process involving the optic canals, eroding the undersurface of the anterior clinoids.

As the pituitary tumor extends beyond the confines of the sella turcica (Fig. 4), it may project inferiorly into the sphenoid sinus and nasopharynx; posteriorly, by destroying the posterior clinoids, dorsum sellae, and clivus; or anteriorly, projecting into the optic canals, sphenoidal fissure, and nasal cavity. Two of our patients presented with nasal masses. Pituitary adenomas may extend into the optic canals, producing decalcification and blurring of the inferior margins of the optic canals. This is in contrast to the diffuse enlargement of the optic canals with maintenance of the sharp margins which is seen more frequently with optic gliomas and neurofibromas of the optic nerves. Aneurysms of the cavernous portion of the carotid artery may produce ipsilateral sellar destruction, widening of the sphenoidal fis-

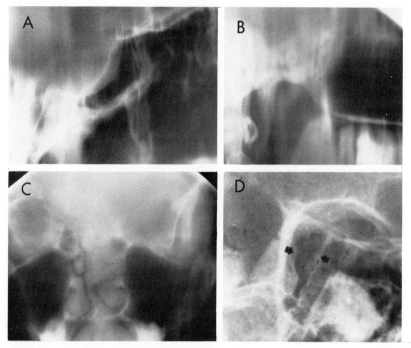

FIG. 4.—Extrasellar extension of pituitary tumors: *A*, destruction of the posterior cli-noids and dorsum sella, as well as the anterior clinoids, by a pituitary adenoma; *B* and *C*, pituitary adenoma extending into the sphenoid sinus and nasal cavity, producing exten-sive destruction of the base of the skull; *D*, projection of a pituitary adenoma into the optic canal and superior orbital fissure. (Courtesy of Dr. N. Leeds, Montefiore Hospital, New York.)

sure, and erosion of the anterior inferior aspect of the anterior clinoids. There may be erosion of the lower and outer wall of the optic canal with destruction of the porous strut of bone which arises from the side of the body of the sphenoid to the lesser wing of the sphenoid to complete the circumference of the foramen. Craniopharyngiomas may also extend into the optic foramina and may be associated with sclerosis of the sellar floor.

Superior extension of pituitary tumors takes place through the dia-phragma sellae, eroding the anterior clinoids from below, thinning and straightening the posterior clinoids and dorsum sellae. These tumors may extend into the suprasellar cistern, hypothalamus, and third ventricle and may eventually obstruct the lateral ventricles at the foramen of Monro. In-creased intracranial pressure from obstruction of the foramen of Monro or obliteration of the arachnoid pathways in the suprasellar cistern is unusual with sellar or parasellar lesions in adults, but may be seen in children. Suprasellar processes including hypothalamic and chiasmatic gliomas, craniopharyngiomas originating in the infundibulum or tuber cinereum, teratoid tumors, ectopic pinealomas, and lesions producing a dilated anterior third ventricle may penetrate into the sella, eroding the anterior and posterior clinoids from above.

Calcification in the sellar and parasellar areas may give some indication of the nature of the lesion. Only 1.2 to 9 per cent of pituitary adenomas are reported to be calcified (Lombardi, 1967). This calcification may be curvilinear when it occurs in the capsule or wall of a cyst or it may be flake-like, usually within the lesion (Fig. 5A). Calcification of craniopharyngiomas is reported to occur in as many as 89 per cent of patients below 15 years of age and in 40 per cent above 15, with an over-all incidence of 56 per cent. The calcification is most frequently flocculent. Craniopharyngiomas are rarely confined to the sella and may be associated with sclerosis of the floor of the sella. Incidence of calcification of optic and hypothalamic gliomas was as high as 50 per cent in one series but was considered rare in another (Lombardi, 1967 [rare]; Ross and Greitz, 1966 [20 per cent]; Lindgren and Di

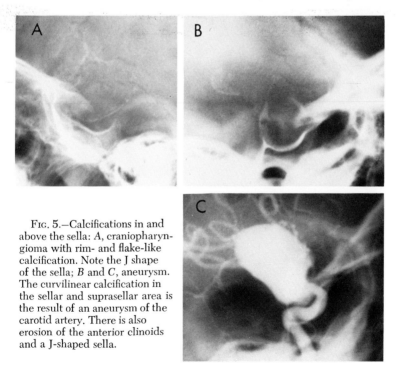

Fig. 5.—Calcifications in and above the sella: *A*, craniopharyngioma with rim- and flake-like calcification. Note the J shape of the sella; *B* and *C*, aneurysm. The curvilinear calcification in the sellar and suprasellar area is the result of an aneurysm of the carotid artery. There is also erosion of the anterior clinoids and a J-shaped sella.

Chiro, 1951 [50 per cent]). Meningiomas may also calcify (6.7 to 14.7 per cent). The possibility of an aneurysm must always be kept in mind when calcification is seen and is of the curvilinear type (Fig. 5B and C).

Angiography

The purpose of vascular studies in the evaluation of sellar and parasellar lesions is to determine the extent of involvement and the nature of the lesion

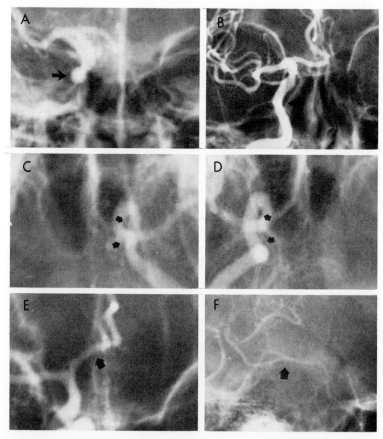

Fig. 6.—Angiographic changes in pituitary tumors: *A*, normal cavernous portion of the internal carotid artery in the AP projection (→); *B*, lateral displacement of the cavernous portion of the carotid artery (AP projection: →) by a pituitary adenoma; *C*, normal cavernous portion of the internal carotid artery: (→) base view; *D*, cavernous portion of the carotid artery, displaced by pituitary adenoma with lateral extension; *E*, elevation of the initial portion of the anterior cerebral artery by a pituitary adenoma with anterior extension; *F*, elevation of the basilar vein of Rosenthal by a pituitary adenoma extending superiorly.

as well as to rule out the existence of an aneurysm (Fig. 5C). There even have been occasional reports of pituitary hyperfunction associated with an aneurysm (White and Ballantine, 1961).

Immediately surrounding the sella turcica is the cavernous sinus. Opacification of this structure may be accomplished by orbital venography and/or jugular venography with the added assistance of subtraction technique (Weidner, Rosen, and Hanafee, 1965; Hanafee, Rosen, Weidner, and Wilson, 1965).

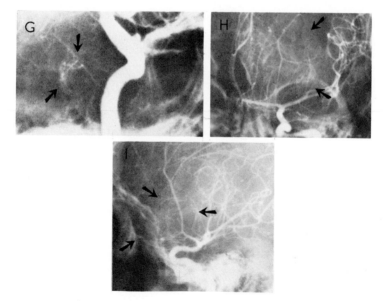

Fig. 6 (*continued*).—G, increased vascularity from the cavernous branches of the carotid artery to a pituitary adenoma (→); H and I, increased vascularity to a large pituitary adenoma which projected superiorly, anteriorly, and inferiorly.

Perhaps a more reliable index of the lateral extension of a pituitary lesion is achieved by opacifying the cavernous portion of the carotid artery as it penetrates the cavernous sinus (Fig. 6A through D). In the anteroposterior projection, the posterior portion of the cavernous segment of the carotid artery lies medially to or superimposed upon the anterior portion. Therefore, lateral displacement of the posterior portion is indicative of lateral extension. A base view of the cavernous portion is even more revealing for the demonstration of lateral displacement.

Suprasellar extension will straighten the supraclinoid portion of the carotid artery as well as displace it laterally. Anterior extension will produce elevation of the anterior cerebral and anterior communicating arteries (Fig. 6E). Superiorly, the anterior choroidal and posterior communicating arteries as well as the mamillary branches may be displaced. The initial portion of the basilar vein of Rosenthal may be elevated (Fig. 6F). Posterior extension into the interpeduncular cistern may displace the basilar artery.

The pituitary gland is supplied by the inferior hypophyseal artery, a branch of the meningohypophyseal trunk originating from the posterior portion of the cavernous segment of the carotid artery. In addition, the superior hypophyseal, which originates from the carotid artery opposite the takeoff of the ophthalmic artery, supplies the anterior and superior aspects of the hypophysis. The capsular branches from the cavernous carotid also contribute to the hypophyseal supply. Pituitary tumors (Fig. 6G and H) may exhibit a vascular blush (Kricheff and Schotland, 1964; Feiring and Shapiro, 1964; Doron and Schwartz, 1965; Lehrer and Richardson, 1969). It has been suggested by Doron and Schwartz (1965) that a vascular blush indicates greater aggressiveness of the lesion, but this was not confirmed by the other authors. Doron, Behar, and Beller (1965) also reported a vascularized myoblastoma of the pituitary, a neoplasm of the embryonic muscle cells. Meningiomas in the area may be associated with increased vascularity. Metastases to the pituitary might be accompanied by a vascular blush.

Pneumoencephalography

Pneumoencephalography is a complementary procedure to angiography and supplies essential information in the diagnosis and management of sellar or parasellar lesions. Pneumoencephalography is primarily used to demonstrate the suprasellar extension of pituitary tumors (Fig. 7A through E). Normally, air injected into the basilar cisterns will temporarily collect behind the transverse arachnoidal membrane (membrane of Liliqvist), a fold of arachnoid extending from the mamillary bodies to the posterior clinoids, which has an anterior concavity. Once the air bypasses this membrane, it outlines the tuber cinereum, which also forms a concavity anteriorly. A suprasellar mass will reverse this contour. Projection of the neoplasm into the suprasellar cistern is best seen in the lateral view in the erect position and in the hyperextended lateral views in the supine position. Tomography is helpful in separating midline from more laterally placed air. At times, air will surround the dome of the suprasellar portion of the tumor. This may be demonstrated by anteroposterior tomograms. Anterior extension may distort the olfactory grooves, displacing them laterally.

Encroachment on the ventricular system is best shown by pneumo-encephalography. The anterior inferior portion of the third ventricle, the chiasmatic and hypophyseal recesses, is blunted when the neoplasm projects superiorly. This too is best demonstrated by tomography in the lateral position with the patient supine and the head hyperextended so the anterior third ventricle and the recesses are maximally filled. If cisternal air is confused with third ventricular air, the brow-up position can be maintained for one or two hours (Mishkin, 1970), since cisternal air is absorbed more quickly than ventricular air. These landmarks may be obliterated by any suprasellar tumor, including meningiomas, which are usually more anteriorly placed, and optic gliomas, which may obliterate the chiasmatic recess or separate the chiasmatic and hypophyseal recesses. Craniopharyngiomas are usually more posterior, since they originate in rests in the hypophyseal stalk or tuber cinereum. Dilatation, tortuosity, or aneurysms of the basilar artery may impinge upon the floor of the third ventricle behind the hypophyseal recess.

If the mass projects into the third ventricle, it may obstruct the foramen of Monro and dilate the lateral ventricles. Positive contrast ventriculography may be used to demonstrate better the involvement of the third ventricle.

Lateral extension of pituitary tumors may displace the temporal horns of the lateral ventricles.

Sellar enlargement may be caused by the downward projection of the subarachnoidal pathways of the suprasellar cistern through an incomplete diaphragma sellae (Fig. 7F). Busch (1951) reported a 5.5 per cent incidence of a large defect in the diaphragma sellae and introduced the term "empty sella." In this condition, the pituitary is usually not absent but is flattened posteriorly. An "empty sella" may be caused by a congenital defect or may result from spontaneous infarction of a pituitary gland or tumor. Following radiation therapy to a pituitary tumor, "empty sella" may result.

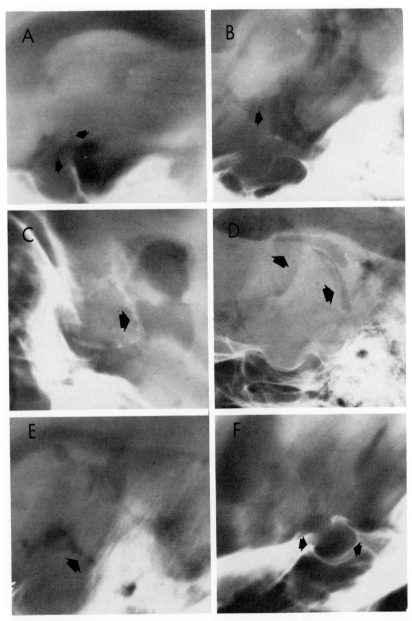

FIG. 7.—Pneumoencephalographic changes: *A*, pituitary adenoma with no evidence of extrasellar extension (→): note the normal concavity anteriorly of the transverse arachnoidal membrane; *B*, straightening of the normal curve of the transverse arach-

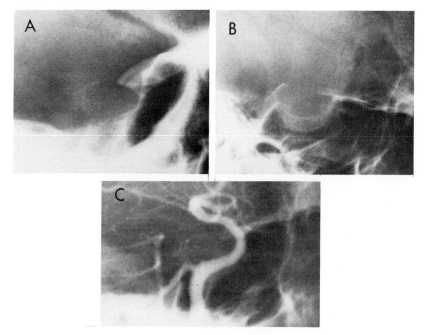

Fig. 8.—Metastasis to the sella turcica and hypophysis: *A*, breast metastasis producing destruction of the dorsum and posterior clinoids. The patient clinically had diabetes insipidus; *B* and *C*, metastatic melanoma. The sella is enlarged because of metastasis to the pituitary. There is an increased vascularity from the cavernous portion of the carotid artery to the pituitary metastasis. The carotid-basilar anastomosis is an incidental finding.

Metastases

Any of the previously described findings may also be found with metastases to the sellar and parasellar areas (Fig. 8). Breast carcinoma is the primary lesion which most frequently metastasizes to the pituitary. Other primaries include prostate, lung, melanoma, lymphoma, and leukemia. Metastases are more frequent to the bony casement than to the pituitary. Metastases are invariably to the posterior hypophysis and then to the anterior hypophysis. Anterior pituitary involvement alone is exceedingly rare (Duchen, 1966; Hägerstrand and Schönebeck, 1969).

---

noidal membrane, produced by superior extension of the pituitary adenoma ($\rightarrow$); *C*, blunting of the chiasmatic and hypophyseal recesses of the anterior inferior portion of the third ventricle by a craniopharyngioma; *D*, elevation and distortion of the third ventricle and aqueduct of Sylvius by a pituitary adenoma extending superiorly; *E*, posterior displacement and distortion of the pons by a pituitary adenoma extending superiorly and posteriorly; *F*, empty sella syndrome; note the air in the sella turcica. The recesses of the anterior inferior third ventricle are normal.

REFERENCES

Arsene, C., Ghitescu, M., Cristescu, A., et al.: Intrasellar aneurysms simulating hypophyseal tumors. European Neurology, 3:321-329, 1970.

Busch, W.: Die Morphologie des Sella Turcica und ihre Beziehungen zur Hypophyse. Virchows Archiv für pathologische Anatomie und Physiologie, 320:437, 1951.

Caplan, R. H., and Dobben, G. D.: Endocrine studies in patients with the "empty sella syndrome." Archives of Internal Medicine, 123:611-619, June 1969.

Conley, L. M.: Radiologic Seminar, CI. Roentgen changes in the sella turcica in pituitary tumors. Journal of the Mississippi State Medical Association, 11:600-601, 1970.

Di Chiro, G., and Nelson, K. B.: The volume of the sella turcica. The American Journal of Roentgenology, Radium Therapy and Nuclear Medicine, 87:989-1008, June 1962.

Doron, Y., Behar, A., and Beller, A. J.: Granular-cell "myoblastoma" of the neurohypophysis. Journal of Neurosurgery, 22:95-99, January 1965.

Doron, Y., and Schwartz, A.: The significance of the angiographic demonstration of tumour vessels in pituitary neoplasms. British Journal of Radiology, 38:356-359, May 1965.

du Boulay, G. H., and Trickey, S. E.: Case reports: Calcification in chromophobe adenoma. British Journal of Radiology, 35:793-795, November 1962.

Duchen, L. W.: Metastatic carcinoma in the pituitary gland and hypothalamus. Journal of Pathology and Bacteriology, 91:347-355, April 1966.

Feiring, E. H., and Shapiro, J. H.: Evaluation of angiography in the diagnosis of suprasellar tumors. The American Journal of Roentgenology, Radium Therapy and Nuclear Medicine, 92:811-828, October 1964.

Friedmann, G., and Marguth, F.: Intraselläre Liquorzysten. Zentralblatt für Neurochirurgie, 21:33-41, 1961.

Friesen, H. G., and Astwood, E. B.: Changes in neurohypophyseal proteins induced by dehydration and ingestion of saline. Endocrinology, 80:278-287, February 1967.

Hägerstrand, I., and Schönebeck, J.: Metastases to the pituitary gland. Acta Pathologica et Microbiologica Scandinavica, 75:64-70, 1969.

Hanafee, W., Rosen, L. M., Weidner, W., and Wilson, G. H.: Venography of the cavernous sinus, orbital veins, and basal venous plexus. Radiology, 84:751-753, April 1965.

Hertzog, E., Bamberger, C., and Guiot, G.: Neuro-radiological aspects of hypophyseal adenoma. Annales de Radiologie (Paris), 13:765, 1970.

Heuser, G., Moderator: Trends in clinical neuroendocrinology. UCLA Interdepartmental Conference. Annals of Internal Medicine, 73:783-807, November 1970.

Kaufman, B.: The "empty" sella turcica—a manifestation of the intrasellar subarachnoid space. Radiology, 90:931-941, May 1968.

Krach, J., and Tamm, J.: Invasiv gewachsenes basophiles Adenom des Hypophysenvorderlappens bei Cushing-Syndrome. Acta Endocrinologica, 43:330-344, 1363.

Kricheff, I. I., and Schotland, D. L.: Tumor stain in pituitary adenoma. *Radiology*, 82:11-13, January 1964.

Krieger, D. T., Krieger, H. P., and Soffer, L. J.: Cushing's syndrome associated with a suprasellar tumour. *Acta Endocrinologica*, 47:185-199, 1964.

Krueger, E. G., and Unger, S. M.: Extrasellar extension of pituitary adenomas: Clinical and neuroradiological considerations. *The American Journal of Roentgenology, Radium Therapy and Nuclear Medicine*, 98:616-630, November 1966.

Krueger, E. G., Unger, S. M., and Roswit, B.: Hemorrhage into pituitary adenoma with spontaneous recovery and reossification of the sella turcica. *Neurology*, 10:691-696, July 1960.

Lee, K. F.: The arterial relations of the diaphragma sellae: Preliminary report. (In preparation.)

Lee, W. M., and Adams, J. E.: The empty sella syndrome. *Journal of Neurosurgery*, 28:351-356, April 1968.

Lehrer, H. Z., and Richardson, D. E.: Meningioma blush in pituitary adenoma. *Acta Radiologica; Diagnosis*, 9:370-378, 1969.

Le May, M.: The radiologic diagnosis of pituitary disease. *Radiologic Clinics of North America*, 5:303-315, August 1967.

Lewtas, N. A.: Symposium on pituitary tumours: (2) Radiology in diagnosis and management. *Clinical Radiology*, 17:149-153, 1966.

Lindgren, E., and Di Chiro, G.: Suprasellar tumors with calcification. *Acta Radiologica*, 36:173-195, September 1951.

Lombardi, G.: *Radiology in Neuro-Ophthalmology*, Baltimore, Maryland: The Williams and Wilkins Co., 1967, 244 pp.

Meador, C. K., and Worrell, J. L.: The sella turcica in postpartum pituitary necrosis (Sheehan's syndrome). *Annals of Internal Medicine*, 65:259-264, August 1966.

Mishkin, M. M.: Juxtasellar mass lesions. *Seminars in Roentgenology*, 5:165-185, April 1970.

Nelson, D. H., and Meakin, J. W.: A new clinical entity in patients adrenalectomized for Cushing's syndrome. (Abstract) *Journal of Clinical Investigation*, 38:1028-1029, 1959.

Ring, B. A., and Waddington, M.: Primary arachnoid cysts of the sella turcica. *The American Journal of Roentgenology, Radium Therapy and Nuclear Medicine*, 98:611-615, November 1966.

Roessmann, U., Kaufman, B., and Friede, R. L.: Metastatic lesions in the sella turcica and pituitary gland. *Cancer*, 25:478-480, February 1970.

Ross, R. J., and Greitz, T. V. B.: Changes of the sella turcica in chromophobic adenomas and eosinophilic adenomas. *Radiology*, 86:892-899, May 1966.

Scatliff, J. H., and Bull, J. W. D.: The radiological manifestations of suprasellar metastatic tissue. *Clinical Radiology*, 16: 66-70, 1965.

Scothorne, C. M.: A glioma of the posterior lobe of the pituitary gland. *Journal of Pathology and Bacteriology*, 69:109-112, 1955.

Sheehan, H. L., and Stanfield, J. P.: The pathogenesis of postpartum necrosis of the anterior lobe of the pituitary gland. *Acta Endocrinologica*, 37:479-510, 1961.

Sheline, G. E., Boldrey, E. B., and Phillips, T. L.: Chromophobe adenomas of the pituitary gland. *The American Journal of Roentgenology, Radium Therapy and Nuclear Medicine*, 92:160-173, July 1964.

Silverman, F. N.: Roentgen standards for size of the pituitary fossa from infancy through adolescence. *The American Journal of Roentgenology, Radium Therapy and Nuclear Medicine*, 78:451-460, September 1957.

Waga, S., Kikuchi, H., Handa, J., and Handa, H.: Cavernous sinus venography. *The American Journal of Roentgenology, Radium Therapy and Nuclear Medicine*, 109:130-137, May 1970.

Weidner, W., Rosen, L., and Hanafee, W.: The neuroradiology of tumors of the pituitary gland. *The American Journal of Roentgenology, Radium Therapy and Nuclear Medicine*, 95:884-889, December 1965.

White, J. C., and Ballantine, H. T., Jr.: Intrasellar aneurysms simulating hypophyseal tumors. *Journal of Neurosurgery*, 18:34-50, January 1961.

Pituitary Adenomas— Surgical Treatment

MILAM E. LEAVENS, M.D.

Department of Surgery, The University of Texas at Houston
M. D. Anderson Hospital and Tumor Institute,
Houston, Texas

SCHLOFFER, in 1906, operated on pituitary adenomas by the transsphenoidal approach. Cushing's earliest verification of an adenoma of the pituitary was in 1909. The patient was an acromegalic farmer, age 38, referred by Dr. C. H. Mayo of Rochester, Minnesota. The patient had headaches and no visual loss. A transsphenoidal partial removal of the adenoma was accomplished. The patient's vision remained intact and he survived 21 years, dying of a coronary at the age of 59.

Hirsch, in 1910, also used the transsphenoidal approach to pituitary tumors. Davidoff (1926) stated that Cushing operated on large pituitary adenomas which extended into the sphenoid sinus. He operated on these patients through the sphenoid sinus but later preferred the transfrontal approach.

Most neurosurgeons of today use the transfrontal approach for pituitary adenomas. Hardy (1971) has recently been an advocate of the transsphenoidal approach to the pituitary gland, and has obtained good visibility using the dissecting microscope and X-ray-T.V. monitoring.

Chromophobe Adenomas

Chromophobe adenomas are tumors which are not hormonally active but which slowly destroy the function of the anterior lobe of the pituitary gland. This results in hypofunction of the target glands (gonad, thyroid, and adrenals). They also produce symptoms by enlarging the sella turcica and growing out of it, causing headaches and visual field defects. They may become huge, growing up into the basofrontal region, the middle fossa, or the sphenoid sinus. Carotid arteriography is indicated in studying these patients to determine the size and direction of growth of the tumor and to rule out other lesions, such as aneurysms or meningiomas, which may mimic chromophobe adenomas. Pneumoencephalography is useful to document the size of the tumors and to rule out hydrocephalus and the empty sella syndrome, both of which may be associated with hypofunction of the pituitary gland.

The usual standard treatment is irradiation (3,000 to 4,000 rads in four weeks) in those patients with little or no visual field defect. Chromophobe adenomas, which are associated with more than just a minimal bitemporal field defect, are generally treated first surgically and then by irradiation. Surgical techniques are indicated if there is a rapid or progressive visual loss or if the diagnosis of chromophobe adenoma is in doubt.

Cushing's series (German and Flanigan, 1964) is remarkable because Cushing operated before the time of blood banks, antibiotics, and cortisone, and yet had a respectable operative mortality rate. He performed transsphenoidal operations on 240 patients with chromophobe adenomas with an operative mortality rate of 5.8 per cent. The operative mortality rate was 4.7 per cent for those patients who were operated on transfrontally. His mortality rate during the last 10 years (205 cases) was 2.4 per cent.

The greatest hazard in the transfrontal operation was postoperative wound hematoma. In the transsphenoidal operation, the greatest hazard was meningitis. Four of Cushing's patients had hematomas, four meningitis, and one hemorrhage. His postoperative results in 247 patients were generally good. In 68 per cent, vision improved or progression of visual loss stopped and the patient returned to a normal occupation. In 18 per cent, postoperative vision was poor or presumably worsened. The best results were obtained in patients with partial involvement of one eye, bitemporal defects, central scotomas, or inferior quadrant defects. The next best results were in those with homonymous hemianopsia. The poorest results were those blind in one or both eyes.

Cushing's late results showed the advantage of the frontal over the transsphenoidal operation, as done at that time, and also the value of combining irradiation with the surgical treatment. The percentages of his chromophobe patients without recurrence after five years were as follows: transsphenoidal, 33 per cent; frontal craniotomy, 57 per cent; transsphenoidal and X-ray, 65 per cent; and frontal craniotomy and X-ray, 87 per cent.

Furst (1966) reported on 131 patients with chromophobe adenomas treated in Sweden from 1921 to 1960. Of these, 110 received surgical therapy; 78 received frontal craniotomies and medium voltage radiation. Nine of these died after craniotomy. Two had progression of tumor less than a year postoperatively and two had recurrences 11 and six years postoperation. Ten patients died four to 12 years after operation without recurrence, and 57 are still living without recurrence (five to 19 years) after operation. Five patients had only a biopsy (frontal) and irradiation. Two of these experienced recurrence (one at eight years) after operation.

Two patients had transsphenoidal operations and irradiation. One patient had a large adenoma which had not recurred seven years after operation. The other was discovered to have a temporal extension of tumor unrecognized before the initial operation, and a second frontal operation was done. Seven had only surgical treatment. Two have had no recurrence after 10 to 30 years. Five have had recurrence one and a half to 13 years after surgery.

The best effect of the operation was on patients with incomplete hemianopsia. If more than one half of the visual field was gone, and especially if the defect was of long standing, the chances of recovery were poor. With combined surgical and irradiation treatment, 84 per cent had sufficient visual capacity to allow them to work.

Svien and co-workers (1965) reported on a series of 71 patients with pituitary chromophobe adenoma treated by frontal craniotomy. Vision was improved in 70 per cent, remained unchanged in 8.6 per cent, and became worse in 21 per cent after craniotomy. Vision returned to normal in about 20 per cent.

Elkington and McKissock (1967) reported on the combined surgical and radiotherapeutic treatment of 260 patients with chromophobe adenomas. The indication for operation was impaired vision. In these patients, frontal craniotomy was combined with radiation—3,000 to 4,000 rads over 28 days. The operative mortality rate was 10 per cent. The operative mortality rate in those with huge suprasellar or parasellar middle fossa extension of tumor was 33 per cent. After surgical treatment, 55 per cent had improved vision and 17 per cent had worse vision.

This high mortality rate with transfrontal removal of these huge tumors is prohibitive. Hardy (1971) operates on the huge suprasellar pituitary adenomas transsphenoidally if the tumor is directly above the sella turcica. He has been able to do this without mortality and has demonstrated that the remaining tumor capsule falls into the sella turcica postoperatively. He does not operate on those tumors that extend far anterior to the sella turcica or those extending into the middle fossa.

Acromegaly

Acromegaly is an interesting syndrome resulting from a growth hormone-secreting, acidophilic adenoma of the pituitary gland. The syndrome was described and named acromegaly (*akron*—extremity, *mega*—large) in 1886 by Pierre Marie, a French neurologist. Acromegaly may be associated with gigantism if the tumor begins before puberty. These tumors enlarge the sella and grow out of the sella turcica into the suprasellar, basofrontal region or into the temporal lobe. Headaches and visual field defects, usually bitemporal, occur.

Davidoff (1926) analyzed 100 acromegalics. The disease began at an average age of 26 (14 to 51 years). The course of development of the syndrome could be divided into three periods. There was an early period of accentuated growth with increase in size of the acral parts (extremities) and usually of the entire body, amounting to actual gigantism. In women, this period was also associated with irregular menses and amenorrhea. The early period lasted three to six years. The second or middle period consisted of the development of neighborhood symptoms caused by an enlarging adenoma. Patients had headaches and fading vision in this period. Sixty-eight per cent had visual field defects at the time of admission. Ninety-three per cent had X-ray evidence of an enlarged sella turcica. In the third or final period of development, secondary symptoms and signs caused by late effects of visceral splanchnomegaly (cardiac, in particular) and the effects on the vascular system developed. The patients tended to have peripheral arteriosclerosis, hypertension, cardiac disease and enlargement, and diabetes mellitus which is difficult to control; all of these contributed to a shortened life expectancy.

Bishop and Briggs (1958) analyzed 100 acromegalics and found that 80 per cent died before the age of 60, usually from cardiovascular causes.

Therefore, it is apparent that there are three reasons to treat acromegalics: (1) to stop or reverse the development of acromegalic features, (2) to relieve secondary signs and symptoms (headache and visual loss), and (3) to prevent the late effects of the disease on the cardiovascular system which shorten the life expectancy of the patient.

Total adenoma removal is the treatment of choice for these patients. In some patients, the adenoma is diffuse, occupying the entire sella turcica. An attempt at total hypophysectomy would be necessary in such a patient to lower the human growth hormone output to zero or to a normal range. In other patients, there may be a microadenoma which can be removed, leaving a normally functioning pituitary gland. Subtotal removal of a diffuse adenoma may improve vision but usually does not alter or help the acromegaly. Total hypophysectomy is contraindicated in young acromegalic women who are still menstruating and who desire pregnancy and children. Total hypophysectomy is also contraindicated in those patients who are mentally defective and lack the intelligence needed to follow instructions regarding replacement therapy (cortisone, thyroid).

Cushing (German and Flanigan, 1964) operated on 77 acromegalics—69 using the transsphenoidal approach, seven the frontal approach, and one using subtemporal decompression. Fifty per cent had supplemental radiation. The early results were: Preoperatively, one-half had serious visual impairment, and 86 per cent had significant improvement postoperatively. Three-fourths had significant headaches preoperatively, and 55 per cent eventually obtained relief from their headaches. The immediate operative mortality rate was 10 per cent. The operative deaths plus five-year deaths equalled 31 per cent. There were 54 deaths after leaving the hospital; one half of these were directly or indirectly related to the tumor. This included intracranial extension of tumor in 13 patients, diabetes in seven, cardiac causes in six, and cerebrovascular disease in four. Sixty-nine survived the operation. Twenty-two reached the age of 60; the oldest was 77. Five are still living 30 years after operation. Cushing did not have cortisone and knew he could not do a total hypophysectomy. His subtotal removal of pituitary adenomas relieved the symptoms of headaches and visual loss but very likely altered the acromegaly little, if at all.

Ray and Horwith (1964) recommend total hypophysectomy with removal of the adenoma and all the glandular tissue in the sella turcica in acromegalics. According to these authors, anything less risks leaving abnormal tissue which might perpetuate the disease and cause recurrence. In their series of 18 patients, most patients had had conventional radiation an average of three years before operation. One patient had received 9,000 rads. All had active acromegaly on the basis of laboratory data at the time of frontal craniotomy for adenoma removal. Nearly all developed some degree of diabetes insipidus after operation which decreased in weeks or months and was rarely permanent. Twelve patients had total hypophysectomy, judged by laboratory tests. There was general improvement in acromegaly.

Hardy (1971) operates on these patients transsphenoidally, removing microadenomas when found. A total hypophysectomy is done if the adenoma is diffuse.

Cushing's Syndrome and Adenomas of the Hypophysis

Cushing, in 1933, presented the hypothesis linking the characteristic endocrinopathy which bears his name with basophilic adenomas of the pituitary gland.

Rovit and Berry (1965) cite 55 cases in the literature, including five of their own, of Cushing's syndrome with nonbasophilic adenomas of the pituitary. They state that most patients with Cushing's syndrome have bilateral adrenal hyperplasia. Fifteen to 20 per cent have adrenal adenomas or carcinoma with autonomous secretory activity; 10 per cent have pituitary tumors, most of which are chromophobe adenomas but not basophilic adenomas. The syndrome is occasionally seen in patients with malignant tumors of the lungs, pancreas, or thymus. Also, many pituitary chromophobe adenomas manifest themselves only after adrenalectomy has been performed. Rovit and Berry postulate that patients may have adrenal hyperplasia, which is secondary to either pituitary adenomas (chromophobe) or to a suprapituitary mechanism. The latter is thought to be a hyperactivity of a pituitary driving mechanism in the limbic system or in the hypothalamus. Hyperactivity of the suprapituitary driving mechanism can result in adrenal hyperplasia, pituitary adenomas, or both.

Chromophobe adenomas formerly were thought to be nonsecretory and nonfunctioning tumors. Schelin (1952) says it is not always possible to demonstrate or exclude secretory function of cells by light microscopy. He has shown that chromophobe adenomas studied by electron microscopy may show sparsely granulated acidophils with signs of secretory function. With this information, it is reasonable to assume that chromophobe adenomas diagnosed by light microscopy in Cushing's syndrome are really functioning, adrenocorticotropic hormone-secreting adenomas.

Increased cortisol activity produces the Cushing's disease picture of plethora, round face, truncal obesity and buffalo hump, purple abdominal striae, hypertension, polycythemia, elevated blood sugar levels, amenorrhea, decreased libido and potency, and osteoporosis. Those caused by pituitary adenomas which secrete adrenocorticotropic hormone (ACTH) may initiate enlargement of the sella turcica, headache, and extrasellar extension with visual field defects.

Rovit and Berry reviewed their five patients and 50 cases in the literature resulting from nonbasophilic adenomas of the pituitary. One-half developed visual symptoms, usually because of extrasellar extension of their adenomas. A third of those with visual symptoms also developed extraocular muscle palsies. In one-fourth, visual symptoms preceded signs of hyperadrenalism. Adrenalectomy either induced or greatly exacerbated the visual symptoms in two thirds of the patients undergoing that procedure.

An interesting hyperpigmentation of flexor creases, surgical scars, areolae, and skin in general, may develop in Cushing's syndrome patients weeks or months after bilateral adrenalectomy with the development of pituitary adenomas. The increased pigmentation is thought to be caused by secretion of melanin-stimulating hormone (MSH) by the pituitary gland.

The surgical treatment for Cushing's disease consists of adrenalectomy in those with adrenal hyperplasia or adrenal tumors. In those with pituitary adenomas, treatment is total hypophysectomy by the transfrontal or transsphenoidal approach. This may be combined with conventional irradiation, but irradiation is not effective alone. Some patients will need both adrenalectomy and hypophysectomy to reverse the Cushing's syndrome and to relieve the headaches and visual changes. The MSH-secreting adenoma may become invasive; therefore, total hypophysectomy should be done, not just selective adenoma removal.

Hypophysectomy for the pituitary adenoma in this condition should be complete and can be done through the transfrontal craniotomy or transsphenoidal hypophysectomy advocated by Hardy (1971). Rand, in 1964, treated a patient with Cushing's disease by cryohypophysectomy (stereotactic freezing of the pituitary). The procedure was unsuccessful, and the patient underwent bilateral adrenalectomy two months later.

Lactation Caused by Prolactin-Secreting Adenoma

Another interesting hyperpituitary syndrome is that caused by a prolactin-secreting adenoma. The syndrome consists of lactation, headache, lack of normal vaginal mucus secretions, and dyspareunia and may have its beginning symptoms following pregnancy and delivery.

In acromegalics, this syndrome apparently is caused by an adenoma which secretes both growth hormone and prolactin. Davidoff (1926), on reviewing charts of 100 cases of acromegaly seen in Boston, found four women with persistently secreting yellowish fluid, resembling colostrum, which had drained from one or both breasts for years. One patient had been pregnant five years previously and had never stopped lactating. Menstruation never resumed, and she became acromegalic.

We have seen this syndrome in two women. One had continued to lactate two years following pregnancy and delivery. She had had a hysterectomy because of fibroids one year following delivery. Visual fields were normal. Skull X-ray films showed a slightly enlarged sella turcica. Pneumoencephalography revealed a pocket of air almost completely filling the sella turcica. Treatment was not recommended for this patient because she seemed to have an active but cystic or infarcted adenoma of the pituitary, with her only symptom being lactation. It was thought best, under the circumstances, to follow up on her periodically and not to add hypopituitarism to a minor symptom.

Four types of secreting pituitary adenomas have been mentioned (HGH, prolactin, ACTH, and MSH). A fifth type has been treated by Hardy (1971). He removed a pituitary adenoma which apparently was secreting thyroid stimulating hormone (TSH) and which was responsible for progressive, malignant exophthalmos. The exophthalmos did not respond to total thyroidectomy but did respond to removal of the pituitary adenoma.

Six patients treated at M. D. Anderson Hospital will be reviewed to illustrate some of the interesting findings and treatments used in various types of pituitary adenomas at this institution.

CASE 1.–This patient illustrates three main points: (1) that chromophobe adenomas do at times recur after combined operation and irradiation, (2) that some adenomas become cystic from intra-adenoma bleeding and can enlarge rapidly, causing rapid visual loss, and (3) that this latter situation represents a surgical emergency.

This 41-year-old woman first had symptoms of amenorrhea at the age of 31. Headaches and bitemporal field defects appeared three years later. In February 1970, at another hospital, a frontal craniotomy and biopsy of the adenoma were done, followed by cobalt irradiation. After irradiation, there was a return of lost vision. Seven months after craniotomy, there was again the reduction in visual acuity and development of visual bitemporal field defects.

She was seen for the first time at M. D. Anderson Hospital in December 1970, 10 months after irradiation. The neurological examination was unremarkable except for notable reduction of visual acuity and a bitemporal field defect (Fig. 1). The preoperative lab work was as follows: T_3, 35 per cent (normal) and thyroxine I, 4 ng. per cent (normal). Skull X-ray films showed a significantly enlarged sella turcica.

Because there had been rapid progression of visual loss over a period of several days, an emergency operation (frontal) was performed on December 30, 1970. The optic nerves and chiasm were compressed by an enlarging chromophobe adenoma which contained a 5-cc. wine-colored fluid cyst. Using Hardy's nucleators, intracapsular removal of the adenoma was accomplished. Notable improvement in vision was evident on the second postoperative day. Pitressin was given for transient diabetes insipidus, and the patient was dismissed on cortisone, 37.5 mg./day, and Cytomel, 50 mcg./day. Six months after operation, visual acuity was 20/30 in both eyes, and there was only a small, residual superior bitemporal field defect (Fig. 1).

CASE 2.–This patient illustrates that patients with chromophobe adenomas may present clinically with eye symptoms and lack symptoms of hypopituitary function. If there is more than a minimal upper bitemporal field

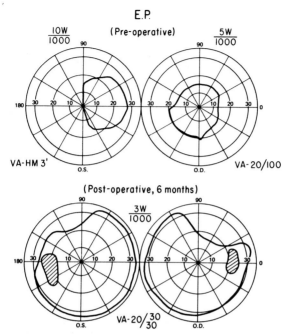

FIG. 1.—CASE 1. Visual acuity and bitemporal field before and after therapy.

defect or if there is significant reduction in visual acuity, surgical decompression should precede irradiation. If surgical decompression can be done before there is complete bitemporal field defect and before there is considerable reduction in visual acuity and optic pallor, the improvement in vision is usually good.

This 51-year-old man developed blurred vision seven or eight months before being seen at M. D. Anderson Hospital. The blurred vision involved the upper outer quadrant of the right eye. Five or six months later, he developed progressive bitemporal field visual field loss. Arteriography, done in another hospital, was unremarkable. He denied having symptoms which might have suggested endocrine hypofunction. His general examination at M. D. Anderson Hospital was essentially normal except for a soft atrophic left testicle. He had a past history of syphilis. His skin and hair did not definitely indicate a hypopituitary state. The positive neurological findings were confined to the eye examination. The visual acuity was 20/50 in the right eye and 20/100 in the left eye. He had notable bitemporal anopsia with the 1-mm. white test object and complete bitemporal anopsia on testing with the 5-mm. red test object (Fig. 2).

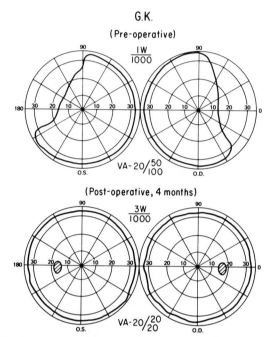

FIG. 2.—CASE 2. Bitemporal field before and after treatment.

Preoperative laboratory studies were as follows: cortisol, 21 ng./100 ml. (normal) and growth hormone, fasting, 0.4 ng./ml. (normal). Skull X-ray films revealed an enlarged sella turcica and a demineralized or eroded dorsum with sharp anterior clinoids. Pneumoencephalography demonstrated suprasellar extension of the adenoma with slight elevation of the third ventricle.

On January 28, 1971, a chromophobe adenoma, which was part soft and part firm and contained 1 cc. of wine-colored liquid, was removed through a frontal craniotomy. The optic nerves and chiasm were elevated by the tumor. One week after craniotomy, the visual acuity was 20/15 in the right eye and 20/30 in the left eye, and fields were normal to a 3-mm. white test object. Postoperative medication included cortisone acetate, 37.5 mg./day; euthyroid #3, one per day; testosterone, 200 mg. intramuscularly every 3 to 4 weeks. Postoperative laboratory work was as follows: cortisol, 3 ng./100 ml. (low) and growth hormone, 0.4 ng./ml. (normal). After operation, irradiation was given in his home town. Four months after operation, visual acuity was 20/20 in both eyes and visual fields were normal (Fig. 2).

CASE 3.—This patient had a large chromophobe adenoma which grew through the floor of the sella turcica and sphenoid sinus, and into the naso-pharynx. The adenoma did not grow in the suprasellar region and therefore did not produce visual symptoms. The adenoma did result in hypogonadal symptoms. Adenomas with a similar growth direction, as in this case, some-times result in a spontaneous cerebrospinal fluid (CSF) rhinorrhea with the danger of meningitis and brain abscess. Such a patient is ideally suited for transsphenoidal removal of tumor before irradiation. In this operative approach, the tumor can be removed and the defect in the floor of the sella turcica can be repaired with cartilage and fascia lata.

A 50-year-old man had onset of symptoms at age 47 with a loss of libido and potency. There was no loss of energy or alteration in skin or trunk or face hair. At age 50, he complained of a stuffy nose and was examined by a physician in his home town. A biopsy of a posterior nasopharyngeal "polyp" was done, and a diagnosis of transitional cell carcinoma of the sphenoid sinus was made. Examination at M. D. Anderson Hospital within a few weeks after the biopsy revealed an obese, middle-aged male with wrinkled, pasty, fine-textured facial skin, suggestive of hypopituitarism. His sense of smell, visual fields, visual acuity, and cranial nerves were intact. Results of the remainder of the neurological examination were normal. Body hair was of normal distribution. Skull X-ray films revealed an enlarged sella turcica, a defect in the floor of the sella turcica, and a mass in the sphenoid sinus. Pneumoencephalography showed an absence of suprasellar extension of the tumor. The pertinent endocrine studies were as follows: T_3 uptake, 27.5 per cent (25 to 35 per cent normal); thyroxine I, 5.8 ng. per cent (3.6 to 6.6 normal); testosterone, 124 ng./100 ml. (400 to 1,000 ng./100 ml. normal); and growth hormone, 1 ng./ml. peak insulin tolerance (low). The outside biopsy slides were considered to be either a chromophobe adenoma or an unclassified tumor.

On June 18, 1971, surgical removal (transsphenoidal) of a large chromo-phobe adenoma was done. The tumor had produced defects in the anterior and posterior walls of the sphenoid sinus and filled the sella turcica and the sphenoid sinus.

The tumor was generally soft. Tissue in the posterior aspect of the sella turcica, which had more the consistency of normal pituitary gland, was left in place to try to preserve some pituitary function, if possible. The dia-phragma sellae was left intact. Diabetes insipidus and rhinorrhea did not develop. The patient received postoperative irradiation of the sella turcica and sphenoid sinus in his home town. Postoperative serum growth hormone was unmeasurable. He returned to work two weeks after operation. He continues on daily maintenance of cortisone acetate.

CASE 4.—This patient illustrates the point that conventional irradiation usually does not control acromegaly, although in this patient there apparently was no progression for a few years following radiation. The treatment of choice is total removal of the adenoma or total hypophysectomy, in some cases. Another point is that when acromegalic features have been present for a number of years and treatment results in lowering the growth hormone level to normal or zero, improvement occurs, but the acromegalic features remain.

A 46-year-old woman had developed irregular menses at age 25. At age 28, she began developing signs of acromegaly with enlargement of the face, nose, extremities, and tongue and separation of the teeth. At age 36, a diagnosis of pituitary adenoma was made at another hospital and irradiation was directed toward the sella turcica. Postirradiation, menses ceased and there was some reduction in soft tissue of the face and extremities. Nine years after irradiation, there was progression of the acromegalic features with enlargement of the hands, forearms, feet, and legs.

Examination at M. D. Anderson Hospital in March 1965 revealed a typical acromegalic 46-year-old woman (Fig. 3). Her facial features were acromegalic, she had large hands and feet, and a heavy growth of hair on her extremities. Visual fields and visual acuity were normal. X-ray studies

FIG. 3.—CASE 4. A typical acromegalic woman.

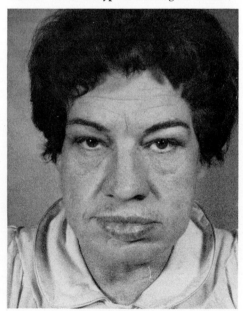

revealed an enlarged sella turcica with a double floor, enlarged frontal sinuses, a large mandible, and large hands and feet.

The pertinent laboratory studies were: ^{131}I uptake was 20 per cent; urinary 17-ketosteroid and 17-OH steroid levels were normal. The serum growth hormone level was 35 ng./ml. (0.4–6.0 ng./ml. normal).

On October 21, 1965, a mixed chromophobe and eosinophilic adenoma was considered totally removed by a frontal craniotomy. The central part of the tumor was necrotic. There was no suprasellar extension. Postoperatively, medical treatment has included daily cortisone and thyroid therapy. She had transient diabetes insipidus, requiring Pitressin nasal insufflation for a few months.

During the first seven months after craniotomy, there was reduction in the size of her hands and feet, and she became able to make a complete fist with her hands. There was also less hair on her extremities. Her tongue and fingers became smaller, and her dress size went from 22½ to 16½. Facial features, although slightly improved, remained acromegalic. Serum growth hormone level was 3.2 ng./ml. (normal) four years following operation. There has been no clinical evidence of progression of her acromegaly, which is considered arrested.

CASE 5.—This case illustrates a patient with Cushing's disease with bilateral adrenal hyperplasia and an ACTH- and MSH-producing chromophobe adenoma of the pituitary gland. The adenoma was probably already present before adrenalectomy, since headaches were occurring at that time. Adrenalectomy was quickly followed by increase in skin pigmentation and increase in headaches, apparently caused by increase in growth of the adenoma. Headaches were relieved and pigmentation reduced after hypophysectomy.

A 38-year-old woman had the onset of Cushing's disease at age 34 with development of joint aches, increase in weight, development of buffalo hump, increase in facial hair, and hypertension. In August 1966, she had one of two hyperplastic adrenals removed in another hospital. There followed some regression of her symptoms for about seven years. Between 1968 and 1970, there was progression of her Cushing's disease with increase in facial hair, rounding of her face, development of prominence of the upper back and abdominal fat pad, increase in weight to 220 lbs., and the appearance of mental depression and emotional instability. In May 1970, she developed progressive, generalized, severe headaches. Her 24-hour urine 17-OH steroid output was 20.6 mg., and the 17-ketosteroid output was 31.6 mg. The serum cortisol level was 56 ng./100 ml. (high).

Examination in September 1970, showed: blood pressure, 170/110 and pulse, 75. She had a moon face, buffalo hump, abdominal fat which was excessive, and excessive hair over the chest and back. Visual fields and acuity were normal.

In January 1971, at M. D. Anderson Hospital, the remaining hyperplastic adrenal was removed. Soon afterward, the patient improved, losing 19 lb. However, within one month after operation, she began gaining weight (11 lb. in two weeks) in spite of a daily intake of 750 to 1,000 calories. Cortisone was reduced two months after operation. There was continued headache and the onset of progressive pigmentation of skin in general. This pigmentation was especially notable in surgical scars, areolae, and skin folds. Visual fields were normal. Skull X-ray films revealed a demineralized dorsum and sharp anterior clinoids. Carotid angiography and pneumoencephalography did not show evidence of suprasellar tumor.

On April 23, 1971, transsphenoidal exposure of the pituitary was accomplished. There was a central, soft chromophobe adenoma present. Total hypophysectomy was done. Postoperatively, there was mild diabetes insipidus. There was also an early, steady reduction in skin pigmentation, and the patient's headaches were relieved. She did not develop CSF rhinorrhea.

Preoperative serum growth hormone (fasting) was 4 ng./ml., and the postoperative growth hormone (fasting) was 0.9 ng./ml. When seen four months after operation, she was not having headaches, and her skin pigmentation was less. Medication included cortisone acetate, 50 mg. per day and euthyroid #2, one tablet per day.

CASE 6.—This patient represents an interesting chromophobe adenoma which had its onset during pregnancy, causing continued lactation after delivery. The patient had a small adenoma embedded in the anterior lobe of the pituitary. This is an ideal situation for transsphenoidal removal since it is possible to remove the adenoma and leave the remaining normal pituitary. This would have been difficult, if not impossible, to do through a frontal craniotomy. After removal of tumor, the patient began menstruating and has had a significant reduction in lactation.

This 21-year-old woman had continued to lactate and had been amenorrheic following pregnancy and delivery at the age of 16. She subsequently developed dyspareunia and decreased libido. At age 20, she began having headaches. There was no visual complaint, excessive thirst, or polyuria. She desired further pregnancies and sought medical treatment for her lactorrhea and infertility.

Examination at M. D. Anderson Hospital revealed normal development of her breasts; however, white milk would drip or squirt from the nipples under pressure. The distribution of body and pubic hair was normal. The 24-hour base line urinary estrogens were extremely low. Thyroid function was normal. The serum cortisol level was normal. The neurological examination, including visual fields, was normal. Skull X-ray films showed a sella turcica increased in size. Carotid angiography and pneumoencephalography were normal.

On April 22, 1971, the pituitary gland was approached transsphenoidally. There was a well-localized semiliquid chromophobe adenoma in the pituitary gland. This was removed, and the remaining normal pituitary was left in the sella turcica. Postoperatively, the patient's headaches ceased. She had diabetes insipidus for a few days. Two months after operation, she had her first menstrual period since her pregnancy five years previously. Her menstrual periods have since consisted of either a small menstrual flow or cramps. Lactation has diminished. She no longer has spontaneous drainage of milk from her breasts or dyspareunia. Postoperatively, urine estrogen levels were normal. The serum prolactin was 250 ng. before and 35 ng. after operation (normal, 10–25 ng./ml.).

Summary

Pituitary adenomas may be divided by light microscopy into chromophobe, acidophilic, basophilic, or mixed adenomas. Pituitary adenomas may be functioning and secrete hormones—or may be nonsecretory, producing endocrine changes by slowly destroying the secretory activity of the normal hypophysis. The common chromophobe adenoma is nonfunctioning. Some chromophobe adenomas are actually secretory and have secretory granules, as seen with special staining under the light microscope or by the electron microscope and may be responsible for hyperpituitary symptoms such as (1) Cushing's disease, (2) hyperpigmentation caused by MSH-producing adenoma, or (3) lactation caused by prolactin-producing adenoma. Basophilic adenomas are extremely rare, remain minute in size, and can also be associated with Cushing's disease. Acidophilic adenomas are growth hormone-producing adenomas, responsible for acromegaly and gigantism. A TSH-producing pituitary adenoma can result in malignant exophthalmos.

Chromophobe adenomas, if producing few or no visual symptoms, may be adequately managed with conventional irradiation. When these tumors produce significant visual loss, are associated with CSF rhinorrhea, or have destroyed the floor of the sella turcica and sphenoid sinus, surgical treatment should be combined with irradiation.

Acidophilic adenomas are best treated surgically with total hypophysectomy or total removal of the adenoma. This may be accomplished by a frontal or transsphenoidal approach or by stereotactic cryogenic techniques. Patients with Cushing's disease with pituitary adenomas and those with MSH-secreting adenomas should be treated surgically with total hypophysectomy. Prolactin-secreting adenomas causing lactation may be effectively treated by removal of the microadenoma, preserving the normal pituitary gland. This can best be accomplished by the transsphenoidal approach to the pituitary gland.

Acknowledgments

I am indebted to Dr. Jules Hardy of Montreal, Canada, who kindly consented to demonstrate his surgical technique of transsphenoidal hypophysectomy at M. D. Anderson Hospital. He performed the operation on the fifth and sixth patients described above, as well as on two other patients (with carcinoma of the breast) not described in the text.

The endocrine evaluations and investigations were studied by the Endocrine Section of The University of Texas at Houston M. D. Anderson Hospital and Tumor Institute.

This study was supported by American Cancer Society Grant No. T-558 and U.S.P.H.S., NIH Grants No. CA 05831-01 and CA 12521-01.

REFERENCES

Bishop, P. M. F., and Briggs, J. H.: Anterior-pituitary gland. Acromegaly. *The Lancet*, 1:735-736, April 1958.

Cushing, H.: Dyspituitarism: Twenty years later, with special consideration of the pituitary adenomas. *Archives of Internal Medicine*, 51:487-557, April 1933.

Davidoff, L. M.: Personal communication.

———: Studies in acromegaly: Anamnesis and symptomatology in 100 cases. *Endocrinology*, 10:461-483, September-October 1926.

Elkington, S. G., and McKissock, W.: Pituitary adenoma. Results of combined surgical and radiotherapeutic treatment of 260 patients. *British Medical Journal*, 1:263-266, February 1967.

Furst, E.: On chromophobe pituitary adenoma. *Acta Medica Scandinavica*, (Supplement) 452:1-111, 1966.

German, W. J., and Flanigan, S.: Pituitary adenomas: a follow-up study of the Cushing series. In Mosberg, W. H., Ed.: *Clinical Neurosurgery*. 1st ed., Baltimore, Maryland, The Williams and Wilkins Co., 1964, Vol. X, pp. 72-81.

Hardy, J.: Transsphenoidal hypophysectomy. *Journal of Neurosurgery*, 34:582-594, April 1971.

Hirsch, O.: Endonasal method of removal of hypophyseal tumors, with report of two successful cases. *The Journal of the American Medical Association*, 55: 772-774, August 1910.

Rand, R. W., Dashe, A. M., Paglia, D. E., Conway, L. W., and Solomon, D. H.: Stereotactic cryohypophysectomy. *The Journal of the American Medical Association*, 189:255-259, July 1964.

Ray, B. S., and Horwith, M.: Surgical treatment of acromegaly. In Mosberg, W.

H., Ed.: *Clinical Neurosurgery,* 1st ed., Baltimore, Maryland, The Williams and Wilkins Co., 1964, Vol. X, pp. 31-59.

Rovit, R. L., and Berry, R.: Cushing's syndrome and the hypophysis. A re-evaluation of pituitary tumors and hyperadrenalism. *Journal of Neurosurgery,* 23: 270-295, September 1965.

Schelin, U.: Chromophobe and acidophil adenomas of the human pituitary gland. A light and electron microscopic study. *Acta Pathologica et Microbiologica Scandinavica,* (Supplement) 158:1-80, 1952.

Schloffer, H.: Zur frage der Operation an der Hypophyse. *Beiträge zur Klinische Chirugie,* 50:767-817, 1906.

Svien, H. J., Love, J. G., Kennedy, W. C., Colby, M. Y., Jr., and Kearns, T. P.: Status of vision following surgical treatment for pituitary chromophobe adenoma. *Journal of Neurosurgery,* 22:47-52, January 1965.

Technique of Transoral, Transnasal, Transsphenoidal Hypophysectomy

R. H. JESSE, M.D., AND M. E. LEAVENS, M.D.

Department of Surgery, The University of Texas at Houston
M. D. Anderson Hospital and Tumor Institute,
Houston, Texas

THE TRANSSPHENOIDAL APPROACH to the sella turcica is advantageous in that it provides rapid access to the pituitary, needs no external incisions, and requires no intracranial manipulation of the brain. Cushing (1932) performed about 75 per cent of his operations for pituitary adenoma using this approach. Few surgeons used the transsphenoidal approach, however, until use of the radiofluoroscope was described by Guiot (1958). When the operating microscope became available, the surgeon was provided with microsurgical methods of dissection and the transsphenoidal approach was revived. Hardy (1971) provided the impetus of combining the radiofluoroscope and the microscope and has designed microsurgical instruments which make the removal of the pituitary much safer for the patient and easier for the surgeon.

The patient is placed in a semisitting position on the operating table, with the head taped in place on an occipital head rest (Fig. 1). The chin is pointed toward the right shoulder so that the head is about 30 degrees off the longitudinal line of the body. The head position is important so that the surgeon can stand comfortably beside the table and direct the microscope in a longitudinal line with the patient's head. A C-arm image intensifier is placed so that the horizontal beam is centered on the sella turcica. A television screen is placed behind the patient's head so that it can be seen by the surgeon over the instrument table. The anesthesiologist places the endotracheal tube in the left corner of the mouth (Fig. 2).

A fascia lata graft measuring about 6 cm. in diameter is taken from the right leg along with a generous portion of the underlying muscle (Fig. 3).

The patient is then preliminarily draped and the nasal cavity, face, and oral cavity are thoroughly washed with soap. Using the syringe with a tonsil

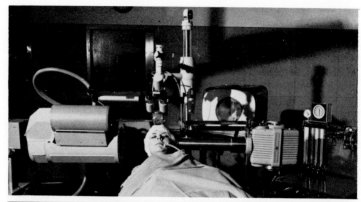

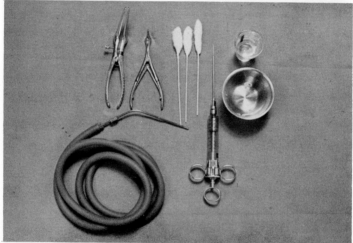

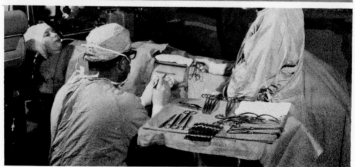

FIG. 1 (*top*).—Position of patient.
FIG. 2 (*center*).—Equipment for anesthesia.
FIG. 3 (*bottom*).—Fascia lata graft obtained.

needle, 1 per cent Xylocaine with adrenalin is injected in the anterior labial gingival fold, in the floor of the nasal cavity, and under the mucosa of the nasal septum. Large swabs are soaked in 10 per cent cocaine, wrung out and placed along the lower portion of the nasal floor and septum. The face is then painted with tincture of benzoin, and an adhesive waterproof drape is placed on the face. A small hole is cut in the drape over the nose and mouth.

FIG. 4 (*top*).—Final draping and incision.
FIG. 5 (*bottom*).—Reflection of mucosa removal of cartilage.

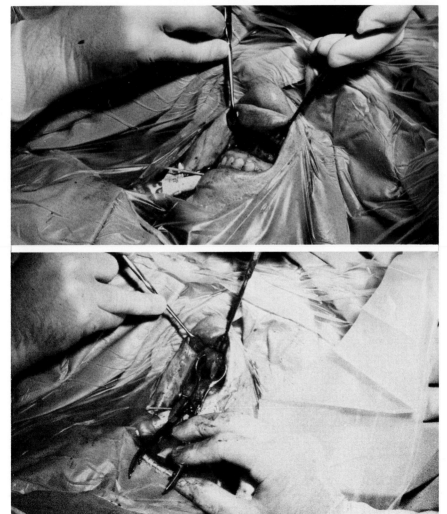

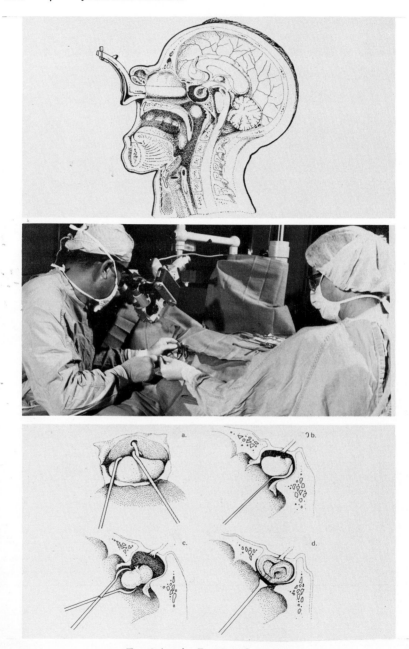

Fig. 6 (*top*).—Position of retractor.
Fig. 7 (*center*).—Operating microscope and camera in position, shown here without its drape.

Fig. 8 (*bottom*).—Removal of total pituitary (see text).

The incision is made in the superior gingival labial sulcus about 4 cm. on either side of the midline (Fig. 4). The incision is carried down to the bone where the periosteum is raised to the anterior choana. The columella is detached from the anterior nasal spine of the maxilla and this spur of bone and the sharp rim of the lateral maxillary bone are rongeured away.

The mucosa is then dissected in turn from off the nasal floor and the septum back to its attachment on the sphenoid bone (Fig. 5). The lower portion of the cartilage of the nasal septum is removed with a swivel knife and preserved for later use. The upper portion of the vomer is removed, exposing the sphenoid bone. The floor of the sphenoid sinus is entered and enlarged so that the promontory of the sella turcica can be seen.

A self-retaining retractor is then inserted in the defect with the tips of its jaws lying at the level of the anterior face of the sphenoid bone (Fig. 6). The operating microscope is focused on the posterior-superior wall of the sphenoid sinus (Fig. 7). The image intensifier is helpful in locating the center of the floor of the sella turcica. A perforation is made in the floor of the sella turcica and the defect is enlarged, exposing the dura. A cruciate incision is then made in the dura. Careful microscopic inspection of the pituitary follows, and, depending on the disease process and the presentation of the tumor, the surgeon decides either to remove a microadenoma and preserve the remaining pituitary gland or to do a total hypophysec-

Fɪɢ. 9.—Incision is closed.

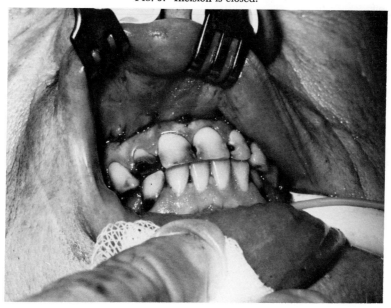

tomy. The microsurgical instruments developed by Hardy aid in separating the pituitary from its capsule (Yasargil, 1969). If the entire gland is to be removed, the stalk is sectioned just above the pituitary gland (Fig. 8a, b, c). Bleeding vessels are carefully coagulated. After removal of the tumor, the fossa is carefully lined with the fascia lata and then packed with muscle (Fig. 8d). The cartilage of the nasal septum is then fashioned slightly bigger than the defect in the floor of the sella turcica and is wedged inside the sella turcica to hold the muscle in place. A square piece of fascia lata is then placed over the posterior-superior wall of the sphenoid sinus and the opening of the sella turcica. The retractors are withdrawn, allowing the mucosa to collapse. Intranasal packing is placed around bilateral nasal airways and the incision is closed with interrupted sutures (Fig. 9). The nasal airways are removed in 24 hours and the nasal packing is removed in 72 hours.

REFERENCES

Cushing, H.: *Intracranial tumours. Notes Upon a Series of Two Thousand Verified Cases with Surgical Mortality Percentages Pertaining Thereto.* Springfield, Illinois, Charles C Thomas, 1932, Vol. XII, 150 pages.

Guiot, G.: *Adenomes hypophysaires.* Paris, France, Marson, 1958, 276 pages.

Hardy, J.: Transsphenoidal Hypophysectomy. *Journal of Neurosurgery,* 34:582-594, April 1971.

Yasargil, M. G.: *Transnasal-Transsphenoidal Approach to the Pituitary Gland.* In Thieme: *Microsurgery Applied to Neurosurgery,* New York, Academic Press, 1969, pp. 180-194.

Pathology of Pituitary Tumors

BRUCE MACKAY, M.B., Ch.B., Ph.D.,
MICHAEL L. IBANEZ, M.D.,
ALBERTO G. AYALA, M.D., and
WILLIAM T. TOBLEMAN, B.A., B.S.

Department of Anatomic Pathology, The University of Texas at Houston M. D. Anderson Hospital and Tumor Institute, Houston, Texas

Adenomas of the anterior lobe are by far the most common tumors of the pituitary gland. They are traditionally classified on the basis of the staining qualities of the tumor cells, but in recent years it has become increasingly apparent that a classification based on the functional characteristics of the adenoma cells would be more meaningful to both pathologist and clinician. This is discussed in the present paper, following a brief review of the main morphologic features of pituitary tumors.

A precis of the embryological development of the pituitary is germane to a consideration of tumors of the gland. In the three-week-old embryo, an outpouching appears in the wall of the oral cavity; this is the craniopharyngeal, or Rathke's, pouch. It expands dorsally, and by the end of the second month has lost its connection with the oral cavity and is in close contact with a downgrowth from the diencephalon, the infundibulum, which forms the posterior lobe and stalk. Cells in the anterior wall of Rathke's pouch proliferate to form the anterior lobe. Some cells migrate upward and around the sides of the infundibular stalk forming the pars tuberalis.

The craniopharyngeal duct is generally obliterated, although remnants of the lumen may persist as small cysts between the anterior and posterior lobes, and the occasional larger pituitary cyst probably develops from this source. Cells resembling those of the anterior lobe may be left behind along the course of the duct, and rarely these proliferate to produce an adenoma. Erdheim (1909) described a case in which an acidophil adenoma, causing acromegaly, was located beneath the sella.

Craniopharyngioma

This tumor is sometimes called an adamantinoma because of its histological resemblance to tumors of the jaw arising from the enamel organ. It could conceivably develop from oral epithelial cells displaced during the dorsal expansion of Rathke's pouch, and Halmi (1966) points out that nests of squamous cells have been observed in the vicinity of the pars tuberalis. The tumor may grow to a considerable size, and although it is nonfunctional, it may nevertheless be responsible for endocrine symptoms

FIG. 1.—Light micrograph of a craniopharyngioma. Parts of three cystic spaces can be seen, with aggregates of squamoid cells present in one. Electron microscopic studies have shown that keratinization is abundant in these tumors. Palisading is evident in the peripheral layer of epithelial cells bordering the cystic spaces (hematoxylin and eosin: × 250).

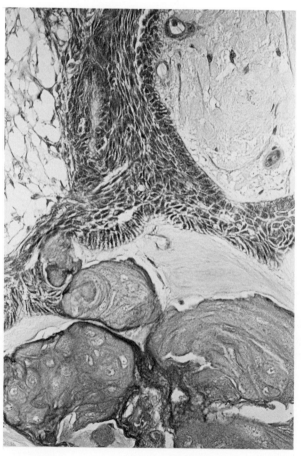

through pressure on the hypothalamic region. Histologically the appearance is characteristic (Fig. 1). Cyst-like spaces of varying size are enclosed by cords and sheets of cells, and the peripheral layer of cells is typically palisaded. The tumors frequently show calcification and ossification, features of radiological significance. Ghatak, Hirano, and Zimmerman (1971) described the fine structure of a craniopharyngioma and confirmed the epithelial nature of the polygonal or elongated cells. They also illustrated keratinization in the epithelial cells but pointed out that this is not the orderly process found in normal epidermal squamous cells.

The craniopharyngioma is a slow-growing tumor, but its anatomic location and often intimate apposition to surrounding tissues make complete removal difficult. Recurrence following resection is frequent.

Posterior Pituitary Tumors

Gliomas of the posterior lobe occur but they are extremely rare neoplasms. Granular cell tumors, whose nature has not yet been elucidated, have been described. Luse and Kernohan (1955) reported the presence of small aggregates of granular cells in more than 6 per cent of pituitary stalks and posterior lobes, and granular cell tumors in this location have been variously called choristomas, pituicytomas, and granular cell myoblastomas (Russell and Rubinstein, 1971).

Anterior Pituitary Adenomas

In histologic sections of the anterior lobe stained with hematoxylin and eosin, three cell types can be distinguished by the staining qualities of the cytoplasm. These are the acidophils, basophils, and chromophobes. The latter group of cells has a pale lilac-appearing cytoplasm. The relative proportions of the cell types vary from one area of a gland to another, but approximately half the cells are generally chromophobic, and acidophils are more plentiful than basophils. The standard classification of the anterior pituitary adenomas has been based on this nomenclature, and the relative incidence of the tumor types parallels that of the normal cells. Russell and Rubinstein (1971) state that approximately 80 per cent are chromophobe, 15 per cent acidophil, and less than 10 per cent basophil adenomas. Certain clinical and pathological features have become associated with each type of adenoma.

The acidophil adenomas are usually small and confined to the sella turcica. Many are associated with the clinical manifestations of hypersecretion of growth hormone. In the syndrome of pluriglandular adenomatosis, in which adenomas are found in the pituitary, parathyroid, and pancreatic islets, the pituitary tumor is frequently an acidophil adenoma (Moldawer, Nardi, and Raker, 1954).

Basophil adenomas also are usually small tumors and rarely produce erosion of the sella turcica. However, the actively secreting tumors may be detected through their endocrine effects before they grow to a large size. Since the time of Cushing's original paper (1932), basophil adenomas have been associated with the syndrome that bears his name, but many patients with Cushing's syndrome have chromophobe adenomas, and the majority have no pituitary tumor.

Fig. 2.—Light micrograph of a chromophobe adenoma. The tumor is composed of sheets of cells exhibiting no pleomorphism and no attempt to form an organoid pattern. Electron microscopic study revealed numerous secretory granules in the cells of this tumor (hematoxylin and eosin: × 250).

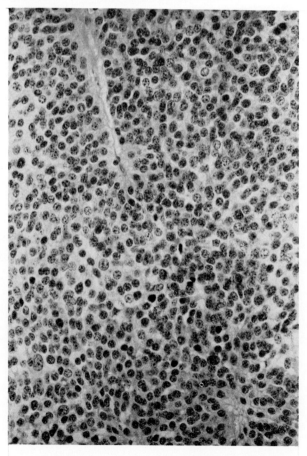

Chromophobe adenomas are the most frequent tumors of the pituitary gland. They may reach a considerable size, expanding the sella turcica and extending beyond its confines in various directions. Suprasellar extension is often observed, presumably because this represents the direction of least resistance, and the bulk of the tumor may be located above the sella. When this occurs, the tumor may have a dumbbell configuration with the waist constricted by the diaphragma sella, and the vessels of the circle of Willis may be deeply embedded in the tumor. Clinical manifestations resulting from pressure on adjacent structures, notably the hypothalamus and the optic chiasma, are frequently described. The floor of the sella may be eroded, and the tumor can initially present in the sphenoid sinus. Lateral extension of a chromophobe adenoma initially compromises the cavernous sinus and its associated cranial nerves. Further growth may progress for a considerable distance over the floor of the cranial fossae.

The histologic pattern of a chromophobe adenoma is variable, but generally the cells are spherical and rather small, appearing as monotonous sheets intersected by vascular channels (Fig. 2). Intermittent bands of connective tissues are present, and growth of the tumor cells along these septa can confer a pseudo-organoid pattern. Russell and Rubinstein (1971) suggest the terms "diffuse" and "sinusoidal" to denote these characteristics but point out that many specimens combine features of both types. Follicular arrangements of anterior pituitary cells are described by Bergland and Torack (1969) in the normal anterior pituitary and in adrenocorticotropic hormone (ACTH) producing adenoma in man.

Pleomorphism may be seen in a proportion of the adenomas, but unless it is accompanied by considerable mitotic activity, it should not be interpreted as proof of an aggressive disposition. The existence of true malignant tumors of the pituitary gland has been questioned (Winkelman, Cassel, and Schlesinger, 1952). The only valid criterion is the presence of distant metastasis; this undoubtedly is rare, but well-documented cases are cited by Russell and Rubinstein (1971).

Nomenclature of Anterior Pituitary Adenomas

It has become apparent in recent years that the traditional nomenclature for the anterior pituitary adenomas could benefit from revision to take into account the precise cell of origin and its functional behavior. Evidence for this has accrued from various sources. A series of studies by light microscopy demonstrated that, with careful fixation of tissue and the use of a selected group of staining procedures, more than the three basic types of cell could be recognized in the normal anterior pituitary. Halmi (1966) provides a tabular summation of several of the more notable contributions.

These light microscopic studies demonstrated that two cell types were included in the acidophil group and that up to three cell types could be distinguished among the basophils. These procedures also revealed staining qualities in many of the chromophobe cells.

Further impetus for a more precise categorization of the anterior pituitary cells came from attempts to correlate the production of a particular hormone with a specific cell type. Since at least six hormones were known to be elaborated by the anterior lobe, it was logical to seek six distinct cell types. Laboratory and clinical observations furnished cumulative data. Fluorescent antibody techniques showed that human growth hormone could be localized in acidophil cells (Leznoff *et al.*, 1960). The histochemical demonstration that basophil cells contain glycoproteins linked these cells with the glycoprotein hormones, thyrotropin and the gonadotropins (Halmi, 1966). Experimental removal of a target organ and subsequent histological study of the pituitary gland will reveal alterations in the appropriate anterior lobe cell. Thus, thyroidectomized rats show degranulation of acidophils, and castration produces alterations in basophils (Halmi, 1966). Clinical observations demonstrated the association of Cushing's syndrome with basophil adenomas; in this syndrome, or following administration of corticosteroids, histologic examination of pituitary tissue reveals accumulation of homogenous material in basophil cells, the so-called Crooke's hyaline change.

Studies of normal anterior pituitary tissue with the electron microscope have been conducted mainly on animal material, and further observations on human glands would be valuable. However, despite differences between species, up to six cell types can be distinguished on the basis of fine structural characteristics. Mikami (1970) provides a detailed discussion of the morphologic features of the various cell types based on his studies of the bovine adenohypophysis; line drawings depicting the fine structure of the cells are included in the publication of Lentz (1971).

The most important criteria are the size and distribution of intracytoplasmic secretory granules (Pooley, 1971). Electron-dense aggregates of secretory material are a well-known morphologic feature of many gland cells, and the mechanism whereby they are produced frequently has been described. Polypeptide secretory material is formed by ribosomes that stud the endoplasmic reticulum, and is then passed along the cisternae of the reticulum to the Golgi complex where it is packaged into small aggregates that appear in electron micrographs as spherical, electron-dense bodies surrounded by a limiting membrane. In this form, the secretion is stored in the cell, and the granules maintain their integrity until they are extruded from the cell in the process of secretion. In contrast, steroid-producing cells contain smooth-surfaced reticulum and no intracytoplasmic secretory granules (Fawcett, Long, and Jones, 1969). In exocrine gland cells, the secretory granules may be quite large. In most endocrine cells, however, the secretory granules are relatively small, fitting within a rather narrow range of diameters for the particular cell type. Differences in these features among the anterior pituitary cells, in conjunction with less reliable criteria such as the size and shape of the cell and the size and location of the Golgi complex and other cytoplasmic structures, provide the morphologic basis for distinguishing the various cell types.

Cells formerly classified as acidophils, and from histochemical studies known to comprise two distinct cell types, are responsible for the production of growth hormone and prolactin. The growth hormone-producing cell contains a large number of secretory granules, most of which are between 300 and 350 mμ in diameter; the Golgi complex is typically large. The granules in the prolactin-producing cell are considerably larger than those of any other anterior pituitary cell, measuring in excess of 600 mμ and varying in shape. Numerous lysosomes, which degrade excess secretion, are an additional feature of the prolactin-producing cell.

Gonadotrophic hormones are produced by basophil cells, and it is probable that separate cell types elaborate follicle-stimulating hormone and luteinizing hormone in the female or interstitial cell-stimulating hormone in the male. Morphologically, distinctions between the two cell types are subtle, and each contains granules in the 250 mμ range.

Thyrotrophic hormone-producing cells are smaller and more angular than the other cell types. The secretory granules are distinctly smaller than those of the various other anterior pituitary cells, with measurements in the range of 100 to 150 mμ. Typically, the granules are located peripherally in the cytoplasm where they form a single line or narrow band just within the cell membrane.

Siperstein and Miller (1970) described the ACTH-producing cell in the rat as having an irregular outline and containing sparse secretory granules which measure between 200 and 260 mμ.

It is apparent, from electron microscopic studies of the anterior pituitary in various species including man, that the term chromophobe, connoting an inactive cell, is a misnomer. The pale-staining cytoplasm indicates a considerable degree of degranulation but this may merely reflect hyperactivity. The argument may be extended to the adenomas. A chromophobe adenoma contains cells which have a reduced content of secretion within the cytoplasm. Secretory granules have been present in every chromophobe adenoma that we have studied with the electron microscope (Figs. 3, 4, and 5) although they may be few in number and lack the electron

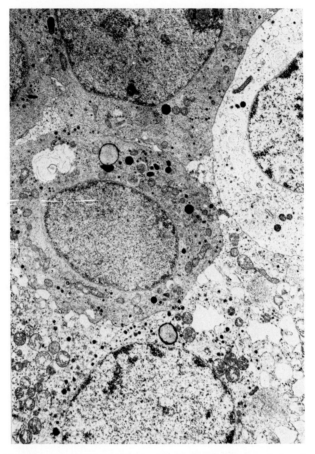

Fig. 3.—Electron micrograph showing several cells of a chromophobe adenoma. Moderate numbers of small, electron-dense secretory granules are present in the cytoplasm of the cells together with occasional larger bodies (× 6,600).

density of granules in normal cells (Fig. 5). In a recent publication, Mc-Cormick and Halmi (1971) report that in a series of 166 pituitary adenomas, 145 from autopsy material and 21 removed surgically, none was unequivocally chromophobic when studied with specially controlled light microscopic staining procedures following careful fixation. They conclude that truly chromophobic adenomas are extremely rare or nonexistent.

To determine whether it would be possible to characterize the cells of an anterior pituitary adenoma on the basis of their morphology, we studied five chromophobe adenomas with the electron microscope, measuring granule size. Our results suggest that this would be an inconstant and probably precarious method of characterization. The number of granules is extremely varied in the adenoma cells compared with those in cells of the normal gland, and some adenoma cells are practically devoid of granules. Also, granule size is more varied in adenoma cells than in normal gland cells, and occasionally two adjacent cells contain granules which

Fig. 4.—Electron micrograph of chromophobe adenoma cells. The profusion of granules is unusual for a chromophobe adenoma, and it is also uncommon to find such a sharp difference between granule diameters in cells of the same tumor. Most of the cells in this particular tumor contained only moderate numbers of granules that were similar in size to the smaller ones illustrated (× 13,000).

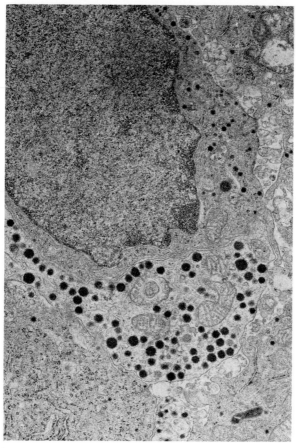

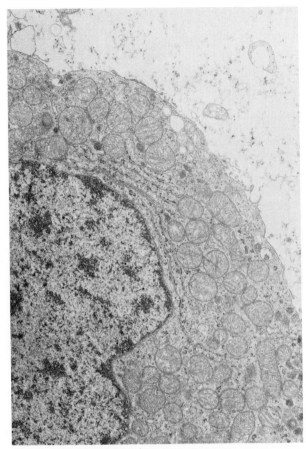

FIG. 5.—The cells of this chromophobe adenoma are larger than normal and contain numerous mitochondria. Secretory granules are present, but they are relatively sparse and of low electron density (× 13,000).

obviously are in entirely different ranges of diameters (Fig. 4). In four of the five adenomas studied, the average granule diameter was intermediate between that of normal thyrotrophs and the larger granules of normal anterior pituitary cells. It has been demonstrated that functioning chromophobe adenomas possess secretory granules that morphologically can be equated with the particular normal gland cell (Russfield, 1967; Peake, McKeel, Jarrett, and Daughaday, 1969; Pasteels, 1972). Paucity of secretory granules and variability in their size may, therefore, reflect dedifferentiation of the tumor cells.

REFERENCES

Bergland, R. M., and Torack, R. M.: An ultrastructural study of follicular cells in the human anterior pituitary. *The American Journal of Pathology*, 57:273-297, November 1969.

Cushing, H.: Basophil adenomas of the pituitary body and their clinical manifestations (pituitary basophilism). *Bulletin of the Johns Hopkins Hospital*, 50: 137-195, March 1932.

Erdheim, J.: Ueber einen Hypophysentumor von ungewöhnlichem Sitz. *Beitraege zur pathologischen Anatomie und zur allgemeinen Pathologie*, 46:233, 1909.

Fawcett, D. W., Long, J. A., and Jones, A. L.: The ultrastructure of endocrine glands. *Recent Progress in Hormone Research*, 25:315-380, 1969.

Ghatak, N. R., Hirano, A., and Zimmerman, H. M.: Ultrastructure of a craniopharyngioma. *Cancer*, 27:1465-1475, June 1971.

Halmi, N. S.: Adenohypophysis. In Greep, R. O., Ed.: *Histology*, 2nd Edition, New York, McGraw-Hill, 1966, pp. 747-760.

Lentz, T. L.: *Cell Fine Structure*. Philadelphia, Pennsylvania, W. B. Saunders Co., 1971, 437 pp.

Leznoff, A., Fishman, J., Goodfriend, L., McGarry, E., Beck, J., and Rose, B.: Localization of fluorescent antibodies to human growth hormone in human anterior pituitary glands. *Proceedings of the Society for Experimental Biology and Medicine*, 104:232-235, June 1960.

Luse, S. A., and Kernohan, J. W.: Granular-cell tumors of the stalk and posterior lobe of the pituitary gland. *Cancer*, 8:616-622, May-June 1955.

Mikami, S.: Light and electron microscopic investigations of six types of glandular cells of the bovine adenohypophysis. Zeitschrift für Zellforschung und mikroscopische Anatomie, 105:457-482, 1970.

Moldawer, M. P., Nardi, G. L., and Raker, J. W.: Concomitance of multiple adenomas of parathyroids and pancreatic islets with tumor of the pituitary: A syndrome with familial incidence. *The American Journal of the Medical Sciences*, 228:190-206, August 1954.

McCormick, W. F., and Halmi, N. S.: Absence of chromophobe adenomas from a large series of pituitary tumors. *Archives of Pathology*, 92:231-238, October 1971.

Pasteels, J. L.: Morphology of prolactin secretion. In Wolstenholme, G. E. W., and Knight, J., Eds.: *Ciba Foundation Symposium—Lactogenic Hormones*. Edinburgh, Scotland and London, England, Churchill Livingstone Publishers, 1972, pp. 241-255.

Peake, G. T., McKeel, D. W., Jarett, L., and Daughaday, W. H.: Ultrastructural, histologic and hormonal characterization of a prolactin-rich human pituitary tumor. *Journal of Clinical Endocrinology and Metabolism*, 29:1383-1393, November 1969.

Pooley, A. S.: Ultrastructure and size of rat anterior pituitary secretory granules. *Endocrinology*, 88:400-411, February 1971.

Russell, D. S., and Rubinstein, L. J.: *Pathology of Tumours of the Nervous System*. 3rd Edition, Baltimore, Maryland, The Williams and Wilkins Co., 1971, pp. 233-242.

Russfield, A. B.: Pituitary Tumors. In Sommers, S. C., Ed.: *Pathology Annual.* New York, Appleton-Century-Crofts, 1967, pp. 314-350.

Siperstein, E. R., and Miller, K. J.: Further cytophysiologic evidence for the identity of the cells that produce adrenocorticotrophic hormone. *Endocrinology,* 86:451-486, March 1970.

Winkelman, N. W., Jr., Cassel, C., and Schlesinger, B.: Intracranial tumors with extracranial metastases. *Journal of Neuropathology and Experimental Neurology,* 11:149-168, 1952.

The Syndrome of Inappropriate
Secretion of Antidiuretic Hormone

FREDERIC C. BARTTER, M.D.

National Heart and Lung Institute,
National Institutes of Health, Bethesda, Maryland

IN THIS PAPER I will discuss one of the malignant tumors which produces hormones. In the broadest sense, we are focusing on cells whose genetic information encodes the message for two "errors" of metabolism. First, they have been "transformed" into cancer cells, having lost, for example, the message for contact inhibition. Second, they are producing peptides they were never meant to produce. As we turn to a detailed consideration of the individual syndromes, we should not lose sight of the broader implications of this relationship. It seems almost certain that peptide production involves derepression of a site of chromosomal DNA which normally is completely repressed in, for instance, a lung cell. There is growing evidence that transformation involves derepression of another site—an oncogene, perhaps—or insertion of new genetic material into selected cell lines.

Does the coexistence of these defects—aberrant hormone production and transformation—in a single cell mean that the same chromosome that codes for peptide hormones also codes for transformation? Alternatively, could it mean that one derepressor serves both sites?

In the syndrome of inappropriate secretion of antidiuretic hormone (SIADH) (Bartter and Schwartz, 1967), an identical physiologic picture can result from two distinct pathophysiologic entities. The first to be recognized (Schwartz, Bennett, Curelop, and Bartter, 1957) was that of the double defect mentioned above. SIADH was found in patients with oat cell carcinoma of the lung and it has been convincingly shown that this tumor cell produces an aberrant peptide closely resembling, and probably identical to, vasopressin.

In the second entity, SIADH results from endogenous secretion of vasopressin from the supraoptico-hypophyseal system in quantities inappropriate for normal physiologic control. To clarify this definition, let us review briefly (1) the action of antidiuretic hormone (ADH) and (2) the normal control of ADH secretion.

A subject deprived of water excretes concentrated urine of low volume. The osmolality of the urine exceeds that of the plasma. Figure 1 shows the effect of an oral water load in such a subject. The absorbed water lowers plasma osmolality, whereupon the volume of urine rises rapidly while its osmolality falls below that of plasma. This last condition defines the situation in which free water is being excreted. The free water is that which would be required to dilute the urinary solute from the osmolality of plasma to that of the hypotonic urine actually being excreted. Vasopressin is known to produce the initial concentrated urine. The inhibition of ADH secretion by hypotonicity of the plasma (specifically, the plasma perfusing the supraoptico-hypophyseal system) represents the most important physi-

Fig. 1.—The effect of a water load on serum and urinary osmolality, urinary volume, osmolar clearance, and free water in a normal subject.

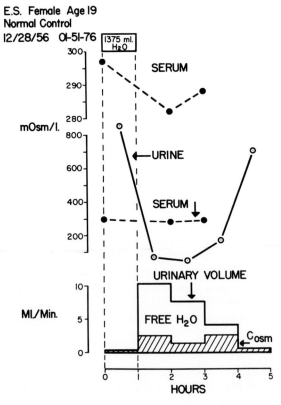

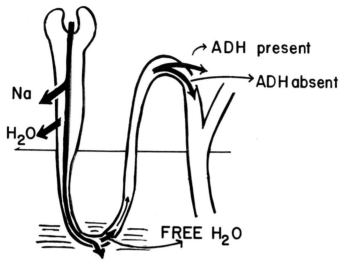

Fɪɢ. 2.—Representation of a nephron, demonstrating the fate of water throughout the tubule.

ologic control mechanism for this system. Figure 2 illustrates the renal action of ADH. Its presence allows back diffusion in the distal tubules (and collecting ducts) of some of the water of dilute urine formed in the ascending limb of the loop of Henle. Excretion of this dilute urine constitutes the response to inhibition of ADH secretion which we have considered. ADH probably has no effect on proximal tubular reabsorption of sodium and water in solution which is isosmotic with plasma. This relationship is important in the differential diagnosis of SIADH (vide infra) because some patients, *e.g.*, cirrhotics, absorb sodium and water excessively in the proximal tubules. This limits the amount of filtrate delivered to the loop for the formation of free water. These patients cannot excrete a water load normally even without ADH.

The effect of exogenous ADH in normal man is illustrated in Figure 3. Pitressin alone has no detectable effects; however, when the subject is given water as well, pitressin causes (1) retention of that water, (2) weight gain, and (3) hyponatremia and hypotonicity of body fluids. Two other sequelae of considerable importance are regularly observed. First, the glomerular filtration rate rises and may increase by 50 per cent or more of control values. Second, aldosterone secretion and excretion decrease. This phenomenon allows a clear separation of the control of aldosterone secretion by body fluid volume from any supposed influence of hyponatremia

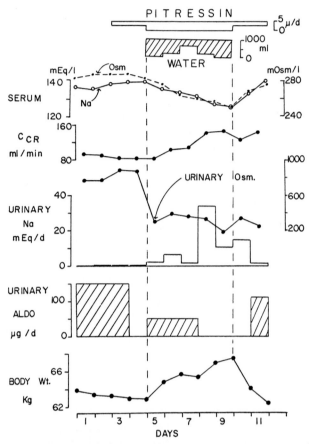

Fig. 3.—The effect of pitressin alone and in combination with a water load on serum sodium concentration and osmolality, creatinine clearance, urinary sodium and aldosterone, and body weight in a normal subject.

per se. The combined effect of an increase in the filtered load of sodium and a decrease in the aldosterone-induced reabsorption of sodium clearly increases urinary sodium excretion and thus aggravates the hyponatremia originally induced by dilution alone. Another sequela of expansion of body fluids such as that induced with vasopressin and water is a decrease in plasma renin activity, despite hyponatremia.

Figure 4 shows studies on a 50-year-old man who presented with vague complaints of periodic episodes of obtundity and confusion. On a diet moderately limited in water, he showed normal values for plasma sodium and osmolality and no detectable metabolic abnormality. When an additional 500 to 800 ml. of water were added to the intake, the sequelae were gain in weight, decrease in plasma sodium and osmolality, and an increase in urinary sodium—precisely those changes that follow the administration of water to normal subjects receiving pitressin tannate. The results suggested that such patients suffered from persistent sustained production of ADH. Because the production apparently continued despite hypotonicity of plasma (the normal inhibitory control stimulus) the production was termed inappropriate. This patient was found to have a bronchogenic carcinoma of the lung.

In another patient with bronchogenic carcinoma and SIADH (Schwartz, Tassel, and Bartter, 1960) (Fig. 5), we wished to assess the relative roles of suppression of aldosterone secretion and of increase of glomerular filtra-

FIG. 4.—The effect of a water load on serum sodium concentration, urinary sodium, serum and urinary osmolality, and body weight in a patient with bronchogenic carcinoma.

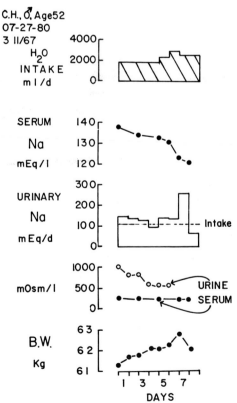

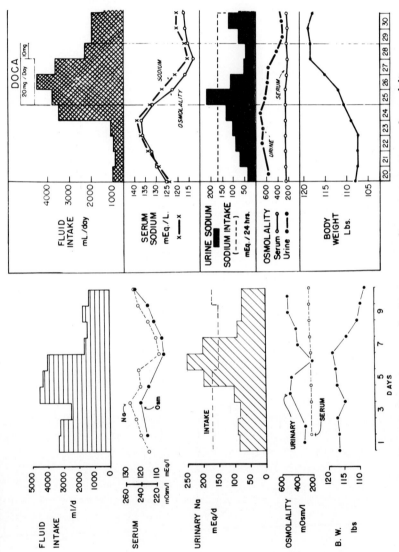

Fig. 5.—The effect of a water load on serum sodium concentration and osmolality, urinary sodium and osmolality, and body weight in a subject with bronchogenic carcinoma; A, water alone; B, water with desoxycorticosterone.

TABLE 1.—ABERRANT PRODUCTION OR INAPPROPRIATE
SECRETION OF ADH

1. Malignant tumors:
   Carcinoma of the lung, duodenum, and pancreas.
2. Central nervous system disorders:
   Meningitis
   Injuries
   Abscess
   Tumor
   Encephalitis
   Porphyria
   Hemorrhage
   Guillain-Barre syndrome
3. Lung diseases:
   Pneumonia
   Tuberculosis
   Cavitation—aspergillosis
4. Idiopathic

tion rate and filtered sodium load in producing sodium loss and hyponatremia. Two studies were run, each consisting of three days of water loading. The role of aldosterone, clearly suppressed in this patient because of his underlying disease, was evaluated by giving desoxycorticosterone (DOCA) to the patient during the second course. It is apparent from the gain of body weight, the plasma hypotonicity, the hyponatremia, and the significant increase in urinary sodium during the first course that the patient was indeed unable to suppress endogenous ADH and consequently showed all the expected effects of the water load. During the second period of water loading (Fig. 5), DOCA was given in quantities large enough to replace any aldosterone whose secretion was suppressed in the first study. During the second study, gain in body weight, hypotonicity, and hyponatremia were more notable than in the first study. Urinary sodium, in contrast, decreased after an initial increase thereby inducing a positive balance over the period of water loading.

The syndrome has subsequently been found in a large number of conditions (Table 1). Only the first category is associated with malignant tumors. The importance of excluding other causes has led to a renewed interest in the water test such as that illustrated in Figure 1.

Response to Water Load in SIADH

The essential features of a normal response to a water load are given in Figure 1. Figure 6 shows a response to the corresponding load in a patient

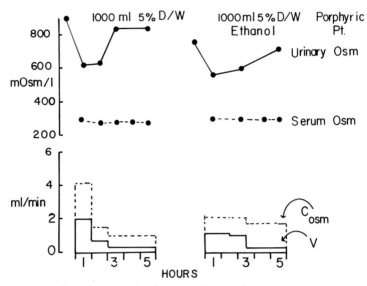

Fɪɢ. 6.—The effect of a water load alone and in combination with ethanol on urinary osmolality, serum osmolality, and urinary volume (V), and on osmolar clearance (ᶜosm) in a patient with porphyria.

with acute intermittent porphyria. The initial value for free water in this patient was negative, *i.e.*, the urine was more concentrated than the plasma. With the water load, the urine remained concentrated, there was no diuresis, and the urinary osmolality never fell to that of the plasma. This was the first indication that patients with acute porphyria suffered from transient inappropriate secretion of ADH (Hellman, Tschudy, and Bartter, 1962). Whereas a failure to show normal diuresis following a water load is generally observed in SIADH, a failure to respond may be observed in the absence of SIADH under certain circumstances. Patients undergoing excessive reabsorption of sodium and water in the proximal tubules may suffer thereby so great a limitation in the formation of free water in the loop that they fail to diurese a water load. Patients with cirrhosis of the liver and those with cardiac failure may develop this complication. In such patients, the limitation of sodium excretion is generally so great as to leave very small quantities of sodium unreabsorbed in the urine. This feature is often of value in distinguishing such patients from those with true SIADH.

The right side of Figure 6 shows the use of alcohol with a water load. Alcohol may block the endogenous secretion and the release of vasopressin. When it does so in a patient with SIADH (it failed in the patient shown in Figure 6), it may serve clearly to distinguish patients in group 1 (Table 1) from those in groups 2 and 3 in whom ADH is produced not by a tumor but by the patient's supraoptico-hypophyseal system under an abnormal stimulus thus far not identified. Figure 7 shows a study performed by Mangos and Lobeck (1964) in a patient with meningitis and hyponatremia who fulfilled the criteria for SIADH. The water load produced virtually no increase in urinary volume but did decrease plasma sodium. In contrast, when the patient received ethanol without a water load, there was a brisk diuresis. This combination of events served to establish that

Fig. 7.—The effect of a water load alone on serum sodium concentration and urine volume (V) in milliliters per minute and of ethanol on the urine volume in a child with meningitis. (Replotted from Mangos and Lobeck, 1964.)

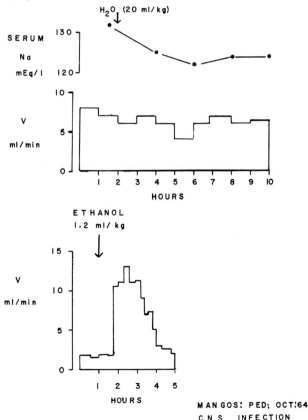

this patient's SIADH resulted from an abnormal endogenous release of vasopressin.

The Essential Features of SIADH

To demonstrate the existence of SIADH it should be necessary only to show concentrations of vasopressin in the plasma compatible with a state of water deprivation in a patient with hyponatremia. As we have seen, the diagnosis can be made with some confidence when certain clinical criteria are met. These classical features are: (1) hyponatremia, (2) urinary solute concentration in excess of plasma concentration even when plasma is abnormally dilute, (3) the presence of sodium in the urine in quantities which

FIG. 8.—The effect of ethanol on serum and urinary osmolality in a patient with myxedema. (Replotted from Goldberg and Reivich, 1962.)

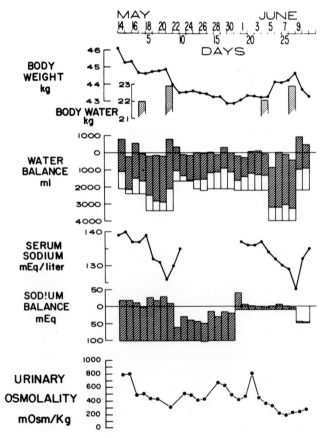

increase with water loading, (4) suppression of plasma renin activity despite hyponatremia, and (5) normal renal function.

It will be immediately apparent that each of these features may be absent in a patient with SIADH so that this syndrome may be easily missed unless sought for by specific testing. (1) Hyponatremia responds to restriction of water in all situations and this, of course, applies to SIADH. The patient may voluntarily avoid water and maintain a normal plasma sodium concentration and osmolality. In such patients, the syndrome is readily unmasked by water loading. (2) When a patient with SIADH is taking liberal amounts of water, the urine may frequently be dilute in relation to plasma as it is, of course, in the normal. The essential feature of SIADH is that urine does not achieve the minimal possible solute concentration for the solute load. Accordingly, enough of the water ingested is retained to expand body fluids and produce the syndrome. (3) Whereas the presence of sodium in the urine and its increase with water loading may be of great diagnostic value, especially in distinguishing the patient with SIADH from the patient with the hyponatremia of cirrhosis or cardiac failure, this feature may be entirely eliminated by restriction of sodium in the diet. In the study shown in Figure 8, for example, a patient with acute intermittent porphyria with SIADH was subjected to water loading on two occasions. During the second study, dietary sodium was restricted. Whereas hyponatremia was readily produced by the water loading, there was no increase of urinary sodium on this occasion. (4) Renin is suppressed in the presence of hyponatremia in SIADH, but such suppression, like the hyponatremia itself, can be obviated by restriction of water. (5) Whereas the finding of normal renal function is useful in eliminating renal failure as a cause of hyponatremia, it is clear that a patient with SIADH may also develop renal damage. Accordingly, no one of the classical features is essential to SIADH.

SIADH in Endocrine and Other Disorders

Certain endocrine disorders frequently produce SIADH when the patient's water intake is excessive. In Addison's disease, it has been shown that the hyponatremia may be associated with concentrations of vasopressin characteristic of a normal subject who is deprived of water and that the plasma ADH decreases as the hyponatremia is cured with water diuresis after administration of cortisol. It is the carbohydrate-active steroid that produces this change, which is unaffected by sodium-retaining steroids (Dingman, Gonzales-Auvert, Ahmed, and Akimura, 1965). The same relationship has been shown for patients with hypopituitarism who char-

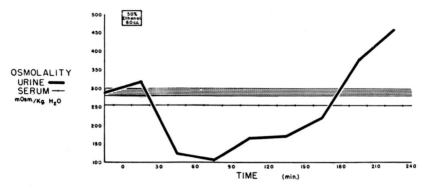

Fig. 9.—The effect of a water load followed by a load of isosmotic mannitol on urinary osmolality and potassium and on serum osmolality and on osmolar and free water clearance in a patient with cirrhosis. Note that the mannitol but not the water increased free water clearance and potassium excretion.

acteristically develop hyponatremia with water loading and who showed diuresis with carbohydrate-active steroids. The stimulus to ADH production in these syndromes has not been established, but it may be related to a decrease in effective blood volume. It has been shown that hypovolemia can stimulate the release of vasopressin (Weinstein, Berne, and Sachs, 1960).

SIADH may be found also in patients with myxedema (Goldberg and Reivich, 1962). The mechanism by which the syndrome is produced in this condition is not clear. The response to alcohol (Fig. 9) makes it likely that it results from endogenous release of vasopressin in quantities inappropriate for a patient with hyponatremia. SIADH of myxedema responds readily to treatment with thyroid hormones. Patients in a postoperative state cannot excrete a water load and readily develop hyponatremia if they are given excessive amounts of water. Since pain and trauma have been shown to induce vasopressin release, it is likely that such a mechanism explains the SIADH of the patient in the postoperative state. Such a response which may be appropriate for the trauma has been termed inappropriate because it persists in the presence of hyponatremia.

Patients with cardiac failure and cirrhosis may fail to excrete a water load normally for reasons not involving ADH, as noted earlier. The reasons involve excessive proximal reabsorption of sodium and water, which can often be demonstrated by infusion of an isotonic load of nonreabsorbable solute. Figure 10 shows the study in a patient with cirrhosis who persistently showed very low urinary sodium values as well as hyponatremia and hypotonicity of plasma which was made worse by infusion of water with metabolizable solute. When the infusion was changed to a solution of mannitol containing no free water, the excretion of free water promptly rose to high values as plasma osmolality rose. It is clear that the normal stimulus to release of ADH should have been increasing with a rise of plasma osmolality. The increase of free water excretion in this patient resulted from the osmotic diuresis with release of isotonic fluid from reabsorption in the proximal tubules and its delivery to distal tubular sites where free water is generated. In strong support of this explanation is the prompt increase of potassium secretion, a distal tubular function dependent upon tubular sodium when the mannitol was given. For our present purposes, it is necessary to state that in addition to this mechanism for hyponatremia, some patients with cirrhosis and cardiac failure may also suffer from true SIADH; *i.e.,* the delivery of solute to the distal tubules may fail to produce a dilute urine despite the formation of more free water which is reabsorbed in the distal tubules. (The increased loss of potassium is, of

Fig. 10.—The effect of changes in sodium and water intakes on body weight, body water, water balance, serum sodium concentration, sodium balance, and urinary osmolality in a patient with porphyria.

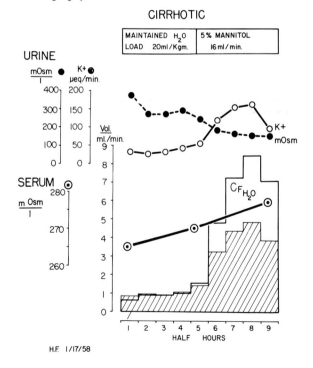

course, still produced.) The expansion of the body fluids (as in cirrhosis) or effective improvement of cardiac function may produce the diuresis of free water in such patients by lowering secretion of ADH.

Summary

The syndrome of inappropriate secretion of antidiuretic hormone (SIADH) may be produced by a tumor secreting vasopressin, a polypeptide with similar chemical and physiological properties from an aberrant source, or by the supraoptico-hypophyseal system secreting vasopressin in quantities inappropriate to plasma tonicity, that is, not suppressed when ingestion of water has induced dilution of plasma.

Two types of SIADH may be distinguished by an alcohol test, since some, but not all, of the patients in the second group show suppression of ADH or vasopressin secretion with alcohol.

The features of this syndrome—hypotonicity of plasma with hyponatremia, urinary solute concentration higher than plasma solute concentration, excretion of sodium in the urine despite hyponatremia, depression of plasma renin despite hyponatremia, and normal renal function—allow ready diagnosis in most cases. Under appropriate circumstances, however, each of these features may be absent in a given patient in a state of moderate deprivation of water and may be unmasked by water loading. Hypopituitarism, myxedema, and Addison's disease may reproduce all the features of this syndrome. The most difficult differential diagnosis concerns a patient with cirrhosis of the liver or cardiac failure with very low urinary sodium. Whereas water loading in such a patient produces or aggravates hyponatremia, it does not appreciably increase urinary sodium. In such patients, hyperabsorption of salt and water in the proximal tubule is extensive. The situation is further complicated by the occasional appearance of the true syndrome in a patient who also shows excessive proximal reabsorption of sodium, characteristic of patients with cirrhosis and ascites or cardiac failure.

REFERENCES

Bartter, F. C., and Schwartz, W. B.: The syndrome of inappropriate secretion of antidiuretic hormone. *The American Journal of Medicine,* 42:790-806, May 1967.

Dingman, J. F., and Gonzalez-Auvert, C., Ahmed, A. B. J., and Akimura, A.: Plasma antidiuretic hormone in adrenal insufficiency. *The Journal of Clinical Investigation,* 44:1041, 1965.

Goldberg, M., and Reivich, M.: Studies on the mechanism of hyponatremia and impaired water excretion in myxedema. *Annals of Internal Medicine,* 56:120-130, January 1962.

Hellman, E. E., Tschudy, D. P., and Bartter, F. C.: Abnormal electrolyte and water metabolism in acute intermittent porphyria. *The American Journal of Medicine,* 32:734-746, May 1962.

Mangos, J. A., and Lobeck, C. C.: Studies of sustained hyponatremia due to central nervous system infection. *Pediatrics,* 34:503-510, October 1964.

Schwartz, W. B., Bennett, W., Curelop, S., and Bartter, F. C.: A syndrome of renal sodium loss and hyponatremia probably resulting from inappropriate secretion of antidiuretic hormone. *The American Journal of Medicine,* 23:529-542, October 1957.

Schwartz, W. B., Tassel, D., and Bartter, F. C.: Further observations on hyponatremia and renal sodium loss probably resulting from inappropriate secretion of antidiuretic hormone. *The American Journal of Medicine,* 26:743, 1960.

Weinstein, H., Berne, R. M., and Sachs, H.: Vasopressin in blood: Effect of hemorrhage. *Endocrinology,* 66:712-718, May 1960.

Hypoglycemia in Pancreatic Tumors: Diagnosis and Treatment

NAGUIB A. SAMAAN, M.D., M.R.C.P., Ph.D.

*Department of Medicine, The University of Texas at Houston
M. D. Anderson Hospital and Tumor Institute,
Houston, Texas*

HYPOGLYCEMIA is a clinical problem, but once the mechanism of its production is established, the treatment is often satisfying. Hypoglycemia in the neonate or young infant is a metabolic error with potentially devastating effects on the brain. Neurologic complications may occur in the adult, but susceptibility to hypoglycemia is much greater in the immature, poorly myelinated brain of the infant. Hypoglycemia may be defined as a clinical state with true blood glucose of less than 20 mg./100 ml. in the premature infant, less than 30 mg./100 ml. in the full-term infant in the first 48 hours of life, and less than 40 mg./100 ml. in an adult or a child after the tenth day of life (Cornblath and Reisner, 1965).

Symptoms of Hypoglycemia

Included among the symptoms of hypoglycemia are: nervousness, trembling, apprehension, perspiration, hunger, faintness, tingling of the fingers and around the mouth, rapid pulse, and palpitation. These symptoms are the results of epinephrine response produced by hypoglycemia. Hypoglycemia may also produce restlessness, mental confusion which may simulate drunkenness, personality changes, hyperactivity, dullness, difficulty in talking, transient hemiparesis, epileptic convulsions, and coma. These symptoms are rapidly reversed by intravenous glucose unless there is brain damage. A few patients may present with a syndrome suggestive of amyotrophic sclerosis, following repeated hypoglycemic episodes (Barris, 1953; Skillern, 1955; Tom and Richardson, 1951).

The recognition of hypoglycemia is based on suspicion, blood glucose determination, and rapid response to the administration of glucose. The key to differential diagnosis is an elimination scheme that automatically resolves the most common problem by clearly distinguishing an islet-cell tumor from ordinary functional hypoglycemia. This is done by determining the age of the patient and whether he has fasting or postprandial hypoglycemia and also by considering the possible causes of hypoglycemia.

Hypoglycemia can be divided into either (1) postprandial hypoglycemia or (2) fasting hypoglycemia. The etiologies of postprandial hypoglycemia are several (Fig. 1). (1) Alimentary hypoglycemia (after gastrectomy or gastric bypass) is characterized by rapid supernormal rise of the blood glucose followed by a rapid fall to subnormal level. (2) Functional hypoglycemia is the most common type of spontaneous hypoglycemia and has been described variously as functional hypoglycemia, nervous hypoglycemia, and reactive hypoglycemia. These patients usually have various manifestations of a hyperactive autonomic nervous system, including hypermobility of the gastrointestinal tract. The symptoms of hypoglycemia wax and wane a great deal with the emotional status of the patient. In this condition, the glucose tolerance test (GTT) is normal except that the glucose level falls below 45 mg./100 ml. at three to four hours. (3) Early diabetes may initiate attacks of hypoglycemia three to five hours after meals. This type of hypoglycemia consists of a delayed hypernormal rise in the glucose level and then a sudden fall to hypoglycemic levels between the third and fifth hours.

Fasting hypoglycemia may be caused by either underproduction or overutilization of glucose.

Fig. 1.—Blood glucose and immunoreactive insulin (IRI) levels during an oral GTT in a patient with insulin adenoma compared with those found in 10 normal subjects.

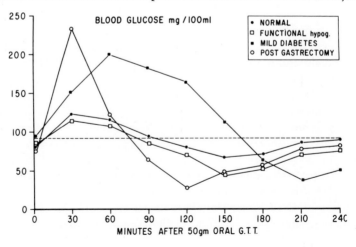

Underproduction of Glucose

Underproduction of glucose may result from hepatic diseases, including circulatory deficiency; cirrhosis and hepatitis; glycogen storage disease (Van Gierke's syndrome); galactosemia, including failure to form glucose 1-phosphate from galactose 1-phosphate; alcohol hypoglycemia; adrenal or pituitary insufficiency; and catecholamine deficiency in children (Broberger and Zetterstrom, 1961) or after the use of ganglion-blocking agents in adults.

HEPATIC DISEASE.—In this disease, there are notable morphological and biochemical abnormalities, and the fasting blood sugar is low while the GTT is of diabetic shape, showing the delayed return to the fasting level (Samaan, Stone, and Eckhardt, 1969). The low fasting blood sugar is caused by decreased ability of the liver to produce glucose. The high blood sugar after intake of glucose is caused by decreased hepatic capacity to store carbohydrates.

Glycogen storage disease (Van Gierke's disease) is associated with a deficiency of glucose-6-phosphatase and the formation of glucose from glycogen. These patients have large quantities of glycogen in the liver and kidneys.

Hereditary disorders of galactose and fructose metabolism also occur and produce hypoglycemia. These patients are unable to utilize galactose and fructose and convert it to glucose or energy.

PITUITARY HYPOFUNCTION AND ADRENOCORTICAL HYPOFUNCTION.—Seldom is hypoglycemia the first manifestation of adrenal or pituitary insufficiency. It is more common to see increased sensitivity to insulin in these conditions. The major mechanism of hypoglycemia in this disorder is decreased glyconeogenesis and defective glycogenolysis.

ALCOHOL HYPOGLYCEMIA.—Ethanol most probably produces hypoglycemia by impeding gluconeogenesis. This type of hypoglycemia is not associated with increased plasma-insulin levels, and the hypoglycemia is unresponsive to intravenous glucagon (Freinkel *et al.*, 1965).

Over-Utilization of Glucose

Over-utilization of glucose may be caused by neoplasms of β cells (benign and malignant), diffuse hyperplasia of β cells, extrapancreatic neoplasms, and exogenous insulin or oral hypoglycemic agents.

ISLET-CELL TUMORS OF THE PANCREAS.—Neoplasms of the islets of Langerhans clinically are the most important cause of hypoglycemia, and the majority of these (85 per cent) are benign adenomata. In about 10 per cent of the cases of insulinomas, two or more tumors are found in the pancreas. They may appear simultaneously, or their appearance may be separated by many years. Multiple tumors occur with greatest frequency in patients with the pluriglandular syndrome.

At least 10 per cent of all insulinomas are malignant. Generally, the metastases from insulinomas resemble in structure the primary tumor from which they originated. The usually accepted criterion of malignancy is the presence of metastasis. The most common site for metastasis is the liver.

The sexes are equally affected with insulinoma. Tumors occur most commonly between the ages of 20 and 50, but at least 30 cases have occurred in children, the youngest being one day old (Bernheim *et al.*, 1961).

Most insulinomas are between 1 and 2 cm. in diameter, but they may be as small as 0.5 mm. or as large as 15 cm. Insulinomas occur throughout the pancreas and are fairly well distributed. When insulinomas lie on the surface of the pancreas, they are characteristically brown, dark blue, or bluish-black because of their extreme vascularity. Rarely insulinomas may be almost white (Priestley, 1962), presumably because of relative avascularity.

DIFFUSE HYPERPLASIA OF THE ISLET CELLS (MICROADENOMATOSIS).—The clinical pictures of patients with microadenomatosis of the islet cells are similar, both clinically and pathologically, to those in which macroscopic tumors are also present.

Pancreatic adenomatosis may not be discovered until necropsy (Frantz, 1944). During life, it is found on microscopic examination (Bickerstaff, Dodge, Gourevitch, and Hearn, 1955; Bell, Samaan, and Longnecker, 1970) of the resected portion of the pancreas following subtotal pancreatectomy undertaken because no macroscopic tumor was palpable *in situ*.

The adenomata vary widely in size from a little larger than a normal islet to a diameter of 2 to 3 cm.; they are spread evenly throughout the pancreas and should be regarded as true multiple neoplasms rather than as hyperplastic islets. Rarely, all the islets are involved, more frequently some are normal, but the majority are enlarged, varying in diameter from 0.2 to 5.0 mm.

Diagnostic Procedures of Hypoglycemia

PROVOCATION OF HYPOGLYCEMIA BY FASTING

Fasting hypoglycemia is established by proving the inability to tolerate fasting. Many patients in whom fasting hypoglycemia occurs can be rendered hypoglycemic merely by withholding food for 12 to 14 hours overnight, or even less. A blood sample taken before breakfast showing a glu-

cose level below 40 mg./100 ml. is suggestive of insulinoma or extrapancreatic tumor in an adult. A number of patients do not develop hypoglycemia
after a short fast, and it is necessary to prolong the period of fasting for 48
to 72 hours. The test should be done in a hospital under strict supervision
to avoid self-administration of insulin in cases of factitious hyperinsulinism, as well as to ensure rapid relief with glucose should severe symptoms
occur. Food is prohibited, but unsweetened fluids *e.g.,* tea and coffee are
allowed *ad libitum.* During waking hours, the patient should exercise, and
blood should be taken regularly for glucose determination. The overnight
or prolonged fast serves to distinguish fasting from reactive hypoglycemia.
Normal people and those with reactive hypoglycemia withstand fasting
well, and the fasting blood glucose falls slightly but seldom to less than 50
mg./100 ml.

ORAL (GTT) AND INSULIN MEASUREMENT

The fasting blood sugar in insulinoma is usually low, but there may be
abnormally high blood sugar in the first two hours followed by a fall to
hypoglycemic level (Figs. 2 and 3), and if the test is prolonged for a few
hours, the patient may go into a coma.

The immunoreactive insulin (IRI) level is usually high at fasting and
during GTT. Occasionally, the IRI level is not high, but with repeated
testing all patients with insulinoma, either benign or malignant, have high
IRI levels (Samols and Marks, 1963). The normal fasting level of IRI is
between 1 to 20 μU./ml. serum at a fasting blood sugar level of 70 to 90
mg./100 ml. Conversely, a fasting insulin level of 20 μU./ml. at a blood
sugar level of 30 mg. is abnormally high (Bell, Samaan, and Longnecker,
1970). A high proportion (10 to 70 per cent) of IRI in patients with insulinoma is usually in the proinsulin form, which can be measured in
radioimmunoassay but which is biologically inactive (Steiner and Oyer,
1967; Steiner *et al.,* 1968). In extrapancreatic tumor-producing hypoglycemia, the IRI level and the insulin-like activity (ILA), either fasting or
during GTT, is usually normal or low (Marks, Auld, and Barr, 1965;
Samaan, Lal, Fraser, and Welbourn, 1965), and the presence of a tumor
in other parts of the body may be evident.

THE TOLBUTAMIDE TOLERANCE TEST

This test has been helpful in the diagnosis of islet-cell tumors in the
adults (Fajans and Conn, 1959). In normal adults, intravenous administration of sulfanilylurea (1 Gm., intravenously) stimulates insulin release

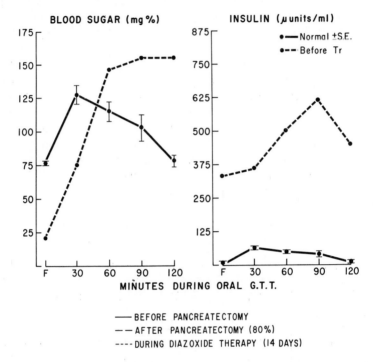

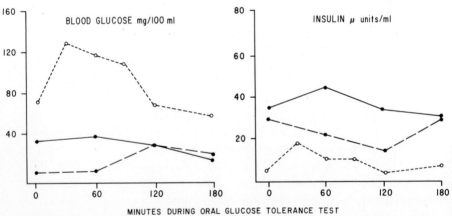

FIG. 2 (*top*).—Blood glucose and insulin levels (IRI) during an oral GTT in a child with microadenomatosis (hyperplasia of the islet cells) before pancreatectomy, 80 per cent pancreatectomy, and diazoxide therapy.

FIG. 3 (*bottom*).—Blood glucose and insulin levels (IRI) during tolbutamide tolerance test (1 Gm., intravenously) in a patient with insulin adenoma compared to those found in seven normal subjects.

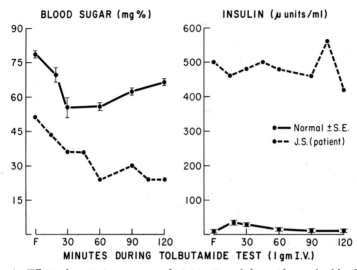

Fig. 4.—Effect of acute intravenous administration of diazoxide on the blood sugar and insulin levels (IRI) compared with saline in a patient with an insulin adenoma. There was a rise of blood glucose after glucose administration and inhibition of insulin release in the peripheral circulation after diazoxide.

with a fall of blood glucose as much as 40 per cent below fasting levels and approaching fasting level in 120 minutes (Fig. 4). Normal children were found to have a decrease in blood glucose as much as 25 per cent below fasting level 15 to 20 minutes following tolbutamide, with return to fasting level in 120 minutes.

Adults with islet-cell tumors characteristically exhibit a greater and more prolonged hypoglycemic response to tolbutamide than do normal persons. Other conditions of increased insulin sensitivity, such as hypopituitarism or liver disease, may also be associated with abnormal hypoglycemic response to tolbutamide. There have been false-negative and false-positive responses to this test (Cunningham, 1964). It can be concluded that the tolbutamide tolerance test with estimations of glucose and serum insulin is advisable. The significance of the results can only be interpreted in conjunction with all the laboratory data plus the clinical course.

SELECTIVE ANGIOGRAPHY

Selective angiography has been used with some success in about 50 per cent of the patients (Olsson, 1969), especially in those with adenomas with numerous vascular channels. Avascular adenomas do not show well with this technique. Since insulinomas are usually small, 1 to 2 cm. in diameter, and do not cause any displacement of the vessels, this test is the least useful for these tumors.

Treatment for Hypoglycemia of Pancreatic Tumor Origin

When possible, surgical therapy should be initiated without delay. In cases where surgical techniques fail (*i.e.*, adenomatosis or metastasis), for patients who are incapable of undergoing major surgical intervention, or during the period of diagnostic assessment, medical therapy should be used. This may include corticoids, human growth hormone (HGH), glucagon zinc retard, diazoxide, and streptozotocin.

CORTICOIDS.—Corticoid therapy has been used for treatment for hypoglycemia; however, it has not been found as effective as diazoxide. Corticoids must be used often and in large doses to be effective, but such doses may bring about severe complications, such as severe gastrointestinal hemorrhage and osteoporosis.

HUMAN GROWTH HORMONE (HGH).—HGH possesses a hyperglycemic effect through increase of gluconeogenesis and peripheral antagonistic effect to the action of insulin. Its use in treatment for hypoglycemia has been without success; moreover, since HGH is of human origin, it is very scarce and impractical.

GLUCAGON ZINC RETARD.—One milligram of the hormone, as commercially available, is usually sufficient to cure paroxysmal hypoglycemia by mobilization of glucose from the liver; its action, however, is of short duration, and the blood sugar level returns to the initial value 90 minutes after the injection.

Investigations into a retarded form of glucagon led to the manufacture of glucagon zinc retard (Kushner, Lemli, and Smith, 1963). The duration of the activity of the product barely exceeded eight hours, but it has been of value in glycogen-storage disease. A disadvantage of zinc glucagon is the need for daily injections. It is now well established that glucagon stimulates insulin secretion from the islet cells of Langerhans; thus it may act as stimulant, which would be undesirable with tumors.

DIAZOXIDE.—Diazoxide is a nondiuretic benzothiadiazine with hypotensive properties. It was soon discovered to produce hyperglycemia and inhibition of ILA in man (Dollery, Pentecost, and Samaan, 1962; Samaan, Dollery, and Fraser, 1963). Diazoxide was then used as a hyperglycemic agent in children with recurrent hypoglycemia caused by intolerance to L-leucine (Drash and Wolff, 1964). The trial was soon followed by its use in hypoglycemia caused by islet-cell tumors. The main action of the drug was found to be inhibition of insulin release from the islet cells (Fajans *et al.*, 1966). The hyperglycemic effect seems to consist of prolongation of postprandial hyperglycemia (Fig. 5). Diazoxide is given orally in a dose of 100 to 800 mg. per day (50-mg. tablets) in adults and 5 to 15 mg./kg. body weight per day in children (pediatric suspension) (Fig. 3).

We found that chronic diazoxide administration, either alone or in combination with chlorothiazide, to patients with insulinoma inhibits the release of regular insulin and to less extent the proinsulin. We also found that the level of "typical" ILA or "suppressible" ILA (biologically and immuno-

Fig. 5 (*top*).—The effect of oral administration of diazoxide and chlorothiazide on the blood sugar and the immunoreactive insulin (IRI) levels is shown. There is a decrease of IRI levels during therapy, but not to the normal levels, while the blood sugar is elevated to above normal.

Fig. 6 (*bottom*).—See text.

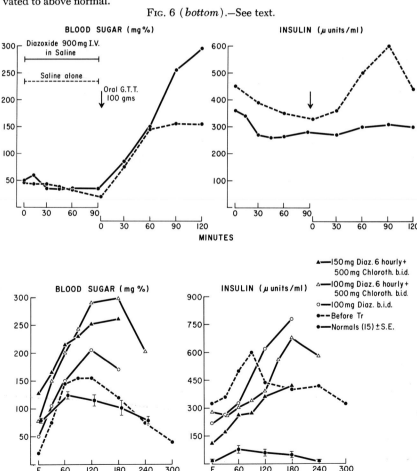

logically active) was significantly less than that measured by the radio-immunoassay of insulin during diazoxide therapy, since most of the radio-immunoassayable IRI measured during diazoxide therapy was in the pro-insulin form which was biologically inactive (Samaan, in preparation). Thus, after diazoxide therapy in insulinoma patients, the IRI level is lowered but remains higher than that seen in normal subjects, although the blood sugar level may still be elevated above normal. This is well illustrated in Figure 6, in a patient who had an insulinoma.

Side effects of diazoxide therapy include nausea and vomiting, hypertrichosis, hyperuricemia, salt and water retention with edema, and decreased immunoglobulin. However, all of these side effects are mild and reversible.

The hypoglycemic effect of diazoxide can be significantly potentiated by the addition of a diuretic of thiazide type. Hypopotassemia, which may result from the use of these two drugs, can be corrected by potassium chloride alone (4 Gm./day) or by potassium chloride plus Aldactone A (spironolactone, 50 mg./day), if potassium chloride alone fails to correct the hypopotassemia.

All the effects of diazoxide are reversible after withdrawal of the drug, and it has no destructive effect on the islet cells.

STREPTOZOTOCIN.—Streptozotocin is an antibiotic extract of Streptomyces achromogenes. When used in animals, it produces selective necrosis of β cells of the islets of Langerhans. It has been successfully used in patients who had malignant metastatic tumors of islet-cell origin which were secreting insulin and gastrin. After therapy, the metastasis regressed almost to the point of disappearing (Murray-Lyon et al., 1968; Cunningham, Quickel, and Lebovitz, 1971). However, the long-term effect of streptozotocin on tumors remains to be determined, since the experience with this drug so far is limited; however, the preliminary results are encouraging.

Streptozotocin is given intravenously in a dose of 1 to 4 Gm. about every three weeks. It is fairly well tolerated. It has a mild renal and hepatic toxicity when given in large doses at frequent intervals.

DIETETIC TREATMENT.—A high protein and low carbohydrate diet is given at frequent intervals. Diet alone cannot prevent the clinical episodes of hypoglycemia, but it does reduce their frequency.

SURGICAL TREATMENT.—The surgical treatment for insulin-secreting tumors of islets of Langerhans is undoubtedly the most satisfactory method. The operative risk involved is increased if the operation has to be repeated. The average mortality rate is 10 per cent.

Complications of pancreatectomy include pancreatic fistula, diabetes mellitus (often transitory), and digestive pancreatic enzyme insufficiency. This requires the provision of large amounts of pancreatic extract in order to assure normal stools and satisfactory weight gain. The requirement for pancreatic extract is less or none if the tumor is only removed and pancreatectomy is incomplete.

Hypoglycemia of pancreatic origin should be diagnosed early to avoid the devastating effect on the brain of the young infant or the severe mental changes and peripheral muscular atrophy in the adult which may occur with the delay in diagnosis. Surgical treatment is the method of choice and should not be deferred too long. Diazoxide is the drug of choice if medical therapy is indicated, while streptozotocin should be tried if malignant insulinoma with metastasis is found.

Acknowledgment

This study was supported by American Cancer Society Grant No. T-558, U.S.P.H.S. CA 05831-01 and CA 12521-01.

REFERENCES

Barris, R. W.: Pancreatic adenoma (hyperinsulinism) associated with neuromuscular disorders. *Annals of Internal Medicine,* 38:124-129, January 1953.

Bell, W. E., Samaan, N. A., and Longnecker, D. S.: Hypoglycemia due to organic hyperinsulinism in infancy. *Archives of Neurology,* 23:330-339, October 1970.

Bernheim, M., Francosi, R., Sacrez, R., Mallet, Guy P., Feroldi, J., Germain, D., Sherrer, M., Ruiton-Ugliengo, M., and Pradon, M.: Hypoglycemie par adenome pancreatique chez une fillette de 8 ans. Intervention. Guerison. *Pediatrie,* 16:330-358, 1961.

Bickerstaff, E. R., Dodge, O. G., Gourevitch, A., and Hearn, G. W.: Adenomatosis of islets of Langerhans. *British Medical Journal,* 2:997-1000, October 1955.

Broberger, O. and Zetterstrom, R.: Hypoglycemia with an inability to increase the epinephrine secretion in insulin-induced hypoglycemia. *The Journal of Pediatrics,* 59:215-222, August 1961.

Cornblath, M., and Reisner, S. H.: Blood glucose in the neonate and its clinical significance. *The New England Journal of Medicine,* 273:378-381, August 1965.

Cunningham, G. C.: Tolbutamide tolerance in hypoglycemic children. *American Journal of Diseases in Children,* 107:417-423, April 1964.

Cunningham, G. R., Quickel, K. E., Jr., and Lebovitz, H. E.: The use of insulin dynamics in the evaluation of streptozotocin therapy of malignant insulinomas. *The Journal of Clinical Endocrinology and Metabolism,* 33:530-536, September 1971.

Dollery, C. T., Pentecost, B. L., and Samaan, N. A.: Drug induced diabetes. *The Lancet,* 2:735-737, October 1962.

Drash, A., and Wolff, F.: Drug therapy in leucine-sensitive hypoglycemia. *Metabolism,* 13:487-492, June 1964.

Fajans, S. S., and Conn, J. W.: An intravenous tolbutamide test as an adjunct in the diagnosis of functioning pancreatic islet cells adenomas. *The Journal of Laboratory and Clinical Medicine*, 54:811-812, November 1959.

Fajans, S. S., Floyd, J. C., Jr., Knopf, R. F., Rull, J., Guntsche, E. M., and Conn, J. W.: Benzothiadiazine suppression of insulin release from normal and abnormal islet tissue in man. *The Journal of Clinical Investigation*, 45:481-492, April 1966.

Frantz, V. K.: Adenomatosis of islet cells, with hyperinsulinism. *Annals of Surgery*, 119:824-844, June 1944.

Freinkel, N., Arky, R. A., Singer, D. L., Cohen, A. K., Bleicher, S. J., Anderson, J. B., Silbert, C. K., and Foster, A. E.: Alcohol hypoglycemia, IV. Current concepts of its pathogenesis. *Diabetes*, 14:350-361, June 1965.

Kushner, R. S., Lemli, L., and Smith, D.: Zinc glucagon in the management of idiopathic hypoglycemia. *The Journal of Pediatrics*, 63:1111-1115, December 1963.

Marks, V., Auld, W. H. R., and Barr, J. B.: Carcinoma of stomach and other nonpancreatic lesions as causes of spontaneous hypoglycemia. *British Journal of Surgery*, 52:925-928, 1965.

Murray-Lyon, I. M., Eddleston, A. L. W. F., Williams, R., Brown, M., Hogbin, B. M., Bennett, A., Edwards, J. C., and Taylor, K. W.: Treatment of multiple-hormone-producing malignant islet cell tumour with streptozotocin. *The Lancet*, 2:895-898, October 1968.

Olsson, O.: Angiographic diagnosis of an islet cell tumor of the pancreas. *Acta chirurgica scandinavica*, 126:346-351, October 1969.

Priestley, J. T.: Hyperinsulinism. *Annals of Royal College of Surgeons (England)*, 31:211-228, April 1962.

Samaan, N. A.: Insulin-like activity and radioimmunoassayable insulin levels in patients with insulin adenoma during diazoxide therapy. (In preparation.)

Samaan, N. A., Dollery, C. T., and Fraser, R.: Diabetogenic action of benzothiadiazines. *The Lancet*, 2:1244-1246, December 1963.

Samaan, N. A., Lal, F., Fraser, R., and Welbourn, R. B.: Insulin assays in two cases of spontaneous hypoglycaemia due to retroperitoneal mesothelioma. *British Medical Journal*, II:195-198, July 1965.

Samaan, N. A., Stone, D. B., and Eckhardt, R. D.: Serum glucose, insulin, and growth hormone in chronic hepatic cirrhosis. *Archives of Internal Medicine*, 124:149-152, August 1969.

Samols, E., and Marks, V.: Insulin assay in insulinomas. *British Medical Journal*, Vol. I:507-510, February 1963.

Skillern, P. G.: Some recent advances in the knowledge of hypoglycemia. *The Journal of Clinical Endocrinology and Metabolism*, 15:826-828, July 1955.

Steiner, D. F., Hallund, O., Rubenstein, A., Sooja, C., and Bayliss, C.: Isolation and properties of proinsulin, intermediate forms, and other minor components from crystalline bovine insulin. *Diabetes*, 17:725-736, December 1968.

Steiner, D. F., and Oyer, P.: The biosynthesis of insulin and a probable precursor of insulin by a human islet cell adenoma. *Proceedings of the National Academy of Sciences of the United States of America*, 57:473-480, February 1967.

Tom, M. I., and Richardson, J. C.: Hypoglycemia from islet cell tumor of pancreas with amyotrophy and cerebrospinal nerve cell changes. A case report. *Journal of Neuropathology and Experimental Neurology*, 10:57-66, January 1951.

Production of Hypoglycemia by Extrapancreatic Tumors

EDGAR S. GORDON, M.D.

Department of Medicine, University of Wisconsin Medical Center,
Madison, Wisconsin

THE CASE REPORT presented in this paper is unusually interesting and is relevant to the topic of endocrine and nonendocrine hormone-producing tumors. In addition to the case report, I propose to speculate briefly on the possible mechanisms involved in the production of hypoglycemia which constitutes such an important aspect of the clinical problem in all such endocrine-activity tumors.

The patient, Mr. W. M., was a 64-year-old white, married, farmer and cattle dealer, first seen at the University Hospitals on June 28, 1965, complaining of "fluid in the chest." A Papanicolaou smear of the fluid showed at this time a few suspicious cells. No etiology for the pleural effusion was established.

The second admission occurred about one week later on July 6, 1965, when the patient returned for further studies. The fluid was still present and revealed no specific findings. X-ray studies at that time, however, showed downward displacement of the left kidney by an ovoid mass, probably located in the left thorax.

The third admission took place one week later, July 12, 1965, when the patient returned for surgical exploration. A thoracotomy performed on July 13 led to partial removal of a large tumor mass, probably weighing in excess of 2 kg., from the left thorax and thought to be attached to the left diaphragm. The tentative diagnosis at that time was rhabdomyosarcoma.

After convalescence at home, the patient was admitted for the fourth time on August 2, 1965, for initiation of therapy consisting of actinomycin D, 5 μg./kg. of body weight daily for 10 days, accompanied by X-ray therapy designed to deliver 4,000 rads over a period of three to four weeks.

The fifth admission was on March 11, 1966, about seven months after therapy had been initiated. At this time, a large recurrence of the tumor

143

was noted at examination. The patient had begun to have episodes of faintness, weakness, and extremely profuse sweating which had begun about four weeks before this admission. These episodes had been identified by his local physician as hypoglycemic in nature, and treatment was initiated with prednisone, continuous high carbohydrate feeding, and regular administration of glucagon.

His terminal course was characterized by continuation of the hypoglycemic episodes, which became gradually more severe, with blood glucose levels recorded as low as 10 mg. per cent. These low levels were accompanied by uncontrollable, violent, psychotic behavior and often by deep coma. The patient responded well throughout his terminal illness to the use of glucagon in doses of 10 mg. per injection, kindly provided without cost by the Lilly Laboratories.

Death occurred at home about six weeks later from superior vena caval obstruction. Autopsy permission was denied.

The histological structure of this tumor is demonstrated in the accompanying photomicrograph (Fig. 1) from which it is apparent that the correct diagnosis is certainly some type of sarcoma, although there has been disagreement among pathologists as to the exact classification.

FIG. 1.—See text.

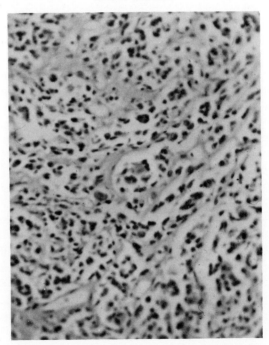

This case appears to be a typical example of the so-called Doege-Potter syndrome, first described by Dr. Karl Doege of Marshfield, Wisconsin, in a patient presenting a clinical problem very similar to the one outlined with this patient. It is apparent that the sharpest focus of interest in all such cases relates to the mechanism by which the hypoglycemia is produced. Widely divergent theories have been proposed in the past, some of which have already been excluded by further investigation. Among those that are no longer seriously considered is the concept that such tumors must represent metaplasia of pancreatic islet tissue in aberrant locations, so that the tumor occurring from such cells retains some capacity to make insulin or related polypeptides. A second theory of passing interest has been the proposal that these tumors, because of their size, have exerted some kind of pressure effect upon a variety of visceral structures, in either the thorax or abdomen, in such a way as to produce autonomic nervous system changes, either adrenergic or cholinergic. Such a concept no longer seems tenable.

Much more serious consideration has been given to the possibility that, because of their large size, the glucose consumption of these tumors may be so great that glucose is removed from the circulation faster than it can be delivered from the liver, thereby producing a clinical hypoglycemic state. Use of glucose by the tumor would probably be chiefly for glycolysis and lactic acid production, so that gluconeogenesis through the Cori cycle would eventually restore liver glycogen. Although this hypothesis seems possible and logical, there is, unfortunately, little factual information to confirm or refute it.

The possibility must also be considered that increases above the usual concentrations of insulin in circulating blood could be produced by an excessive discharge of leucine from the tumor into the circulation. Since both leucine and tryptophane have been known to produce hypoglycemia in human beings, even though their mechanisms of action are different, any large flux of such amino acids might easily produce a hypoglycemic episode.

It is now generally recognized that the most probable correct explanation applies to the capacity of these tumors to produce insulin or an insulin-like material, which circulates in the blood to produce an atypical insulin hypoglycemia. A currently available collation of all the tumors of this type, reported in the literature by Laurent, Debry, and Floquet (1971), has indicated that the basis of the hypoglycemia is truly hormonal, even though the mode of production by the tumor of this insulin-like material remains unknown.

In this presentation, I shall concentrate on the possibility that these tumors are producing either insulin or an insulin-like material which circulates in the blood to produce hypoglycemia. It is of major importance that most of the investigators who have attempted to measure the circulating insulin by radioimmunoassay have been unsuccessful, and this finding by itself tends to diminish the possibility that true insulin is being produced in an ectopic focus of neoplastic tissue. In considering insulin-like activity, there is again wide divergence of opinion. Some investigators have been able to demonstrate the presence of a hypoglycemic factor which is passively transferable to animals, as indicated by the development of a significant degree of hypoglycemia in the recipient animal. Other investigators have failed to demonstrate this; it seems probable that both types of experiments may be valid, indicating that more than one process may be involved in the production of this phenomenon. All of these conflicting data cause even more confusion since the exact chemical identity of insulin-like activity in the human being, as well as in animals, has not been identified.

Perhaps the most interesting of these proposed hypotheses is the so-called "deletion defect" theory of Gellhorn. This hypothesis rests upon the basic concept that all body cells must contain the genetic information necessary for synthesis of all body proteins, including polypeptide hormones such as insulin. The fact that insulin normally is produced only in pancreatic beta cells is believed to be caused by suppression or deletion of this genetic potential in all other body cells. Any factor, therefore, which modifies or reduces this deletion in other cells should theoretically extend the biosynthesis of insulin to tissues and organs that do not normally produce insulin. If the neoplastic process, in the course of its chaotic protein metabolism should be able to suppress this deletion phenomenon, we might have a reasonable explanation for the ectopic production of this and other polypeptide hormones.

This hypothesis, which may be applied to any enzyme or protein in the animal body, seems a logical explanation for the ectopic production of protein (and other) hormones. Unfortunately, it still leaves many questions to be answered, and the failure to demonstrate circulating insulin or insulin-like activity in excessive amounts in these patients weighs heavily against immediate acceptance of this theory.

REFERENCE

Laurent, J., Debry, G., and Floquet, J.: *Hypoglycaemic Tumours*. Amsterdam, Excerpta Medica, 1971, 230 pp.

Hypercalcemia Associated with Malignant Diseases

W. P. L. MYERS, M.D.

*Department of Medicine, Memorial Hospital for Cancer and Allied
Diseases; Division of Medical Research, Sloan-Kettering
Institute; and Cornell University Medical College,
New York, New York*

OF THE VARIOUS METABOLIC derangements observed in the course of malignant diseases in man, the occurrence of hypercalcemia is at the same time intriguing and potentially lethal. Although the exact incidence is not known, it has been generally estimated that about 10 to 20 per cent of patients may develop this disorder at some time during the course of their disease.

Patients may manifest this complication in a variety of ways, including symptoms and findings related to the gastrointestinal tract (anorexia, nausea, vomiting, constipation), central nervous system (somnolence, lethargy, coma, and rarely, bizarre, combative behavior), kidneys (polyuria with attendant polydipsia, hyposthenuria, and at times renal failure and azotemia), and heart (occasionally tachycardia, arrhythmias, shortened QT interval, and ST-T wave abnormalities). In addition to the problems in clinical management that hypercalcemia causes, it has also proved to be of considerable research interest from the standpoint of what it tells us about tumor growth and function.

It is the purpose of this paper to review some aspects of hypercalcemia associated with malignant disease and its management.

Clinical Occurrence

Although hypercalcemia may be associated with a wide variety of tumors, it has been found to be most often associated with cancers of the breast, lung, kidney, head and neck, and cervix and in patients with lymphomas, leukemias, and myeloma. As shown in Table 1, in a retrospective

147

TABLE 1.—TYPES OF MALIGNANT TUMORS
ASSOCIATED WITH HYPERCALCEMIA*

PRIMARY TUMOR	NUMBER OF PATIENTS
Breast	225
Lymphoma	33
Lung	29
Kidney	18
Head and Neck†	16
Leukemia	13
Cervix	12
Myeloma	11
Prostate	11
Neuroblastoma	9
Melanoma	8
Rhabdomyosarcoma	8
Thyroid	7
Miscellaneous tumors	30
Total	430

*Adapted from Myers, 1960.
†Head and neck cancers: larynx 4, tonsil 3, tongue 3, and 2 each floor of the mouth, nasopharynx, and salivary gland.

review of 430 patients who had hypercalcemia associated with malignant tumors, more than half had breast cancer (Myers, 1960). The large preponderance of patients with breast cancer and hypercalcemia reflects not only the fact that the tumor is common but also that it is the only neoplasm in the group where treatment may actually be responsible for the development of hypercalcemia (*i.e.*, treatment with androgens, estrogens, and progestins).

Most patients with hypercalcemia and cancer have X-ray evidence of skeletal metastases. Of the 430 patients in the study cited, 334 had positive skeletal X-ray films; in 40 the X-ray study was not done. Some patients (56 in this series) have no radiographic evidence of skeletal metastases. It has been stated that squamous cell cancer of the lung is the tumor most commonly associated with hypercalcemia in the absence of bone metastases (Muggia and Heinemann, 1970), but we have observed this association often in the lymphomas as well. In our study of 29 patients with lung cancer, 26 had skeletal surveys and only five were negative for metastases, whereas of 33 patients with lymphomas, 26 had skeletal surveys and 10 were negative. Of course, skeletal surveys do not in themselves exclude the presence of bone metastases—a point stressed by Lafferty (1966) in establishing diagnostic criteria for a diagnosis of ectopic hyperparathyroidism (pseudohyperparathyroidism). We have studied another group of 38 patients without radiographic evidence of bone metastases, 20 of whom came to autopsy; of these, seven were found histologically to have bone metastases. The exact incidence of bone metastases at autopsy, of course, will vary, depending on how thorough postmortem examination of the skeleton is. If positive for extrinsic cells (Hyman, 1955), bone marrow aspiration during life may be useful in establishing the presence of metastases, but obviously a negative aspiration does not exclude the possibility of metastases.

Patients with cancer who have hypercalcemia, hypophosphatemia, hypercalciuria, and negative skeletal surveys may have these findings solely because of cancer (ectopic hyperparathyroidism) or coexistent primary hyperparathyroidism. Thus the presence of a breast mass and hypercalcemia does not necessarily mean one is related to the other but may well indicate a combination of cancer and primary hyperparathyroidism (Fig. 1). Of 50 consecutive patients with primary hyperparathyroidism seen at

Fig. 1.—Coexistence of primary operable breast cancer and primary hyperparathyroidism (53-year-old woman; Memorial Hospital). Note the biochemical features of hyperparathyroidism which were unaffected by the radical mastectomy and reversed only upon removal of a parathyroid adenoma.

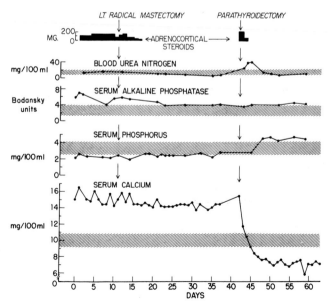

Memorial Hospital, 12 had active coexistent cancer (Fahey and Myers, unpublished data). The problem of differentiating primary hyperparathyroidism from ectopic hyperparathyroidism can be very difficult, but two clinical points may be helpful: If the patient had subperiosteal bone resorption, especially if combined with radiographic evidence of a renal stone, he most probably has primary hyperparathyroidism since these X-ray findings are not features of ectopic hyperparathyroidism. In addition, hypophosphatemia appears to be more common in patients with certain types of tumors than with others. As shown in Figure 2, hypophosphatemia is more likely to accompany the hypercalcemia of cancer of the lung or kidney than the lymphomas, myeloma, or breast cancer. Its occurrence in hypercalcemic patients with these latter diseases should arouse suspicion of coexistent primary hyperparathyroidism (Fig. 1). An interesting and promising approach to the distinction of these two entities lies in the possible immunological differentiation between native parathyroid hormone and that produced ectopically (Riggs, Arnaud, Reynolds, and Smith, 1971). If further work substantiates this initial report, the diagnostic dilemma currently posed by these patients will be resolved.

With respect to the histologic types of tumors, it appears that hypercalcemia as well as the syndrome of ectopic hyperparathyroidism may occur with virtually any histologic type of tumor. Some authors have pointed out

FIG. 2.—The occurrence of hypophosphatemia (2.9 mg./100 ml. or less) according to tumor type in cancer patients with hypercalcemia. Note that modest increases in blood urea nitrogen did not mask hypophosphatemia in some patients.

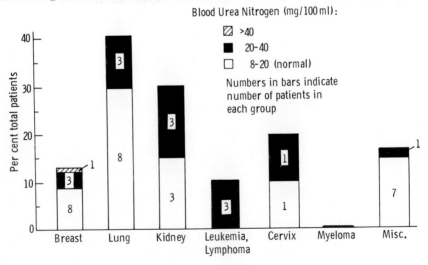

that in lung cancer, oat cell tumors are associated with the ectopic production of adrenocorticotropin while squamous cell cancers appear to be associated with production of parathyroid hormone (Omenn, Roth, and Baker, 1969). We have studied 28 patients with lung cancer and hypercalcemia whose lesions were classified into the following histologic types: oat cell— 1, squamous—6, epidermoid—11, adenocarcinoma—7, and mixed epidermoid and glandular—3. Only five of these patients had hypercalcemia and hypophosphatemia—that is, chemical hyperparathyroidism—but they were scattered among all histological groups except oat cell and adenocarcinoma (Myers, 1968). This is partial corroboration of the experience of others, but there is considerable variation among pathologists in histologic classification so that it does not seem possible at this point to link histological type and nonparathyroid hyperparathyroidism with any degree of certainty.

Mechanisms of Hypercalcemia

Initially, it was postulated that intraskeletal tumors simply eroded the surrounding bone and that the displaced calcium entered the blood faster than it could be cleared by the kidney, with resultant hypercalcemia (Laszlo *et al.*, 1952; Pearson, West, Hollander, and Treves, 1954). This concept was basically descriptive for it gave no hint as to how a given tumor could actually erode bone.

Figure 3 diagrammatically represents some possibilities concerning the production of hypercalcemia as related to the various components of calcium homeostasis. If one assumes a daily dietary calcium intake of about 1 gm., approximately 0.4 gm. is absorbed, and the remainder, 0.6 gm., contributes the major fraction of fecal calcium. The latter is also contributed to by endogenous secretion of calcium (0.2 gm.). In addition, calcium is also being constantly filtered by and reabsorbed from the kidney, with approximately 0.15 to 0.20 gm. being excreted normally per 24 hours. Finally, calcium is constantly being laid down and resorbed from bone at a rate of about 0.4 to 0.5 gm. per 24 hours.

It can be postulated that hypercalcemia might result either from increased entry of calcium into the extracellular space or decreased exit from it. Thus, one might observe enhanced absorption from the gastrointestinal tract, increased bone resorption, or increased renal reabsorption (Fig. 1, arrows 1, 2, 3) in one instance, or decreases of endogenous secretion, bone accretion, and renal filtration in another (Fig. 1, arrows 1 ', 2 ', 3 '). Finally, it might be postulated that there was an increased binding affinity of serum proteins for calcium or some fundamental alteration of the bone-extracellular calcium equilibrium.

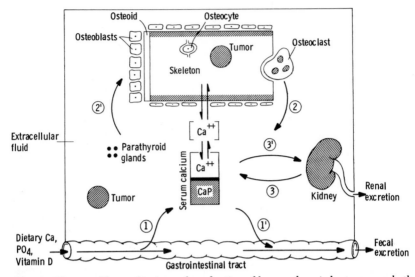

Fɪɢ. 3.—The possible mechanisms of production of hypercalcemia by tumors, whether intra- or extraskeletal, are shown in this diagram of calcium homeostasis. The body is represented as a rectangle within which the skeletal mass (approximately 1,000 gm. calcium in the adult) is shown as an "internal rock" surrounded by extracellular fluid (containing about 1 gm. calcium). The shaded portion of the skeleton is exchangeable bone. The serum calcium is shown in the center, partitioned into ionized, complexed, and protein-bound fractions. The linear half-arrows define an equilibrium between bone and extracellular ionized calcium and between the latter and the ionized calcium of the serum. The curvilinear arrows indicate directions of calcium movement into and out of the extracellular compartment: ① and ①′ indicate absorption from and endogenous secretion into the gastrointestinal tract, respectively; ② and ②′ define resorption from and accretion into the skeleton; ③ and ③′ indicate the processes of reabsorption from and filtration by the kidney. There are many hormonal and biochemical influences that modify these processes, but for the sake of simplicity they have been omitted from this diagram. (Adapted from Myers, 1962.)

Most of these possibilities have been examined, with the following findings:

(1) Balance studies (Myers, 1962) and radiocalcium data (Spencer, Lewin, and Samachson, 1969; Myers, unpublished data) have shown neither enhanced calcium absorption of gastro-intestinal calcium nor decreased endogenous secretion in patients with cancer hypercalcemia.

(2) Calcium has been shown to have a profound effect on renal function (Zeffren and Heinemann, 1962; Epstein, 1968), and the data with respect to the role of the kidney in the pathogenesis of hypercalcemia have indicated that renal mechanisms may play a role in some patients but not in others. Thus, it has been reported in a patient with multiple myeloma

that there is an increased clearance of calcium and a decreased tubular reabsorption during hypercalcemia, changes which were reversed with successful management of the hypercalcemia (Myers, 1962). In contrast, an increased tubular reabsorption of calcium in three patients with other types of cancer associated with hypercalcemia (types of cancer are not specified except that none were multiple myeloma) has been reported (Nordin and Peacock, 1969). Until this matter has been investigated further, it is not possible to state categorically what role, if any, the kidney plays in the hypercalcemia of cancer patients even though one might surmise a role similar to that in primary hyperparathyroidism in those cancer patients manifesting the syndrome of ectopic hyperparathyroidism.

(3) Studies of calcium accretion and resorption were performed (Myers *et al.*, 1968) in 20 patients, 16 with cancer and four with primary hyperparathyroidism, and the results are shown in Figure 4. The patients were divided into four groups: five patients with normocalcemia, eight with hypercalcemia, three with ectopic hyperparathyroidism, and four with primary hyperparathyroidism. The patients in the first two groups all had X-ray evidence of bone metastases, whereas the patients with ectopic hyperparathyroidism had negative bone X-ray films and otherwise fulfilled the diagnostic criteria for this entity (Lafferty, 1966). The patients with primary hyperparathyroidism were surgically proved to have this condition. The patients were hospitalized on the metabolic ward and studied under conditions of metabolic balance for calcium, phosphorus, and nitrogen. After dietary adjustment, 50 μCi of ^{47}Ca were administered, and blood samples were obtained at repeated intervals for 14 days. Stool, urine, and blood aliquots were analyzed for radioactivity and for stable calcium. Determinations of plasma-specific activity, accretion and resorption rates of calcium, and exchangeable calcium pools were calculated according to the method of Bauer, Carlsson, and Lindquist (1957).

The findings in these patients were as follows:

(1) Patients with cancer, bone metastases, and normocalcemia were found to have normal accretion and resorption rates of calcium, slightly lower-than-normal exchangeable pools, and decreased turnover rates of calcium.

(2) The development of hypercalcemia in patients with cancer and bone metastases was attended by an enhanced rate of accretion and an even greater increase in resorption rate with a consequent rise in turnover.

(3) Patients with cancer and the syndrome of ectopic hyperparathyroidism had normal rates of calcium accretion and decreased total body retention of the isotope, in contrast to the generally increased rates of accretion in those with primary hyperparathyroidism. When considered in

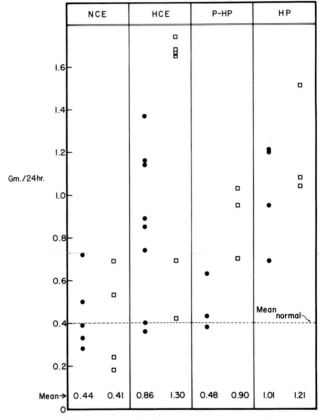

Fɪɢ. 4.—Accretion and resorption of calcium as measured in 16 patients with cancer and four patients with primary hyperparathyroidism by means of ^{47}Ca or ^{85}Sr. NCE = normocalcemic patients; HCE = hypercalcemic patients; P-HP = patients with pseudo-hyperparathyroidism (ectopic hyperparathyroidism); HP = patients with primary hyperparathyroidism. The black circles represent the values for accretion rates of calcium and the open squares the values for resorption rates. In a few instances, it was only possible to measure accretion rates alone. Each dot and square represents values obtained in one patient. The mean values are shown numerically at the bottom of each column, the first figure being the mean accretion rate and the second the mean resorption rate.

the light of the accretion and excretion rates, the specific activity curves were consistent with enhanced turnover of calcium in primary hyperparathyroidism while excretion was the predominant factor in ectopic hyperparathyroidism.

The difference noted in patients with ectopic versus primary hyperparathyroidism may not be borne out by further experience since it appears that occasionally patients with primary hyperparathyroidism may also have normal rates of calcium accretion. However, the data summarized above and in Figure 4 indicate that increased resorption of calcium from bone is central to the production of hypercalcemia in cancer patients, whether the tumor is intra- or extraskeletal; a decreased rate of accretion does not appear to be a factor since it was not observed in any of the patients.

ROLE OF PARATHYROID GLANDS

Considering further the matter of enhanced resorption of calcium, it has been postulated that tumors might elaborate a substance that would stimulate the patient's own parathyroid glands to become overactive and that the hypercalcemia in fact would be caused by this and not by some osteolytic tumor product (Stone, Waterhouse, and Terry, 1961). Although some studies have suggested that parathyroid hyperplasia may be observed in these patients (Klemperer, 1923; Kohout, 1966), other studies of parathyroid glands in cancer patients with hypercalcemia have revealed no significant differences in gland weights or in histologic appearance when compared to normal persons and to cancer patients with normocalcemia (Anderson, Rothschild, and Myers, 1962).

Additional support for the concept that the parathyroids are not central to the production of cancer hypercalcemia came in the course of a study of a patient whose data are shown in Figure 5. The patient was a 42-year-old woman who had been treated seven years previously by radium and X rays for an epidermoid cancer of the cervix. Subsequently, she developed metastatic disease, initially to the right kidney (which was resected) and then to the liver. She was found to have hypercalcemia, hypercalciuria, hypophosphatemia, and a negative skeletal survey. Because of these findings and the persistence of hypercalcemia despite treatment, the possibility of a coexistent parathyroid adenoma was considered, and a neck exploration was undertaken. Four normal parathyroid glands were found, but in an effort to control the hypercalcemia, all four glands were removed. As can be seen in Figure 5, there was no reduction of the serum calcium level, and she died 18 days postoperatively of hypercalcemia, despite the absence of her parathyroid glands. The resected glands were normal in weight and histological appearance, and at autopsy, there was no evidence of accessory parathyroid tissue. The bones showed no evidence of tumor invasion but did show osteoclastic resorption. The data clearly suggested that the patient's own parathyroid glands were not responsible for her hypercalcemia but rather that the tumor elaborated a substance similar to or identical with native parathyroid hormone (PTH).

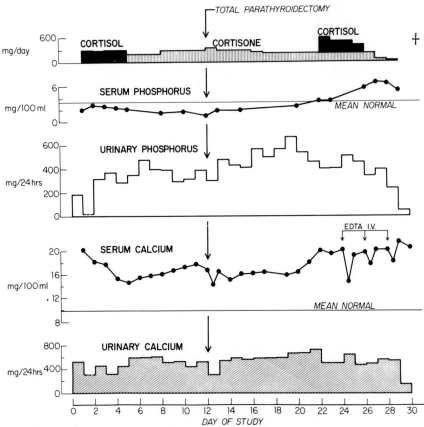

Fɪɢ. 5.—Calcium and phosphorus data from a 42-year-old woman with metastatic carcinoma of the cervix (Memorial Hospital). Note the absence of any significant effect on the serum calcium by treatment with cortisol and cortisone. Note also that the hypercalcemia continued, despite total parathyroidectomy, and ultimately led to the patient's death 18 days postoperatively. EDTA = di-sodium ethylenediaminetetraacetate.

Ectopic Production of Parathyroid Hormone

To pursue the possibility that the patient whose data are shown in Figure 5 had a tumor that synthesized parathyroid hormone ectopically, an effort to extract the hypercalcemic principle from the tumor was undertaken. At autopsy, the tumor was found primarily located in the patient's liver (the liver weighed 2,500 gm., 80 per cent of which was estimated to be tumor). Frozen tumor tissue was defatted, the resultant tissue powder was extracted with 0.2 N HCl, and the supernatant was ultimately precipitated with trichloroacetic acid (TCA). This TCA material was examined for (1) biological activity in an in vitro system utilizing radiocalcium-labeled embryonic rat bones in organ culture (Fell and Mellanby, 1952; Gaillard, 1961), and (2) immunological activity by radioimmunoassay (Sherwood, O'Riordan, Aurbach, and Potts, 1967).

In the organ culture experiments, 19-day-old rat embryo bones were cultured in a medium which was half chemically defined and half heat-inactivated rat serum. The bones were cultured at 37.5° C in an atmosphere of 5 per cent CO_2 and 95 per cent air for three days. They were subcultured every 24 hours, and at the end of 72 hours the explants were examined grossly and microscopically. The explants had been prelabeled with [47]Ca by injecting the mother on the sixteenth day of pregnancy. They were counted after 72 hours of culture to determine the degree of radiocalcium release. Each experimental bone had its paired control bone.

The extract prepared from the patient's tumor was added to the culture medium in one set of experiments, and for comparison, purified bovine parathyroid hormone was added to the medium in another set. Osteoclastic resorption of trabecular bone and fibroblastic proliferation were observed in the explants exposed to parathyroid hormone, and a qualitatively similar response was observed in the explants exposed to the extract of human cervical carcinoma. Addition of 10 μg. of purified bovine parathyroid hormone led to a mean radiocalcium loss of 40 per cent at 72 hours as compared to paired control bones, whereas addition of 1.25 mg. of a partially purified extract of the cervical cancer led to a 30 per cent loss of radiocalcium from the explants. Since the tumor extracted was from massive deposits in the patient's liver, we controlled these observations with normal liver tissue which led to no radiocalcium release.

These data were interpreted as demonstrating biologic activity of the tumor extract qualitatively similar to that seen in the same test system with purified bovine parathyroid hormone. Finally, the tumor extract was analyzed for parathyroid hormone by radioimmunoassay and was found to have immunologic cross-reactivity with antibovine parathyroid hormone.

Some workers have criticized immunoassay data on the grounds that what one might be analyzing could be native parathyroid hormone which was "trapped" by the tumor. Clearly, this could not be the case in the patient cited since the prior total parathyroidectomy excluded the possibility of the tumor "trapping" native hormone. We therefore interpret these data as indicating that the patient's tumor was able to elaborate a substance that biologically and immunologically was similar to or identical with native parathyroid hormone.

Other Humoral Products

The elaboration of humoral products by tumors has been widely reported in recent years, and several reviews have been published (Bower and Gordan, 1965; Myers, Tashima, and Rothschild, 1966; Liddle *et al.*, 1969). Of pertinence to the problem of hypercalcemia are studies suggesting that osteolytic phytosterols may be synthesized by human breast cancers and thus be responsible for the hypercalcemia observed in this tumor (Gordan *et al.*, 1966). Patients with breast cancer and hypercalcemia do not usually have hypophosphatemia, as noted above, and there was good reason to think that some tumor product other than parathyroid hormone was being elaborated by breast cancer tissue. However, recent work has revealed that phytosterols may be found in breast cancers from normocalcemic patients as well as in cancers of other tissues, and there is, therefore, some question as to the possible role of these sterols in the hypercalcemic state of cancer (Rice, 1969). In addition, the elaboration of a breast tumor product demonstrating cross-reactivity with antibovine parathyroid hormone by immunoassay has been described (Mavligit, Cohen, and Sherwood, 1971). Also, studies of bone resorption in tissue culture have led to the demonstration that the lysosomes of bone cells and their hydrolytic enzymes are involved in the processes of bone resorption (Vaes, 1968). Conceivably, tumors might elaborate these enzymes directly, rather than stimulate their production by bone cells via the ectopic production of parathyroid hormone, as the principal way in which they induce resorption of bone. A further possibility is that tumors might in some fashion interfere with calcitonin so that the normal regulatory control of this hormone is lost. This is pure speculation, however, since the exact role of calcitonin in serum calcium regulation in the adult is poorly understood, and there is no evidence thus far that there is any defect in calcitonin metabolism in cancer patients with hypercalcemia. It appears that there is still much to be learned with respect to tumor products and hypercalcemia.

Treatment for Hypercalcemia

Regardless of what this metabolic complication is telling us about tumor growth and function, the occurrence of hypercalcemia can be a life-threatening event, and immediate measures to reverse it are usually indicated. An approach to treatment is outlined in Table 2. Although some of the treatment modalities may be effective against hypercalcemia of other causes, they are considered here solely in the context of the treatment for hypercalcemia caused by cancer.

TABLE 2.—TREATMENT FOR THE HYPERCALCEMIA
OF CANCER PATIENTS

General Measures
 (a) Reduce calcium intake.
 (b) Promote calcium output:
      intravenous fluids (saline), diuretics.
 (c) Avoid protracted immobilization.

Nonspecific Measures
 (a) Corticosteroids.
 (b) Phosphate, sulfate.
 (c) Dactinomycin, mithramycin.
 (d) Di-sodium ethylenediaminetetraacetate.
 (e) Calcitonin.
 (f) Dialysis.

Specific Measures
 (a) Surgical removal of tumor.
 (b) Castration in breast cancer patients.
 (c) Stop androgens, estrogens, progestins.
 (d) Chemotherapy: tumor-specific if possible, corticosteroids.
 (e) Radiation therapy.

GENERAL MEASURES

Reduction of calcium intake is usually of little importance since the patients often suffer from anorexia, nausea, vomiting, and polyuria, all of which combine to limit intake and promote output. Also, the source of the calcium is the skeleton rather than the diet; however, it is wise to reduce intake to avoid any aggravation of the situation. Protracted immobilization may also aggravate the condition. Usually the patients are so sick that there is no question of ambulation, but normal turning in bed is often adequate. However, if the patient is immobilized because of pathological fractures or severe bone pain, the hypercalcemic state may well be intensified. Measures such as pinning of fractures, rather than casting, and relief of bone pain are obvious steps to avoid this.

With respect to intravenous fluid therapy, it is important to restore normal hydration since these patients are often water depleted from vomiting, poor intake, and polyuria. It had been our earlier observation that one could not "superhydrate" these patients and "wash out" calcium to correct hypercalcemia. However, the advent of newer potent diuretics has led to a reconsideration of this viewpoint. It has been demonstrated that the intravenous administration of large doses of furosemide can result in notable calcium diuresis with restoration of normocalcemia in some patients (Suki *et al.*, 1970). This approach is illustrated by data (Fig. 6) which indicate that vigorous treatment with furosemide was able to reverse the hypercalcemia which occurred in the course of medroxyprogesterone therapy of a woman with metastatic breast cancer. It must be remembered, however, that this treatment should not be undertaken unless a laboratory is available to provide measurements of the losses of other urinary electrolytes (sodium, potassium, and magnesium), which must be replaced as the treatment proceeds.

The composition of intravenous fluid therapy should obviously be directed at correcting any electrolyte abnormalities coexisting with hypercalcemia (such as hypokalemic alkalosis, which we have frequently seen in association with cancer hypercalcemia). In addition, the administration of sodium chloride has been used to promote the excretion of calcium (Kleeman, Bohannon, Berstein, Ling, and Maxwell, 1964). The relationship of the excretion of sodium and calcium is depicted in Figure 7. The study was done in a normocalcemic patient who was subjected to a seven-day period of severe sodium restriction. Urinary sodium decreased virtu-

Fig. 6.—Reversal of hypercalcemia by furosemide in a 53-year-old patient with metastatic cancer of the breast (Memorial Hospital). The hypercalcemia, thought to have been caused by medroxyprogesterone, was corrected despite continuation of this hormone. Note the large urinary volumes induced by this treatment.

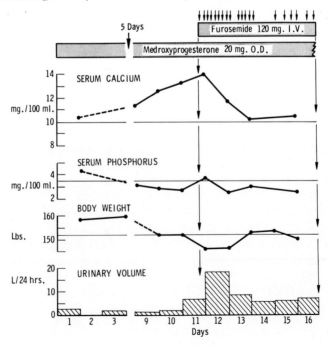

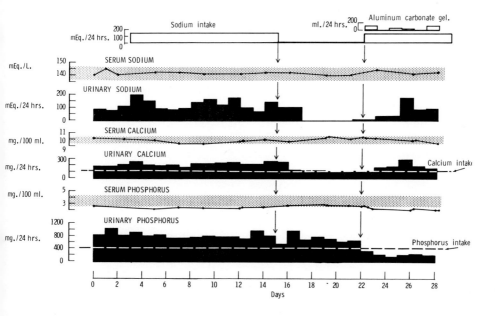

Fɪɢ. 7.—Serum and urinary concentrations of sodium, calcium, and phosphorus in a 46-year-old man who had essential hypertension (Memorial Hospital). Note the approximately 50 per cent reduction in urinary calcium with marked dietary sodium restriction and its reversion to control values on restoration of dietary sodium. The effects of aluminum carbonate gel on serum and urinary phosphorus are also shown.

ally to zero in response to this challenge, and the urinary calcium, without any change in the calcium intake, decreased by approximately 50 per cent. With the resumption of normal sodium intake, calcium in the urine rose again to control levels. The administration of isotonic saline to hypercalcemic patients is based on such evidence and can be shown to induce greater urinary losses of calcium than is possible by dextrose in water alone.

Nonspecific Measures

There is a variety of substances that have been used in the management of hypercalcemia. Some act nonspecifically on calcium homeostasis while others act in ways not yet understood. However, all of the nonspecific measures should be used only to gain time pending the administration of specific antitumor therapy, since hypercalcemia will tend to recur in the absence of control of the underlying malignant condition. Also, if the hypercalcemia is mild to moderate (14 mg./100 ml. or less) and the patient is not particularly symptomatic, it is reasonable to proceed directly with specific therapy. Nonspecific therapy, therefore, is generally reserved for patients with pronounced hypercalcemia, for those who are symptomatic and for those in whom it is anticipated that there will be a long delay in the onset of a therapeutic effect from a given antitumor measure.

CORTICOSTEROIDS.—Corticosteroids have been used for many years with varying degrees of success (Myers, 1958; Thalassinos and Joplin, 1970). Although there is some evidence that corticosteroids are tumor inhibitory in certain situations and as such are therefore also listed under specific measures discussed below, they are also capable of profoundly altering calcium homeostasis, and it is possible that their mechanism of action in cancer hypercalcemia may be related to these effects. As a practical matter, they have proved most useful in the hypercalcemia of breast cancer, multiple myeloma, and lymphosarcoma. When they first came into use, there was little else to try, and they were used widely and often proved to be ineffective. Our present view is that they should be the first line of treatment for hypercalcemia associated with the tumors noted, if the hypercalcemia is severe or symptomatic and if one anticipates a delayed onset of an antitumor effect from specific treatment. Corticosteroids may be tried in other tumors, but often valuable time is lost waiting for a beneficial response, and it is often best to consider some other form of treatment in these instances.

PHOSPHATE AND SULFATE.—The use of inorganic phosphate in the management of hypercalcemia has been known for many years (Bulger, Dixon, Barr, and Schregardus, 1930), but the recent studies of Goldsmith and Ingbar (1966) form the basis of the current use of phosphate. Phosphate therapy causes reduced renal calcium excretion, in contrast to sulfate and corticosteroids which usually lead to calcium diuresis after acute administration. The mechanism whereby phosphate causes lowering of the serum calcium appears to be its inhibition of bone resorption (Raisz and Niemann, 1969). The response to phosphate is dose related. Thus, in a study of 21 patients, the mean maximum decreases in serum calcium following various doses of disodiummonopotassium phosphate (dissolved in 1 L. of 5 per cent dextrose in water administered intravenously over six to eight hours) were as follows: 25 millimols—1.1 mg./100 ml.; 50 millimols—2.4 mg./100 ml.; 75 millimols—4.1 mg./100 ml.; and 100 millimols—6.1 mg./

100 ml. (Fulmer, Dimich, Rothschild, and Myers, 1972). The duration of the calcium-lowering effect also appears to be dose related in that the larger quantities of administered phosphate produced significantly longer periods of lowered concentrations of serum calcium. Although there has been some concern that phosphate administration leads to an increased risk of metastatic calcification, our observations indicate that at autopsy there is about the same degree of soft tissue calcification as is found in patients with hypercalcemia not treated with phosphate. This experience has been borne out by others (Thalassinos and Joplin, 1968). However, the use of intravenous phosphate in patients with azotemia is generally contraindicated in view of adverse effects reported under these circumstances (Shackney and Hasson, 1967).

Intravenous sulfate is usually given as a solution of 38.9 Gm. of hydrated sodium sulfate dissolved in 1 L. of 5 per cent dextrose in water (Chakmakjian and Bethune, 1966). This solution contains 200 mEq. of sodium per liter. Infusions of sulfate lead to calcium diuresis, but in our experience with use of sulfate in seven instances of hypercalcemia, the maximum serum calcium-lowering effect (observed at the end of the infusion) averaged only 1.9 mg./100 ml., and rises to pretreatment serum calcium levels occurred within 18 to 24 hours. Because of these limitations and the occasional development of hypernatremia with its use, we have not found sulfate infusions to be as useful a nonspecific treatment method as phosphate infusions.

DACTINOMYCIN AND MITHRAMYCIN.—These agents were first discovered as having tumor inhibitory properties, and initially it was thought that their action in the reversal of hypercalcemia was dependent on these properties. However, more recent studies have indicated that they may block the action of parathyroid hormone on bone and that reversal of hypercalcemia may occur at doses that would not be expected to have any antitumor effect. Thus, single doses of 2 mg. of dactinomycin have been observed to ameliorate or reverse hypercalcemia, with the effect sometimes lasting as long as a week (Muggia and Heinemann, 1970). Similarly mithramycin has been reported as causing reversal of hypercalcemia 48 hours after single doses of 25 gamma/kg. (Perlia *et al.*, 1970). Our experience with these chemical agents in the management of hypercalcemia has produced variable results, but in general, we have observed restoration of normocalcemia primarily with the administration of doses in the antitumor range. However, this has not been uniformly so, as is shown in the study illustrated in Figure 8. The patient, a 57-year-old man with bronchogenic carcinoma and the syndrome of ectopic hyperparathyroidism, was studied under conditions of metabolic balance. After a two-week control period, mithramycin was administered intravenously in a dose of 12.5 gamma/kg./ day. It can be seen that this treatment, although not sufficient for an antitumor effect, nevertheless caused a reversal of hypercalcemia to normal attended by a sharp reduction in hypercalciuria and hyperphosphaturia. However, the benefit was short lived, and when the treatment was at first interrupted and then stopped, a prompt recurrence of hypercalcemia, hypercalciuria, and hyperphosphaturia was observed. Despite this and other similar experiences, the single-dose administration of dactinomycin or mithramycin may well have a place in the acute treatment for the hypercalcemia of cancer. Of the two agents, dactinomycin is probably preferable because of the hemorrhagic complications that may occur with mithramycin, although with the small single doses noted, no complications should be observed with either agent. At this stage of our knowledge, it must be emphasized that these agents should be considered only for the management of cancer hypercalcemia.

OTHER NONSPECIFIC MEASURES.—These include the administration of disodium ethylenediaminetetraacetate (di-sodium EDTA), calcitonin, and dialysis.

Di-sodium EDTA has been used effectively for many years in the treatment for hypercalcemia (Spencer *et al.*, 1956; Myers, 1956). This chelating agent complexes calcium in the circulation and fosters calcium excretion. In essence, it binds excess calcium and renders it inert from a physiological point of view, but whether actual lowering of the concentration of serum calcium is observed or not depends upon the method used for its measurement. Thus, measurement of serum calcium by atomic absorption spectrometry will reveal no decrease since this method measures calcium bound to EDTA as well as that not bound. However, concentrations of serum calcium measured by complexometric methods (usually automated) will reveal a decrease because they will not measure the calcium that is bound to EDTA. Such measurements will show gratifying reductions of the serum calcium, but in one sense these reductions are artifacts while in another they represent decreases in a physiological sense. As a general rule we have not exceeded doses of 90 to 100 mg./kg./day with a maximum adult dose being 6 gm./day given as an effusion (500 ml. 5 per cent dextrose in water) over periods of one to four hours. It can be calculated that 6 gm. of di-sodium EDTA will lower the serum calcium about 4 mg./100 ml. in a 70-kg. patient with an estimated extracellular space of 14 L. The administration of di-sodium EDTA is not without hazard because if given too rapidly hypocalcemia and hypotension may result. For this reason we have always recommended that a physician be in attendance during an infusion to monitor the Chvostek and Trousseau signs and the blood pressure. The infusion

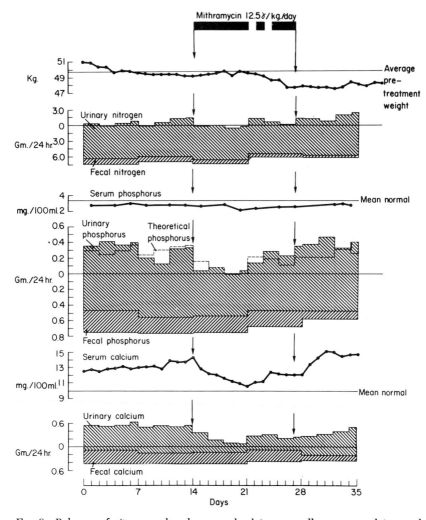

Fig. 8.—Balances of nitrogen, phosphorus, and calcium as well as serum calcium and phosphorus concentrations in a 57-year-old man with bronchogenic carcinoma and the syndrome of ectopic hyperparathyroidism (Memorial Hospital). The balance data are plotted according to the usual convention; that is, the intake is plotted from the zero line downward and the output from the intake line upward, fecal excretion first and then urinary excretion. The shaded areas above the zero line indicate negative balances. The theoretical phosphorus balance is based on calcium and nitrogen. Note the beneficial but transient effects of mithramycin on the level of serum calcium.

must be stopped promptly with any indication of hypocalcemia or hypotension. Conversely, the infusion cannot be given too slowly or no decrease in serum calcium will occur, since the rate of bone resorption must be exceeded by the rate of EDTA administration in order to cause the temporary disequilibrium needed to observe a fall in serum calcium. Although others have noted renal toxicity associated with prolonged use of EDTA, we have not observed this during short periods (*i.e.*, a few days) of its use, and we have tended to use it in those patients requiring intravenous therapy for hypercalcemia where the use of intravenous phosphate has been contraindicated, such as in azotemia.

Experience with the use of calcitonin in the management of cancer hypercalcemia is limited, but there have been some brief observations indicating that it can cause temporary reductions of hypercalcemia (Foster, 1966). Its role must be determined by further investigation. Similarly, although the concentration of serum calcium can be regulated by dialysis and although both hemodialysis (Eisenberg and Gotch, 1968) and peritoneal dialysis (Maxwell, Rockney, Kleeman, and Twiss, 1959) have been applied to the problem of hypercalcemia, the existence of simpler and equally effective alternative methods of treatment has precluded their wider use. Certainly, if the patient has renal failure associated with hypercalcemia and requires dialysis for the management of the renal failure, the hypercalcemia can be corrected in the process.

SPECIFIC MEASURES

Since hypercalcemia in the last analysis is caused by tumor growth or function, it is obvious that specific antitumor measures are central to the lasting control of this metabolic derangement. Surgical intervention still represents the most effective and rapid treatment modality, and there have been numerous reports of reversal of hypercalcemia with surgical removal of tumors (Lafferty, 1966; Myers, 1968). Surgical procedures not only should be applied to localized resectable lesions but also should be considered in regional disease, if feasible, as a rapid way to control the bulk of the tumor. Complete reversal of hypercalcemia following resection of cancer is usually quite prompt, *i.e.*, within the first 24 to 48 hours. Incomplete or partial reversal suggests incomplete removal of the tumor and failure to modify the hypercalcemia altogether indicates that the serum calcium elevation has some other cause (Fig. 1). Recurrence of a tumor following surgical resection is often heralded by the reappearance of hypercalcemia, and a careful search for recurrent cancer is always indicated in such patients.

Indirectly related to surgical resection of a tumor is the surgical modification of the hormonal environment in patients with hormonally dependent tumors, notably breast cancers. Thus, hypercalcemia might be corrected by surgical ablation of the ovaries or adrenals. However, if the hypercalcemia is cyclical with the menstrual period, one could anticipate that it will usually be reversed with cessation of the menstrual period (Pearson, West, Hollander, and Treves, 1954), and castration need not be undertaken during the actual hypercalcemic phase.

The question arises as to whether hypercalcemia should be corrected by nonspecific measures before operation. This will depend on the magnitude of the disorder. Patients with levels of serum calcium above 17 mg./100 ml. and those who are symptomatic will probably benefit from some attempt to control the serum level preoperatively, but in general, patients with hypercalcemia seem to tolerate anesthesia and surgical procedures quite well. The possibility that hypokalemia coexists with hypercalcemia must always be considered and, if present, should be corrected preoperatively.

Of major importance in the specific treatment for hypercalcemia is an awareness that the patient with breast cancer might be suffering from hypercalcemia induced by treatment with androgens, estrogens, or progestins, all of which have been reported to cause this disorder. Continuation of these hormones in the presence of hypercalcemia is hazardous, even though in rare instances normocalcemia has been restored despite continuation of sex steroid therapy. In our present state of knowledge, however, such continued treatment poses an unnecessary risk to the patient.

Specific antitumor treatment in the form of chemotherapy has been reported to be attended by restoration of normocalcemia in those patients whose tumors are responsive to the agents administered. The implication of reversal of hypercalcemia is that either tumor growth or function or both were altered by the drug. In trials of new chemotherapeutic agents, reversal of hypercalcemia and hypercalciuria may provide objective biochemical evidence of an antitumor effect even in the absence of a visible change in a tumor mass, although simultaneous regression of visible tumor has often been observed (Myers, 1960). The chemotherapeutic agent of choice is the one known to be effective against the tumor causing the hypercalcemia, although in the absence of such indication, an intravenous alkylating agent may be of help. Corticosteroids have been listed in Table 2 under the section on specific antitumor measures because, at times, objective regression of disease occurs in response to their administration. This is particularly true in breast cancer and, at times, in multiple myeloma.

Finally, radiation therapy may be the means whereby tumor regression with restoration of normocalcemia is achieved. The successful use of radiation in cancer hypercalcemia was reported nearly 25 years ago by Albright and Reifenstein (1948). It has been found to be useful not only when administered externally but also when applied by interstitial means (Myers, Tashima, and Rothschild, 1966). The main disadvantage of this form of treatment is the somewhat delayed onset of the beneficial effect. However, symptomatic hypercalcemia can always be temporarily controlled by nonspecific means pending the onset of a full therapeutic effect from radiation. Conceivably, the rapid destruction of a radiosensitive tumor could be associated with intensification of hypercalcemia by massive release of a bone-resorbing tumor product, but to my knowledge this has not been reported.

Conclusions

The problem of hypercalcemia has been considered in the context of ectopic hormone production by cancer. Some biologic and immunologic evidence has been presented to indicate that at least some tumors are capable of inducing hypercalcemia by elaboration of a substance similar to or identical with parathyroid hormone. In addition, a review of the clinical occurrence and management of hypercalcemia has been presented. It has been thought that such "whispers of nature" as presented here suggest that genetic information common to all cells is unmasked as part of the process of conversion from the normal to the malignant state. Better understanding and, ultimately, control and prevention of this conversion are the promise of the future in cancer research.

Acknowledgments

The author wishes to express his gratitude to his colleagues Drs. E. O. Rothschild, E. J. Greenberg, and Alexandra Dimich for their valuable participation and contributions in the studies cited in this chapter. Thanks are also due to Mrs. Vilma Carney and Mrs. Rosalie Rau for their careful and precise technical assistance and to Mrs. Kathleen Murphy and Miss Angela Calandrella for their patience and help in the preparation and typing of this manuscript.

This work was supported in part by research grants CA-08748 and CA-07303 from the National Cancer Institute and by contract AT(30-1)910 from the Atomic Energy Commission.

REFERENCES

Albright, F., and Reifenstein, E. C., Jr.: *The Parathyroid Glands and Metabolic Bone Disease.* Baltimore, Maryland, The Williams & Wilkins Co., 1948, pp. 92-93.

Anderson, H. C., Rothschild, E. O., and Myers, W. P. L.: A study of the parathyroid glands and bone in cases of hypercalcemia associated with malignant tumors. *Clinical Research Proceedings*, 10:238, 1962.

Bauer, G. C. H., Carlsson, A., and Lindquist, B.: Bone salt metabolism in humans studied by means of radiocalcium. *Acta medica scandinavica*, 158:143-150, 1957.

Bower, B. F., and Gordan, G. S.: Hormonal effects of nonendocrine tumors. *Annual Review of Medicine*, 16:83-118, 1965.

Bulger, H. A., Dixon, H. H., Barr, D. P., and Schregardus, O.: The functional pathology of hyperparathyroidism. *The Journal of Clinical Investigation*, 9:143-190, August 1930.

Chakmakjian, Z. H., and Bethune, J. E.: Sodium sulfate treatment of hypercalcemia. *The New England Journal of Medicine*, 275:862-869, October 1966.

Eisenberg, E., and Gotch, F. A.: Normocalcemic hyperparathyroidism culminating in hypercalcemic crisis—treatment with hemodialysis. *Archives of Internal Medicine*, 122:258-264, 1968.

Epstein, F. H.: Calcium and the kidney. *The American Journal of Medicine*, 45:700-714, November 1968.

Fahey, T. J., Jr., and Myers, W. P. L.: Unpublished data.

Fell, H. B., and Mellanby, E.: The effect of hypervitaminosis A on embryonic limb-bones cultivated in vitro. *Journal of Physiology*, 116:320-349, 1952.

Foster, G. V., Joplin, G. F., MacIntyre, I., Melvin, K. E. W., and Slack, E.: Effect of thyrocalcitonin in man. *The Lancet*, 1:107-109, January 15, 1966.

Fulmer, D. H., Dimich, A. B., Rothschild, E. O., and Myers, W. P. L.: Treatment of Hypercalcemia. Comparison of intravenously administered phosphate, sulfate, and hydrocortisone. *Archives of Internal Medicine*, 129:923-930, June 1972.

Gaillard, P. J.: Parathyroid and bone in tissue culture. In Greep, R. O., and Talmage, R. V., Eds.: *The Parathyroids*. Springfield, Illinois, Charles C Thomas, 1961, pp. 20-48.

Goldsmith, R. S., and Ingbar, S. H.: Inorganic phosphate treatment of hypercalcemia of diverse etiologies. *The New England Journal of Medicine*, 274:1-7, January 6, 1966.

Gordan, G. S., Cantino, T. J., Erhardt, L., Hansen, J., and Lubich, W.: Osteolytic sterol in human breast cancer. *Science*, 151:1226-1228, 1966.

Hyman, G. A.: A comparison of bone marrow aspiration and skeletal roentgenograms in the diagnosis of metastatic carcinoma. *Cancer*, 8:576-581, May-June 1955.

Kleeman, C. R., Bohannan, J., Bernstein, D., Ling, S., and Maxwell, M. H.: Effect of variations in sodium intake on calcium excretion in normal humans. *Proceedings of the Society of Experimental Biology and Medicine*, 115:29-32, 1964.

Klemperer, P.: Parathyroid hyperplasia and bone destruction in generalized carcinomatosis. *Surgery, Gynecology and Obstetrics*, 36:11-15, 1923.

Kohout, E.: Serum calcium levels and parathyroid glands in malignant disorders. *Cancer*, 19:925-934, July 1966.

Lafferty, F. W.: Pseudohyperparathyroidism. *Medicine*, 45:247-260, 1966.

Laszlo, D., Schulman, C. A., Bellin, J., Gottesman, E. D., and Schilling, A.: Mineral and protein metabolism in osteolytic metastases: Report to the Council on Pharmacy and Chemistry from the Committee on Research. *The Journal of the American Medical Association*, 148:1027-1032, 1952.

Liddle, G. W., Nicholson, W. E., Island, D. P., Orth, D. N., Abe, K., and Lowder, S. C.: Clinical and laboratory studies of ectopic humoral syndromes. *Recent Progress in Hormone Research*, 25:283-314, 1969.

Mavligit, G. M., Cohen, J. L., and Sherwood, L. M.: Ectopic production of parathyroid hormone by carcinoma of the breast. *The New England Journal of Medicine*, 285:154-156, July 15, 1971.

Maxwell, M. H., Rockney, R. E., Kleeman, C. R., and Twiss, M. R.: Peritoneal dialysis. I. Technique and applications. *The Journal of the American Medical Association*, 170:917-924, 1959.

Muggia, F. M., and Heinemann, H. O.: Hypercalcemia associated with neoplastic disease. *Annals of Internal Medicine*, 73:281-290, August 1970.

Myers, W. P. L.: Clinical aspects and management of hypercalcemia. *Medical Clinics of North America*, 40:871-885, May 1956.

———: Cortisone in the treatment of hypercalcemia in neoplastic disease. *Cancer*, 11:83-88, January 1958.

———: Hypercalcemia in neoplastic disease. *A. M. A. Archives of Surgery*, 80: 308-318, February 1960.

———: Studies of serum calcium regulation. *Advances in Internal Medicine*, 11:163-213, 1962.

———: Hormonal manifestations. In Watson, W. L., Ed.: *Lung Cancer*. St. Louis, Missouri, The C. V. Mosby Company, 1968, pp. 488-503.

———: Unpublished data.

Myers, W. P. L., Rothschild, E. O., Carney, V., Kaplan, N., Greenberg, E. J., Dimich, A., and Weber, D.: Tumor-induced hypercalcemia: radiocalcium and bone culture studies. *Calcified Tissue Research* Supplement, 2:63-64, August 1968.

Myers, W. P. L., Tashima, C. K., and Rothschild, E. O.: Endocrine syndromes associated with nonendocrine neoplasms. *Medical Clinics of North America*, 50:763-778, May 1966.

Nordin, B. E. C., and Peacock, M.: Role of kidney in regulation of plasma-calcium. *The Lancet*, 2:1280-1282, December 13, 1969.

Omenn, G. S., Roth, S. I., and Baker, W. H.: Hyperparathyroidism associated with malignant tumors of nonparathyroid origin. *Cancer*, 24:1004-1012, 1969.

Pearson, O. H., West, C. D., Hollander, V. P., and Treves, N. E.: Evaluation of endocrine therapy for advanced breast cancer. *The Journal of the American Medical Association*, 154:234-239, 1954.

Perlia, C. P., Gubisch, N. J., Wolter, J., Edelberg, D., Dederick, M. M., and Taylor, S. G., III: Mithramycin treatment of hypercalcemia. *Cancer*, 25:389-394, February 1970.

Raisz, L. G., and Neimann, I.: Effect of phosphate, calcium, and magnesium on bone resorption and humoral responses in tissue culture. *Endocrinology*, 85: 446-452, September 1969.

Rice, B. F.: Discussion of paper by Liddle, G. W., Nicholson, W. E., Island, D. P., Orth, D. N., Abe, K., and Lowder, S. C.: Clinical and laboratory studies of ectopic humoral syndromes. *Recent Progress in Hormone Research*, 25:283-314, 1969.

Riggs, B. L., Arnand, C. D., Reynolds, J. C., and Smith, L. H.: Immunologic differentiation of primary hyperparathyroidism from hyperparathyroidism due to nonparathyroid cancer. *The Journal of Clinical Investigation,* 50:2079-2083, October 1971.

Shackney, S., and Hasson, J.: Precipitous fall in serum calcium hypotension, and acute renal failure after intravenous phosphate therapy for hypercalcemia. Report of two cases. *Annals of Internal Medicine,* 66:906-916, May 1967.

Sherwood, L. M., O'Riordan, J. L. H., Aurbach, G. D., and Potts, J. T., Jr.: Production of parathyroid hormone by nonparathyroid tumors. *The Journal of Clinical Endocrinology and Metabolism,* 27:140-146, January 1967.

Spencer, H., Greenberg, J., Berger, E., Perrone, M., and Laszlo, D.: Studies on the effect of ethylenediaminetetraacetic acid in hypercalcemia. *The Journal of Laboratory and Clinical Medicine,* 47:29-41, January 1956.

Spencer, H., Lewin, I., and Samachson, J.: Absorption of calcium in patients with neoplasia and hypercalcemia. (Abstract) *Proceedings of the American Association for Cancer Research,* 10:86, 1969.

Stone, G. E., Waterhouse, C., and Terry, R.: Hypercalcemia of malignant disease: Case report and a proposed mechanism of etiology. *Annals of Internal Medicine,* 54:977-985, May 1961.

Suki, W. N., Yium, J. J., von Minden, M., Saller-Herbert, C., Eknoyan, G., and Martinez-Maldonado, M.: Acute treatment of hypercalcemia with furosemide. *The New England Journal of Medicine,* 283:836-840, October 15, 1970.

Thalassinos, N., and Joplin, G. F.: Phosphate treatment of hypercalcemia due to carcinoma. *British Medical Journal,* 4:14-19, October 1968.

————: Failure of corticosteroid therapy to correct the hypercalcemia of malignant disease. *The Lancet,* 2:537-538, September 12, 1970.

Vaes, G.: The role of lysosomes and of their enzymes in the development of bone resorption induced by parathyroid hormone. In Talmage, R. V., Belanger, L. F., and Clark, I., Eds.: *Parathyroid Hormone and Thyrocalcitonin (Calcitonin).* New York, New York, Excerpta Medica Foundation, 1968, pp. 318-328.

Zeffren, J. L., and Heinemann, H. O.: Reversible defect in renal concentrating mechanism in patients with hypercalcemia. *The American Journal of Medicine,* 33:54-63, July 1962.

Androgens and Erythropoietin Production

RAYMOND ALEXANIAN, M.D., AND
EDMUND GEHAN, PH.D.

*Departments of Medicine and Biomathematics, The University
of Texas at Houston M. D. Anderson Hospital and
Tumor Institute, Houston, Texas*

ERYTHROPOIETIN is a hormone that regulates red blood cell production according to tissue requirements for oxygen. Increased erythropoietin production constitutes one of several major homeostatic adjustments to oxygen need. Changes in blood flow and in the kinetics of oxygen dissociation from hemoglobin constitute two other important physiologic adaptations to anemia or hypoxia.

This report emphasizes clinical studies of (1) the erythropoietin response to anemia in men and women and (2) the effect of androgenic hormones on erythropoietin production. Whether the erythropoietin response to anemia is more precisely expressed when anemia is defined from the red cell mass or from the hematocrit has not been clarified. The relationship of an individual's sex to the erythropoietin level during anemia and the quantitative effect of large doses of androgenic hormones on erythropoietin production also have not been clearly defined. Results indicated that the correlation of erythropoietin with hematocrit was equally as precise as when correlated with the red cell volume. Men showed a four-times higher level of erythropoietin than women for all degrees of anemia. Large doses of certain androgenic hormones induced more than a fivefold further stimulation of erythropoietin production in three fourths of anemic patients with bone marrow failure.

Methods and Materials

This report includes an analysis of erythropoietin measurements in 73 patients with chronic anemia from bone marrow disease, in 35 normal volunteers, and in eight hypogonadal men. All were older than 20 years, the

173

median age being 61 in anemic patients and 33 in normal subjects. Among the anemic individuals, 53 per cent were men; of our normal volunteers, 83 per cent were men. Diagnoses in anemic patients included lymphoma and leukemia (24), multiple myeloma (23), idiopathic refractory anemia (13), myelofibrosis (9), and other solid tumors (4). No patient with renal failure, as defined by a creatinine clearance < 30 ml./minute, was included. Patients with a hemolytic rate greater than two times normal, as defined by erythrokinetic studies, were also excluded. No studies were done within two weeks of red cell transfusions or within two months of chemotherapy for malignant disease. All hypogonadal men had been subjected to prior hypophysectomy for chromophobe adenoma and were receiving replacement thyroid and cortisol therapy, but not testosterone. Control patients included either normal volunteers or patients with indolent cancers and normal red cell volumes, *i.e.*, red cell volume > 950 ml./M^2 for men or > 850 ml./M^2 for women. Red cell volume was measured with ^{51}Cr-tagged red cells; the hematocrit was determined in triplicate by the microtechnique from venipunctured blood samples.

Erythropoietin production was evaluated from the urinary erythropoietin excretion (Alexanian, Vaughn, and Ruchelman, 1967). Urine was collected during a 24-hour period from each subject, frozen immediately, and injected in measured aliquots into groups of polycythemic mice. (These animals have notably depressed endogenous red cell production, and slight elevations in red cell production after low doses of injected erythropoietin are more easily detected.) Red cell production in assay animals was quantified with radioactive iron, and results were converted to Standard B erythropoietin units from the linear portion of a standard dose-response curve. For normal subjects and patients with mild anemia, 24-hour urine samples were concentrated for bioassay; for patients with severe anemia, appropriate dilutions of urine were evaluated. Urinary erythropoietin excretion was expressed in Standard B units/day as previously described (Alexanian, Vaughn, and Ruchelman, 1967). The minimum detectable amount of erythropoietin detected in each assay animal was .05 unit, and the minimum detectable urinary excretion was 0.3 unit/day. Serum erythropoietin concentration was also measured in some patients by the daily injection of 0.1 ml. of serum or serum dilutions for three consecutive days into groups of polycythemic mice. The minimum detectable serum erythropoietin concentration by this method was 0.2 units/ml.

Results

Erythropoietin excretion was correlated with simultaneous measurements of red cell volume and hematocrit in 19 men with chronic steady-state anemia and in 21 normal men before and after phlebotomy. Figure 1 confirms an approximate tenfold rise in erythropoietin for each hematocrit decline of about 10 Vol. per cent or red cell volume decline of about 300 ml./M^2. The reproducibility was similar when values for erythropoietin were correlated with the hematocrit or with the red cell volume (Fig. 1); the proportion of the total variation, explained by the regression equation for hematocrit (0.81), was similar to that for red cell volume (0.74). As a result, hematocrit measurements were considered acceptable for evaluating the degree of anemia in subsequent correlations with erythropoietin excretion.

Erythropoietin excretion was compared with hematocrit in normal and anemic subjects, but separately for men and women. Curves were calculated from 93 measurements in 68 men and from 54 measurements in 40 women. A formula of log EP = 3.74 − .083 (hematocrit) was calculated from the data for men, and a formula of log EP = 3.78 − .100 (hematocrit) conformed with the data for women. The slopes of these curves did not differ significantly (P > 0.2). Figure 2 demonstrates that men had an approximately fourfold greater erythropoietin excretion than did women for all levels of anemia. This difference was significant at the .10 level but not at the .05 level. The erythropoietin excretion for hypogonadal men was less than for normal men (P < .05) and fell within the range found in normal women.

The effect of two different androgenic hormones on erythropoietin excretion was evaluated separately in men and women. Fluoxymesterone (kindly provided by Upjohn Co., Kalamazoo, Michigan) was given in a daily dose of 0.25 mg./kg. to 20 women, and in a dose of 1 mg./kg. to 22 men. Oxymetholone (kindly provided by Syntex Co., Palo Alto, California) was given in a daily dose of 1 mg./kg. to nine women, and in a dose of 5 mg./kg. to 15 men. Minor side effects occurred in most patients (muscle cramps, fluid retention, virilization), and doses were adjusted periodically in order to administer the maximum dose tolerated by each patient. No patient was maintained on less than 10 mg./day of fluoxymesterone or less than 50 mg./day of oxymetholone. All erythropoietin values measured after at least one month of therapy were included. Figure 3 includes 119 measurements in 63 individuals and demonstrates an approximately sevenfold elevation in the urinary excretion of erythropoietin for both men and women with androgen treatment. There was no apparent difference in the capacities of fluoxymesterone and oxymetholone to produce a significant erythropoietin elevation. An erythropoietin excretion appropriate for a hematocrit about 10 Vol. per cent lower than measured was produced by these androgens.

In order to control the effect of anemia alone on erythropoietin excre-

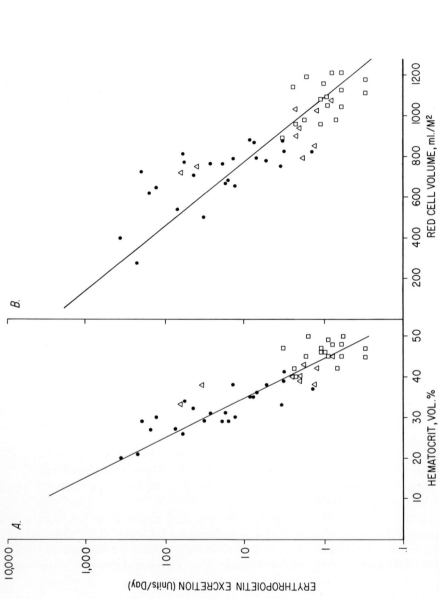

Fig. 1.—Relationship of urinary erythropoietin excretion to 50 simultaneous measurements of hematocrit (*A*) and red cell volume (*B*) in 40 normal and anemic men. Closed circles show values in patients with chronic anemia from marrow failure, squared symbols indicate ... in normal men at least one week after phlebotomy.

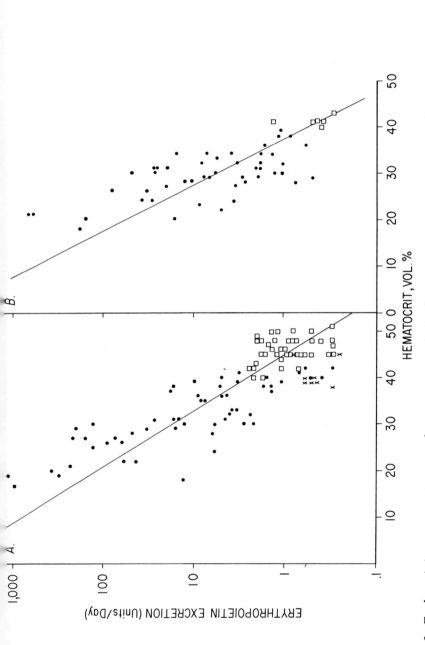

FIG. 2.—Erythropoietin response to increasing hematocrit in men (*A*) and women (*B*). Curves were calculated from 93 measurements in 68 men with normal pituitary function and from 54 measurements in 40 women. Values for anemic patients are shown with closed circles, for normal subjects with open squares, and for hypogonadal men with crosses.

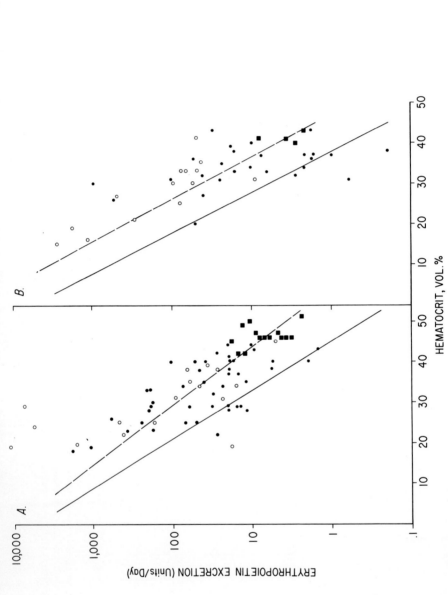

FIG. 3.—Erythropoietin excretion after large doses of oral androgens. The dashed lines were calculated from 75 values in 33 men (A) and from 44 values in 29 women (B) after at least one month of treatment. Values after fluoxymesterone are shown with closed circles and those after oxymetholone with open circles. Measurements for normal individuals after fluoxymesterone are shown with closed squares.

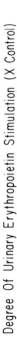
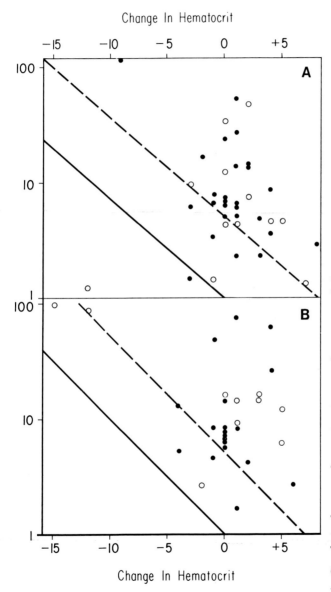

Fig. 4.—Correlation between changes in urinary erythropoietin and changes in hematocrit for 38 studies in 32 men (*A*) and 29 studies in 29 women (*B*) treated with either fluoxymesterone (closed circles) or oxymetholone (open circles). The solid lines indicate the predicted degree of urinary erythropoietin elevation from anemia alone, a five-fold elevation being represented by the dotted lines. Values to the right of the dotted lines indicate more than a fivefold enhancement of erythropoietin.

tion, a more detailed analysis of the magnitude of erythropoietin stimulation was conducted in 37 men and 29 women, before and after one month of androgen treatment. The magnitude of erythropoietin stimulation, *i.e.*, times control, was correlated with the change in hematocrit for each patient. Figure 4 demonstrates the extent of erythropoietin stimulation in most patients, to a degree that could not be accounted for by changes in

Fɪɢ. 5.—Summary of curves for normal and anemic men and women, before and after androgenic hormones. Solid lines conform with control studies and dashed lines with erythropoietin values after androgens. The slopes of all regression lines were similar (P > 0.2).

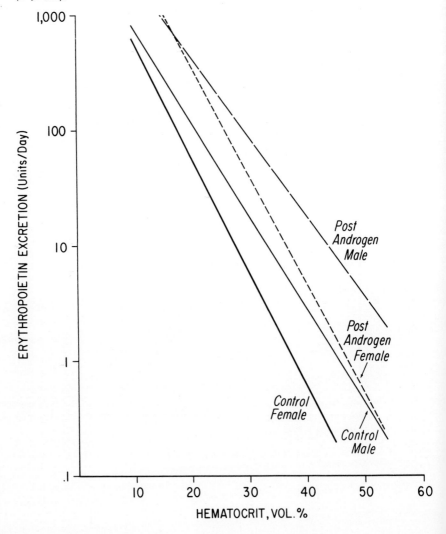

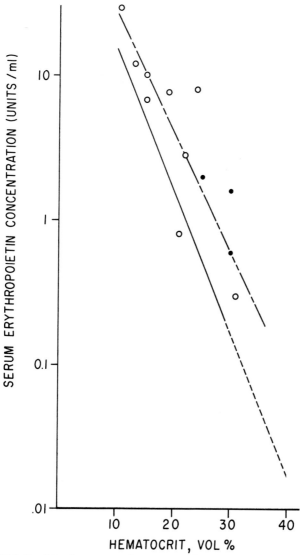

FIG. 6.—Relationship of serum erythropoietin to hematocrit. The solid line was calcu-lated from basal measurements in 14 patients with bone marrow failure. The dotted extension is a linear extrapolation of this line below our minimum detectable erythro-poietin concentration of 0.2 units/ml. The dashed line was fitted to 12 measurements at least one month after large doses of fluoxymesterone (closed circles) or oxymetholone (open circles).

hematocrit. There was a marked variability in the degree of erythropoietin stimulation among patients. The frequency of a fivefold enhancement of urinary erythropoietin in women (83 per cent) was similar to the incidence in men (78 per cent). Figure 5 summarizes all curves, comparing urinary erythropoietin with hematocrit for men and women, before and after androgens. There was no difference between the slopes of these regression lines (P > 0.2).

Serum erythropoietin was measured in 19 anemic men before and/or after treatment with androgenic steroids. Figure 6 correlates these results with the hematocrit. Erythropoietin was not detectable in serum unless the hematocrit was less than 30 Vol. per cent. Androgens induced about a two- to threefold stimulation of erythropoietin concentration, but this difference was not significant (P > 0.1).

Discussion

This study was designed to compare red cell volume and hematocrit as an index of anemia for correlations with erythropoietin level, to clarify the role of an individual patient's sex on the erythropoietin response to anemia, and to demonstrate quantitatively the changes that exogenous androgens produce in erythropoietin production. Erythropoietin production was evaluated from the urinary erythropoietin excretion, although it was recognized that the latter represented less than 2 per cent of the daily production (Alexanian, 1969a). Patients with hemolytic anemia or severe renal disease were excluded in order to define these relationships clearly in patients with bone marrow failure. Urine, rather than plasma, was used more frequently for bioassay because of the greater sensitivity of the urinary method. Thus, urinary erythropoietin was almost always quantified in normal human beings, but serum erythropoietin was not detected reproducibly unless the hematocrit was less than 30 Vol. per cent when the urinary excretion was about 20 times normal. This was possible because the entire 24-hour urinary excretion of erythropoietin, but only a small volume of serum, could be injected into polycythemic mice. (Larger serum volumes destroy the red cells of assay animals so that their polycythemic state is lost.)

A logarithmic increase in erythropoietin was found for increasing degrees of anemia, confirming the results of many other investigators (Hammond, Shore, and Movassaghi, 1968; Adamson, 1968). Expressing the degree of anemia, in terms of either the hematocrit or the red cell volume, provided a similar degree of reproducibility for the correlation with erythropoietin excretion. In view of the greater simplicity and precision of hematocrit measurements, the appropriateness of the erythropoietin response to anemia in human beings without splenomegaly is probably best evaluated by comparing the erythropoietin excretion with the hematocrit. This conclusion is most pertinent to patients with disorders that produce higher-than-normal levels of erythropoietin (hypoxia-, cyst-, or tumor-induced erythrocytosis) or depressed levels (renal disease, hypogonadism, and possibly chronic infection).

In normal and anemic subjects, there was notable variability in the erythropoietin level for a specific hematocrit, *i.e.,* more than tenfold. Even in the same subject, six consecutive values for urinary erythropoietin excretion varied by 300 per cent. Much of this variation was attributed to the imprecision of the bioassay method and emphasized the need for better erythropoietin assay techniques. Lange has developed an immunoassay procedure for erythropoietin quantitation which offers promise for future studies (Lange, McDonald, and Jordon, 1969). Variations between subjects in the renal production of the renal erythropoietic factor (Gordon, 1968), in the renal clearance of erythropoietin, and in the other known adaptations to anemia, *i.e.,* blood flow and oxygen dissociation from hemoglobin, also contribute to the distinct variability in erythropoietin excretion between individuals. These observations suggest that abnormalities in erythropoietin production might be defined more reliably from a combination of indices of tissue-oxygen supply. For example, concurrent assessments of hematocrit, cardiac output, and oxygen dissociation from hemoglobin may provide a clearer insight into tissue-oxygen supply than one of these parameters alone.

The effect of an individual's sex on the erythropoietin response to anemia was evaluated in a large number of subjects. Men demonstrated a higher erythropoietin excretion than women for varying degrees of anemia. In addition, erythropoietin values for hypogonadal men fell within the range for women, indicating that the mild anemia in these patients probably resulted from decreased erythropoietin production. These findings conform with previous studies that showed higher urinary erythropoietin levels in normal adult males in comparison with women or prepubertal boys (Alexanian, 1966) and support the extensive literature documenting the close relationship between androgenic hormones and erythropoiesis (Steinglass, Gordon, and Charipper, 1941). Thus, in comparison with women, greater androgen production not only accounts for the higher hematocrit and red cell volume of normal men but also provides a greater erythropoietin level for a specific degree of anemia in men with bone marrow disease. In this regard, no well-defined clinical studies have evaluated erythropoietin levels in those endocrinopathies associated with increased endogenous androgen production, such as certain adrenal or ovarian disorders.

The direct relationship between androgens and erythropoietin production was studied further by evaluating the effect of maximal doses of fluoxymesterone and oxymetholone on the urinary excretion and serum concentration of erythropoietin. These drugs were chosen because of the convenience of oral administration and their reported efficacy in patients with chronic anemia from bone marrow failure. Previous chromatographic studies had ruled out the likelihood that the excretion of androgen metabolites, rather than of erythropoietin, accounted for the activity noted in our polycythemic mice (Alexanian, Vaughn, and Ruchelman, 1967). Results confirmed a notable stimulation of erythropoietin level with these drugs with a shift in the log erythropoietin/hematocrit relationship. Thus, even when basal erythropoietin levels were elevated in anemic patients, further marked increments resulted from androgen therapy. No apparent difference was found in the capacity of either fluoxymesterone or oxymetholone to stimulate erythropoietin production in man. These findings are similar to the effect of androgens on erythropoietin in anemic animals (Fried, Rishpon-Meyerstein, and Gurney, 1967), conform with the stimulation of the "renal erythropoietic factor" by androgens in rodents (Gordon, 1968), and explain the occasional efficacy of androgens in the treatment of patients with anemia caused by bone marrow disorders (Gardner, 1961). Unfortunately, the severity of the bone marrow defect prevented any elevation in red cell production in most of our treated patients, a conclusion that applied particularly to the patients with the most severe degrees of marrow failure and the highest erythropoietin levels (Alexanian, 1969b).

Conclusion

The urinary erythropoietin excretion and the serum concentration were evaluated in 116 human beings, of whom 35 were normal volunteers, 8 were hypogonadal men, and 73 had a variety of bone marrow diseases. A logarithmic increase in erythropoietin was confirmed for increasing degrees of anemia. Elevations in serum concentration were not detected reproducibly until the urinary excretion had increased to about 20 times normal. The reproducibility of results was similar when erythropoietin excretion was correlated with either hematocrit or red cell volume. The wide variation in erythropoietin among different patients for a specific hematocrit emphasized the need for improved techniques for erythropoietin assay and for better assessments of tissue oxygen supply. Men, whether normal or anemic, had an approximately fourfold greater erythropoietin excretion than women or hypogonadal men for a specific hematocrit. Large doses of androgenic hormones usually induced a definite stimulation of erythropoietin, even when basal levels were elevated. These observations demonstrate that the occasional stimulation of erythropoiesis by androgenic hormones in man is probably mediated to a major degree by erythropoietin. Despite maximal erythropoietin production, the severity of the marrow defect prevented any improvement in red cell production in most anemic patients treated with androgens.

Acknowledgments

The authors appreciate the technical assistance of Brenda Doherty and Terry Smith in conducting these studies and analyses. Dr. Judith Nadell of Syntex Research, Palo Alto, California, provided the oxymetholone for this study.

This work was supported by Grants No. AM 09155 and CA 12014 from the U. S. Public Health Service.

REFERENCES

Adamson, J. W.: The erythropoietin/hematocrit relationship in normal and polycythemic man: Implications of marrow regulation. *Blood: The Journal of Hematology*, 32:597-609, October 1968.

Alexanian, R.: Correlations between erythropoietin production and excretion. *The Journal of Laboratory and Clinical Medicine*, 74:614-622, October 1969a.

———: Erythropoietin and erythropoiesis in anemic man following androgens. *Blood: The Journal of Hematology*, 33:564-572, April 1969b.

Alexanian, R., Vaughn, W. K., and Ruchelman, M. W.: Erythropoietin excretion in man following androgens. *The Journal of Laboratory and Clinical Medicine*, 70:777-785, November 1967.

———: Urinary excretion of erythropoietin in normal men and women. *Blood: The Journal of Hematology*, 28:344-353, September 1966.

Fried, W., Rishpon-Meyerstein, N., and Gurney, C. W.: The effect of testosterone on erythropoiesis of WW mice. *The Journal of Laboratory and Clinical Medicine*, 70:813-819, November 1967.

Gardner, F. H., and Pringel, J. C.: Androgens and erythropoiesis. In preliminary and clinical observations. *Archives of Internal Medicine*, 107:112-128, June 1961.

Gordon, A. S.: Hormonal relations to erythropoiesis. In *Plenary Session Papers, XII Congress International Society of Hematology*, New York, New York, 1968, pp. 288-303.

Hammond, D., Shore, N., and Movassaghi, N.: Production, utilization, and excretion of erythropoietin: I. Chronic anemias. II. Aplastic crisis. III. Erythropoietic effects of normal plasma. *Annals of the New York Academy of Sciences*, 194:516-527, March 1968.

Lange, R. D., McDonald, T. P., and Jordon, T.: Antisera to erythropoietin: Partial characterization of two different antibodies. *The Journal of Laboratory and Clinical Medicine*, 73:78-90, January 1969.

Steinglass, P., Gordon, A. S., and Charipper, H. A.: Effect of castration and sex hormones on the blood of rats. *Proceedings of the Society of Experimental Biology and Medicine*, 48:169-177, October 1941.

Carcinoid Tumors:
The Diagnostic Spectrum

HAROLD BROWN, M.D.

Department of Medicine, Baylor College of Medicine,
Houston, Texas

In 1930, Sir Maurice Cassidy presented to the Clinical Section of the Royal Society of Medicine a patient who suffered from severe flushing attacks of five years' duration and recurrent attacks of watery diarrhea. The skin showed numerous dilated venules over the nose and cheeks. There was a harsh systolic murmur down the left sternal edge, and the liver was large and irregular. The skin changes were so striking that a water color drawing was made and a photograph of this was published with the case report entitled "Abdominal Carcinomatosis with Probable Adrenal Involvement." This was the first published description of the syndrome later described by Thorson, Biorck, Bjorkman, and Waldenstrom (1954) and by Isler and Hedinger (1953), who recognized the association of this bizarre syndrome with a metastasizing carcinoid tumor of the ileum.

I have always been curious about how such a striking clinical syndrome could have escaped description for the 45 years since Oberndorfer's description of the carcinoid tumor in 1907. The features of the classical carcinoid syndrome described in the first publications were as follows: 1. Vasomotor phenomena—flush and telangiectasia. 2. Intestinal hyperperistalsis and diarrhea. 3. Right-sided valvular disease with collagen deposits on the endocardium. 4. Bronchial constriction.

The carcinoid flush is the most striking feature of the classical syndrome. Varying in frequency and intensity, it is most prominent on the face and upper part of the torso. The flushes are red, frequently with a cyanotic hue. The patients develop a fixed erythema which may undergo exacerbations. There is often venous telangiectasia. The flushes may come on spontaneously but are often stimulated by excitement, alcohol, or defecation. Many patients who produce large amounts of serotonin develop a transient red-orange discoloration on the skin in areas where it has been rubbed.

It appears now that the flush is not produced or accompanied by increased serotonin levels in the blood. During the flushing episode, there appear to be increased levels of circulating bradykinin or related peptides in the plasma. Bradykinin is formed from the action of kallikrein, an enzyme liberated by certain carcinoids, on a circulating alpha$_2$-globulin.

The output of kallikrein from the tumor may be stimulated by catechols, and this reaction can be blocked by alpha-adrenergic blocking agents (Adamson, Grahame-Smith, Peart, and Starr, 1971). The use of subpharmacologic doses of intravenous epinephrine to provoke a flush and hypotension may be a useful diagnostic maneuver in patients suspected of having a carcinoid tumor (Levine and Sjoerdsma, 1963; Peart, Robertson, and Andrews, 1959).

Patients with the carcinoid syndrome often have intestinal hyperperistalsis, and they will have frequent diarrheal stools, abdominal cramps, and borborygmi. Exacerbation of the intestinal spasm may produce transient small bowel obstipation which usually responds to conservative management. The hyperperistalsis will respond to the serotonin antagonist, methysergide, and to p-chlorophenylalanine, an experimental drug which impairs the synthesis of serotonin by blocking the hydroxylation of tryptophan (Engelman, Lovenberg, and Sjoerdsma, 1967). It is interesting that this compound has little effect on the flushing episodes. We should be mindful that hyperperistalsis may be present in certain patients who are not producing excessive amounts of serotonin and may be absent in many with considerable serotonin production. The role of prostaglandins, gastrin, and the kinins in the syndromes invites further investigation.

In about half of the patients with long-standing carcinoid symptomatology, a peculiar type of valvular heart disease with collagen deposits on the endocardium, particularly on the right side of the heart, has been seen. These patients have murmurs of pulmonic and/or tricuspid stenosis and, rarely, of regurgitation. Occasionally, the lesions are seen in the left heart, particularly when the humoral substances from the tumor have access to the left heart without prior circulation through the lung.

Bronchial constriction is rather uncommon, having been seen in only 15 per cent of the carcinoid patients in our series.

About the same time that the carcinoid syndrome was recognized, Lembeck (1953) isolated serotonin, or 5-hydroxytryptamine, from carcinoid tumors; later, Sjoerdsma, Weissbach, and Udenfriend (1956) worked out the metabolic pathway and showed that 5-hydroxyindoleacetic acid (5-HIAA) measurements in the urine could be used to detect patients with carcinoid tumors.

As can be seen from Figure 1, serotonin is derived from dietary or en-

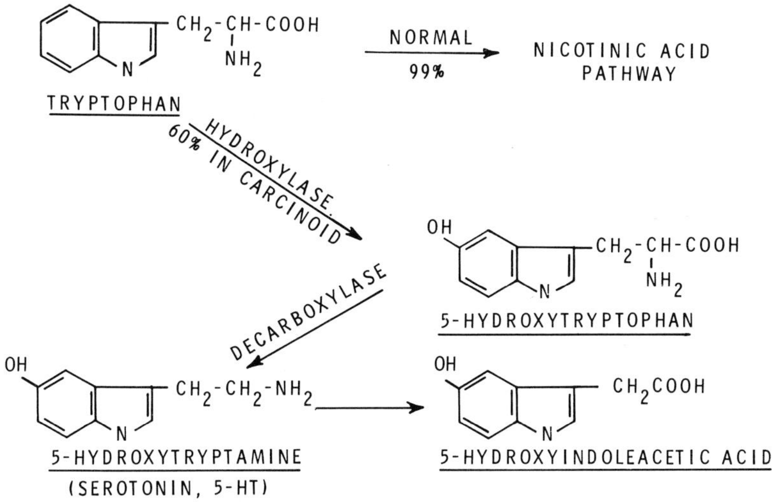

Fig. 1.—Serotonin metabolism.

dogenous tryptophan. Sjoerdsma, Weissbach, and Udenfriend (1955) found that as much as 60 per cent of dietary tryptophan is converted to urinary 5-HIAA in this disorder, in contrast to about 1 per cent conversion in normal persons.

Thus in 1959, William Bean summed up our knowledge of the carcinoid syndrome in a postscript to a paper (Bean and Funk, 1959):

> "This man was addicted to moanin',
> confusion, edema and groanin',
> intestinal rushes, great tricolored blushes,
> and died from too much serotonin."

In the classical carcinoid syndrome, the most practical laboratory test to make the diagnosis has been estimation of the urinary 5-HIAA excretion, which normally ranges from 2 to 8 mg. per day. Patients with diarrhea may have modest elevations of up to 25 mg. per day (Kowlessar, Williams, Law, and Sleisinger, 1958).

The usual screening test for elevated 5-HIAA levels in the urine (Sjoerdsma, Weissbach, and Udenfriend, 1955) is subject to a number of errors (Pitkanen, Airaksinen, Mustala, and Paloheimo, 1962). The phenothiazine drugs suppress the color reaction with nitrosonaphthol and may result in falsely low excretion values (Ross, Weinstein, and Kabakow, 1958). This problem can be circumvented by fluorimetric analysis of extracted 5-HIAA (Udenfriend, Weissbach, and Brodie, 1958).

TABLE 1.—Characteristics of Carcinoid Syndrome Produced by Tumors Occurring at Different Sites*

	MIDGUT Ileal	FOREGUT Bronchial	FOREGUT Gastric	HINDGUT Rectal
Flush	Brief, multiple	Prolonged, severe with facial edema, lacrimation, fever	Bright red, generalized	Carcinoid syndrome very rare
Metastases	Usually in abdomen	Osteoblastic and skin as well as abdomen	Usually in abdomen	Abdomen, but osteoblastic and skin common
Histology	Usually typical argentaffin	Tendency to trabecular pattern; may be very atypical		Tendency to trabecular argentaffin
Metabolic features	Indole secretion largely serotonin	May secrete other polypeptide hormones; symptoms respond to corticosteroids	Frequently secrete 5-hydroxytryptophan and histamine; increased incidence of peptic ulcer	Serotonin secretion very rare

*Modified from Williams and Sandler, 1963.

Falsely high values for 5-HIAA in the urine with the colorimetric determination of 5-HIAA (Udenfriend, Titus, and Weissbach, 1955) can be seen in patients who ingest phenacetin and related drugs, P-hydroxyacetanilide, or n-acetyl-p-aminophenol. Ingestion of mephenesin, used as a muscle relaxant and/or tranquilizer, and methocarbamol (Robaxin) (Honet, Casey, and Runyan, 1959) or glyceryl guaiacolate (Sjoerdsma, 1958), used as an expectorant (Quibron and Robitussin), gives a color reaction similar to 5-HIAA with the nitrosonaphthol reagent. Here again, fluorimetric analysis will give the correct values. I know of two patients who were subjected to a laparotomy for a carcinoid tumor because of falsely high values for 5-HIAA in the urine.

The classical carcinoid syndrome, which was described in the early reports, is typical of those patients who had metastasizing carcinoids of the ileum with massive tumor deposits in the liver. It soon became apparent that there are many variations on this theme, and a much broader spectrum of the carcinoid syndrome has evolved. Williams and Sandler (1963) have suggested that the embryologic origin of the carcinoid tumors will correlate with their histologic pattern and endocrine and clinical behavior as outlined in Table 1.

Tumors arising from all levels of the gastrointestinal tract, from stomach to rectum and including the appendages of gallbladder and pancreas, have been reported with the carcinoid syndrome. The syndrome is also seen with bronchial adenomas and oat cell carcinomas of the lung, as well as tumors of the ovary, testis, thyroid, and thymus (Table 2).

In looking at the totality of carcinoid tumors, it is obvious that only a small fraction of the tumors are associated with hormonal activity. Most of the carcinoid tumors are found by the surgeon at laparotomy or autopsy. In reports of 3,011 gastrointestinal carcinoids collected by Crowder, Judd, and Dockerty (1967), only 103 had the carcinoid syndrome—about 3 per cent (Table 3). The incidence of carcinoid tumors, as reported from Malmö, Sweden, where the system allows for adequate statistics, was

TABLE 2.—SITES OF CARCINOID TUMORS

G-I tract (stomach to rectum)
Lung	Bronchial adenomas, oat cell carcinoma
Pancreas	α-cell
Gallbladder	
Ovary	
Testis	
Thyroid	
Thymus	

TABLE 3.—Reported Carcinoid Tumors of the
Gastrointestinal Tract*

Primary Site	Cases	Carcinoid Syndrome
Stomach	90	8
Duodenum	124	4
Gallbladder	8	0
Jejunum	49	10
Ileum	813	70
Meckel's diverticulum	33	4
Appendix	1,340	5
Cecum	40 }	
Colon	28 }	5
Rectum	486	1
Total	3,011	107

*Crowder et al., 1967.

found from carefully performed autopsies to be 1.1 per cent for gastro-intestinal carcinoids and 0.1 per cent for bronchial carcinoids. In cases found at operation, there was less than one gastrointestinal carcinoid found per 100,000 cases. About one half of these were found in the appendix (Linell and Mansson, 1966).

Variants of the Carcinoid Syndrome

Patients with gastric carcinoids tend to have vivid red, patchy flushes, particularly with eating. These patients excrete, in their urine, histamine and relatively large amounts of 5-hydroxytryptophan and serotonin with only moderately increased amounts of 5-HIAA (Oates and Sjoerdsma, 1962).

Patients with bronchial carcinoids may have much more prolonged and incapacitating flushes, conjunctivitis, lacrimation, and facial edema. Symptoms in such patients may respond dramatically to large doses of cortico-steroids (Melmon, Sjoerdsma, and Mason, 1965). Bronchial adenomas or carcinoids are frequently associated with other endocrine disorders such as multiple endocrine adenomatosis with hyperplasia or tumors of the pituitary, parathyroids, pancreas, and adrenals. The carcinoids or carcinoid-related tumors may be the source of ectopic ACTH, MSH, and other humoral substances (Table 4).

Bronchial carcinoids may be small, and the pulmonary density may be overlooked even when the patient is symptomatic (Melmon, Sjoerdsma, and Mason, 1965; Strott, Nugent, and Tyler, 1968). The response to cortico-

TABLE 4.—HUMORAL SUBSTANCES ELABORATED BY
TUMORS CAUSING CARCINOID SYNDROME

Serotonin (5-hydroxytryptamine)
5-Hydroxytryptophan
Histamine
Kallikrein—to form lysyl-bradykinin and bradykinin
ACTH
MSH
Catecholamines
Insulin
Prostaglandins
CRF ?

steroid therapy or the increased secretion of 5-HIAA should intensify the search for the tumor, which might still be removed surgically.

It is well to remember that the carcinoid syndrome has been described in patients in whom increased serotonin production could not be demonstrated. In such patients, one might attribute the carcinoid manifestations to the ubiquitous prostaglandins or kinins (Oates *et al.*, 1964; Sandler, Karim, and Williams, 1968) which have not been extensively looked for but have been identified in several varieties of carcinoid tumors. It is possible that the carcinoid manifestations may depend upon the interaction of two or more of the humoral substances. This concept could also be invoked to explain the situation of those patients with carcinoid tumors and excess serotonin production, but without carcinoid symptoms.

In recent years, the concept of the carcinoid tumor has broadened even further. By the use of electron microscopy, Bensch, Corring, Pariente, and Spencer (1968) established in normal bronchial epithelium and mucous glands the presence of cells similar in appearance to Kultschitzky's or argentaffin cells of the intestine. These cells contain characteristic cytoplasmic granules, referred to as neurosecretory-type granules, which are similar to those present in intestinal argentaffin cells. Bronchial carcinoids or adenomas and oat cell carcinomas contain similar neurosecretory granules. These neurosecretory granules were shown to consist of a dense aggregation of very fine argentaffin granules. These workers suggested that the oat cell carcinomas of the lung and the bronchial carcinoids are related tumors, both derived from the Kultschitzky-type cells normally found throughout the bronchial tree, with the oat cell carcinoma being the more malignant type. These same neurosecretory granules are also found in the cells of the pancreatic islets and in carcinoma of the thymus. Thus, there is evidence for a common cell origin of the tumors capable of producing the carcinoid syndrome. Weichert (1970) has also emphasized the similarities of the cells of neuroectodermal origin which are capable of producing the carcinoid syndrome, multiple endocrine adenomatosis, and ectopic peptide hormones, and has pointed out that all of the peptide-secreting endocrine glands receive cells from the neural ectoderm.

Thus, we have come full circle back to the ideas expressed by Masson a half-century ago. He described the argentaffin reaction in both carcinoid tumors and enterochromaffin cells and considered carcinoids to be endocrine tumors of argentaffin cell origin (Masson, 1928). He also hypothesized a neural crest origin for argentaffin cells.

The humoral substances, which have been shown to be elaborated by tumors causing the carcinoid syndrome, are listed in Table 4.

I have recently added the corticotrophin releasing factor (CRF) as another hormone that may be produced by the carcinoid tumor. In a number of reports of patients with the ectopic ACTH syndrome, it was noted that certain patients responded to metyrapone, the 11-β-hydroxylase inhibitor, which would be difficult to reconcile unless the hypothalamic-pituitary system remained intact in these patients (Meador et al., 1962; Miura et al., 1967; Strott, Nugent, and Tyler, 1968; Jones, Shane, Gilbert, and Flink, 1969; Brown and Lane, 1965). The responsiveness of the hypothalamic-pituitary-adrenal system in these cases raised the possibility that these tumors secrete another hormone which maintains the secretion of ACTH from the pituitary in the presence of the hypercorticism produced by the ectopic ACTH. To support this hypothesis, peptides with CRF-like activity have been reported in two cases of the ectopic ACTH syndrome (Upton and Amatruda, 1971). It is of great interest that all of the reported patients with the ectopic ACTH syndrome and the anomalous response to metyrapone had carcinoid tumors, or tumors such as oat cell carcinomas of the lung, and certain thymic carcinomas which are often indistinguishable, to the pathologist, from carcinoid tumors (Cohen, Toll, and Castleman, 1960).

In addition, Liddle et al. (1969) found in their collected series of cases with the ectopic ACTH syndrome that about 6 per cent showed suppression of corticosteroid output with dexamethasone therapy; these cases were bronchial adenomas or thymomas which are certainly carcinoid related.

It should be apparent from the preceding discussion that our concept of the carcinoid tumor has broadened considerably—perhaps to a point that the definition covers a confusing variety of situations. We now include tumors whose histology bears only a remote resemblance to carcinoid tumors and, of course, many which do not secrete serotonin. There is strong suggestion, however, that these tumors are related by a common derivation from Kulschitzky's cells which seem to have potential for secreting a variety of amine and polypeptide hormones. It is likely that other secretions will be shown to develop from these tumors to explain the occurrence of acromegaly and pleuriglandular adenomatosis in association with such tumors (Williams and Celestin, 1962).

Thus, in a given tumor, the clinical syndrome of the broadening carcinoid spectrum will depend upon the variety and amount of hormones produced, as well as the location, size, and rapidity of the tumor growth.

Acknowledgments

Supported by a grant (RR-134) from the General Clinical Research Centers Program of the Division of Research Resources, National Institutes of Health.

REFERENCES

Adamson, A. R., Grahame-Smith, D. G., Peart, W. S., and Starr, M.: Pharmacological blockade of carcinoid flushing provoked by catecholamines and alcohol. *American Heart Journal*, 81:141-142, January 1971.

Bean, W. B., and Funk, D.: The vasculocardiac syndrome of metastatic carcinoid. A. M. A. *Archives of Internal Medicine*, 103:189-199, February 1959.

Bensch, K. G., Corrin, B., Pariente, R., and Spencer, H.: Oat-cell carcinoma of the lung. *Cancer*, 22:1163-1172, December 1968.

Brown, H., and Lane, M.: Cushing's and malignant carcinoid syndromes from ovarian neoplasm. *Archives of Internal Medicine*, 115:490-494, April 1965.

Cassidy, M. A.: Abdominal carcinomatosis with probable adrenal involvement. *Proceedings of the Royal Society of Medicine*, 24:139-141, October 10, 1930.

Cohen, R. B., Toll, G. D., and Castelman, B.: Bronchial adenomas in Cushing's syndrome: Their relation to thymomas and oat-cell carcinomas associated with hyperadrenocorticism. *Cancer*, 13:812-817, July-August 1960.

Crowder, B. L., Judd, E. S., and Dockerty, M. B.: Gastrointestinal carcinoids and the carcinoid syndrome: Clinical characteristics and therapy. *Surgical Clinics of North America*, 47:915-927, August 1967.

Engelman, K., Lovenberg, W., and Sjoerdsma, A.: Inhibition of serotonin synthesis by para-chlorophenylalanine in patients with the carcinoid syndrome. *The New England Journal of Medicine*, 277:1103-1108, November 23, 1967.

Honet, J. C., Casey, T. V., and Runyan, J. W., Jr.: False-positive urinary test for 5-hydroxyindoleacetic acid due to methocarbamol and mephenesin carbamate. *The New England Journal of Medicine*, 261:188-190, July 23, 1959.

Isler, P., and Hedinger, C.: Metastasierendes Dunndarmcarcinoid mit schweren, vorwiegend das rechte Herz betreffenden Klappenfehlern und Pulmonalstenose—ein eigenartiger Symptomenkomplex? *Schweizerische medizinsche Wochenschrift*, 83:4-7, January 3, 1953.

Jones, J. E., Shane, S. R., Gilbert, E., and Flink, E. B.: Cushing's syndrome induced by ectopic production of ACTH by a bronchial carcinoid. *The Journal of Clinical Endocrinology and Metabolism*, 29:1-5, January 1969.

Kay, S., and Wilson, M. A.: Ultrastructural studies of an ACTH-secreting thymic tumor. *Cancer*, 26:445-452, August 1970.

Kowlessar, O. D., Williams, R. C., Law, D. H., and Sleisenger, M. H.: Urinary excretion of 5-hydroxyindoleacetic acid in diarrheal states, with special reference to non-tropical sprue. *The New England Journal of Medicine*, 259:340-341, August 14, 1958.

Lembeck, F.: 5-Hydroxytryptamine in a carcinoid tumour. *Nature*, 172:910-911, November 14, 1953.

Levine, R. J., and Sjoerdsma, A.: Pressor amines and the carcinoid flush. *Annals of Internal Medicine*, 58:818-828, May 1963.

Liddle, G. W., Nicholson, W. E., Island, D. P., Orth, D. N., Abe, K., and Lowder, S. C.: Clinical and laboratory studies of ectopic humoral syndromes. *Recent Progress in Hormone Research*, 25:283-314, 1969.

Linell, F., and Mansson, K.: On the prevalence and incidence of carcinoids in Malmö. *Acta medica scandinavica*, (Supplement) 445:377-382, 1966.

Masson, P.: Carcinoids (argentaffin-cell tumors) and nerve hyperplasia of the appendicular mucosa. *The American Journal of Pathology*, 4:181-211, May 1928.

Meador, C. K., Liddle, G. W., Island, D. P., Nicholson, W. E., Lucas, C. P., Nuckton, J. G., and Luetscher, J. A.: Cause of Cushing's syndrome in patients with tumors arising from "nonendocrine" tissue. *The Journal of Clinical Endocrinology and Metabolism*, 22:693-703, July 1962.

Melmon, K. L., Sjoerdsma, A., and Mason, D. T.: Distinctive clinical and therapeutic aspects of the syndrome associated with bronchial carcinoid tumors. *The American Journal of Medicine*, 39:568-581, October 1965.

Miura, K., Sasaki, C., Katsushima, I., Ohtomo, T., Shigeyuki, S., Demura, H., Torikai, T., and Sasano, N.: Pituitary-adrenocortical studies in a patient with Cushing's syndrome induced by thymoma. *The Journal of Clinical Endocrinology and Metabolism*, 27:631-637, May 1967.

Moertel, C. G., Beahrs, O. H., Woolner, L. B., and Tyce, G. M.: "Malignant carcinoid syndrome" associated with noncarcinoid tumors. *The New England Journal of Medicine*, 273:244-248, July 29, 1965.

Oates, J. A., Melmon, K., Sjoerdsma, A., Gillespie, L., and Masou, D. T.: Release of a kenin peptide in the carcinoid syndrome. *The Lancet*, 1:514-517, March 7, 1964.

Oates, J. A., and Sjoerdsma, A.: A unique syndrome associated with secretion of 5-hydroxytryptophan by metastatic gastric carcinoids. *The American Journal of Medicine*, 32:333-342, March 1962.

Oberndorfer, S.: Karzinoide Tumoren des Dunndarms. *Frankfurter Zeitschrift für Pathologie*, 1:426-432, 1907.

Peart, W. S., Robertson, J. I. S., and Andrews, T. M.: Facial flushing produced in patients with carcinoid syndrome by intravenous adrenaline and noradrenaline. *The Lancet*, 2:715-716, October 31, 1959.

Pitkanen, E., Airaksinen, M. M., Mustala, O. O., and Paloheimo, J.: Observations on the specificity of the urinary 5-hydroxyindoleacetic acid determination with 1-nitroso-2-naphthol. *The Scandinavian Journal of Clinical and Laboratory Investigation*, 14(6):571-577, 1962.

Ross, G., Weinstein, I. B., and Kabakow, B.: The influence of phenothiazine and some of its derivatives on the determination of 5-hydroxyindoleacetic acid in urine. *Clinical Chemistry,* 4:66-76, February 1958.

Sandler, M., Karim, S. M. M., and Williams, E. D.: Prostaglandins in amine-peptide-secreting tumours. *The Lancet,* 2:1053-1054, November 16, 1968.

Sjoerdsma, A., Weissbach, H., and Udenfriend, S.: Simple test for diagnosis of metastatic carcinoid (argentaffinoma). *The Journal of the American Medical Association,* 159:397, September 24, 1955.

Strott, C. A., Nugent, C. A., and Tyler, F. H.: Cushing's syndrome caused by bronchial adenomas. *The American Journal of Medicine,* 44:97-104, January 1968.

Thorson, A., Biorck, G., Bjorkman, G., and Waldenstrom, J.: Malignant carcinoid of the small intestine with metastases to the liver, valvular disease of the right side of the heart (pulmonary stenosis and tricuspid regurgitation with septal defects), peripheral vasomotor symptoms, bronchoconstriction, an unusual type of cyanosis. A clinical and pathologic syndrome. *American Heart Journal,* 47:795-817, June 1954.

Udenfriend, S., Titus, E., and Weissbach, H.: The identification of 5-hydroxy-3-indoleacetic acid in normal urine and a method for its assay. *The Journal of Biological Chemistry,* 216:499-505, October 1955.

Udenfriend, S., Weissbach, H., and Brodie, B. B.: Assay of serotonin and related metabolites, enzymes, and drugs. In Glick, D.: *Methods of Biochemical Analysis.* New York, Interscience Publishers, Inc., 1958, Vol. VI, pp. 95-130.

Upton, G. V., and Amatruda, T. T., Jr.: Evidence for the presence of tumor peptides with corticotropin-releasing-factor-like activity in the ectopic ACTH syndrome. *The New England Journal of Medicine,* 285:419-424, August 19, 1971.

Weichert, R. F., III: The neural ectodermal origin of the peptide-secreting endocrine glands. *The American Journal of Medicine,* 49:232-241, August 1970.

Williams, E. D., and Celestin, L. R.: The association of bronchial carcinoid and pluriglandular adenomatosis. *Thorax,* 17:120-127, June 1962.

Williams, E. D., Karim, S. M. M., and Sandler, M.: Prostaglandin secretion by medullary carcinoma of thyroid. *The Lancet,* 1:22-23, January 6, 1968.

Williams, E. D., and Sandler, M.: The classification of carcinoid tumours. *The Lancet,* 1:238-239, February 2, 1963.

Surgical Management of Carcinoid Tumors

RICHARD G. MARTIN, M.D.

Department of Surgery, The University of Texas at Houston
M. D. Anderson Hospital and Tumor Institute,
Houston, Texas

THE FOLLOWING FACTS are essential to remember when managing patients with carcinoid tumors.

I. All carcinoid tumors are malignant. Metastasis is by both the lymphatics and the blood stream. Although some tumors do not metastasize and seem to behave in a benign fashion, they are all potentially malignant and if allowed to remain, they will in time exert their malignant potential. Size alone may not be the determining factor as to whether the lesion has already metastasized. In our series, a small primary lesion metastasized to the breast, simulating breast carcinoma and yet at autopsy, the primary lesion was very small and located in the appendix. Because these lesions metastasize both by way of the lymphatics and the blood stream, in performing any surgical procedure, one must plan to control disease in regional lymph nodes, and must examine the patient thoroughly for distant metastases, especially to the lungs and bones.

II. Surgery is the treatment of choice whenever possible. Because these lesions are potentially malignant and develop in the argentaffin cells of the gastrointestinal tract, they usually lend themselves well to resection, including, whenever feasible, resection of the regional lymph nodes. X-ray therapy may be of help in controlling the pain caused by bony metastasis, and chemotherapy may be of some value in controlling symptoms produced by the so-called carcinoid syndrome when large masses of tumor are unresectable. Often, the surgical procedure required is a gastrectomy or intestinal resection. If the lesion is in the tip of the appendix, one may frequently perform only an appendectomy; however, if it is at the base of the appendix, a right hemicolectomy should be performed. No matter where in the appendix the tumor is, if lymph nodes seem to be enlarged, then right hemicolectomy is necessary. If the lesion is in the rectum, an abdominal perineal resection is indicated, unless the tumor is very low where it can be easily excised and observed closely. Thus, the primary lesion and the lymphatic drainage areas may be removed.

III. Many lesions are associated with other cancers. It is for this reason that, in most series, the appendix is most often the primary site because the lesion is often found incidentally at the time of laparotomy for other causes. This is especially true in the gynecology service. Also, appendiceal lesions usually seem to occur in a younger age group because they are found before they produce symptoms. In our series of 75 cases, 20 had other primary lesions present (Table 1). It was also noted that 17 cases were found incidentally at the time of autopsy and thus had not produced any symptoms. Some of the other primary tumors include chondrosarcoma of the bone, lymphoma, polycythemia, and carcinomas of the cervix, endometrium, ovary, breast, colon, lung, and ureter. The highest percentage of cases with second primaries were those cases in which the carcinoid tumor was located in the ileum and secondly, the appendix. Thus, laparotomy should include a complete exploration of the celomic cavity, removing any suspicious lesions, and obtaining a diagnosis by frozen section at the time of operation whenever possible.

IV. Carcinoid tumors usually appear submucosally. They develop in the so-called Kultschitsky's cells in the crypts of Lieberkühn. Often, they may be hard to diagnose, especially in the rectum. On digital examination, a small nodule felt submucosally may indicate the possibility of a carcinoid tumor. These lesions are usually hard and smooth. If they are low and small, under 2 cm., they may be removed locally. There may be some difficulty in determining whether the lesion is a carcinoid or a carcinoma.

TABLE 1.—PATIENTS WITH CARCINOID TUMORS BY SITE,
TYPE OF FINDING, OTHER PRIMARY LESION
AND AVERAGE AGE

SITE	NUMBER	INCIDENTAL OR AUTOPSY	OTHER PRIMARY LESIONS	AVERAGE AGE YRS.
Ileum	21	5	8	54.2
Rectum	17	0	3	55.4
Appendix	19	10	5	35.7
Lung	7	0	1	51.0
Colon	5	1	2	57.0
Stomach	4	1	1	48.0
Unknown	2	0	0	59.0
Total	75	17	20	

Electron microscopic study may be required to make the final diagnosis.

Electron microscopy is an excellent method of diagnosing carcinoid tumors because the granules show prominently, confirming the diagnosis. Those lesions showing argentaffin granules are easy to identify when using silver stain, but very frequently in rectal and stomach tissue, the granules do not appear, thus making the diagnosis more difficult. As stated, it may be difficult to differentiate between carcinoid and adenocarcinoma of the rectum.

Such a patient in our series had a biopsy of a low rectal lesion performed at the time of delivery and was referred to our institution for adenocarcinoma of the rectum. On reviewing the slides, our pathologist made the diagnosis of carcinoid tumor. The patient was therefore sent home to be observed again six weeks later and again two months after the initial visit. However, on reviewing the slides again, some areas of adenocarcinoma were noted. It was then decided that this patient had both carcinoid tumor and adenocarcinoma of the rectum. A rectal examination at the time of her return two-month follow-up visit revealed two nodules above the biopsy area. These were considered metastatic lymph nodes. An abdominal-perineal resection was performed. There was no further evidence of adenocarcinoma of the rectum; however, the two positive lymph nodes were histologically diagnosed as carcinoid.

V. Metastatic disease may produce the presenting signs and symptoms, such as a lymph node in the neck, a nodule in the umbilicus, or pain in a bone with evidence of a bone lesion. A search for the primary lesion is made in patients presenting with these various areas of metastasis. Usually, the metastatic site is excised for biopsy purposes. If a diagnosis of a carcinoid tumor has been confirmed, complete X-ray examination of the gastrointestinal tract is necessary, including a barium enema and upper GI and small bowel studies. Most frequently, the primary site will be found in the small bowel, especially in the terminal ileum. One of our patients presenting with bone metastasis had a vague pain in the left hip for two years before a biopsy was obtained. The patient is doing well; however, it is suspected from increasing 5-hydroxyindoleacetic acid (5-HIAA) levels that she is developing the carcinoid syndrome.

VI. Patients of all ages may develop carcinoid tumors. These patients may survive long periods of time, even with inoperable lesions. Some of our patients have survived with metastasis as long as 10 years, and some as long as 14 and 15 years after the primary lesion was diagnosed. It is therefore most important that a correct diagnosis be made and that the primary lesion be removed when possible, along with any metastatic disease that can reasonably be resected.

TABLE 2.—PATIENTS WITH CARCINOID SYNDROME AND
ELEVATED 5-HIAA LEVEL

SITE	NUMBER	BENIGN	MALIGNANT	SYNDROME +5-HIAA
Ileum	21	4	13	5
Rectum	17	10	4	0
Appendix	19	12	1	1
Lung	7	4	3	1
Colon	5	1	3	1
Stomach	4	1	2	0
Unknown	2	0	1	1
Total	75	32	27	9

VII. The carcinoid syndrome, consisting of an elevated 5-HIAA level, hot skin flushes, throbbing of the fingers, breathing difficulty, cardiopulmonary symptoms, and diarrhea, may be present in a few patients. It occurred in 9 of our 75 patients (Table 2). Those patients developing the so-called syndrome died from the disease. Chemotherapy has been used, especially in the form of liver infusion, in certain cases in which there was nonresectable disease with some regression of the symptoms. However, as soon as use of the drug 5-fluorouracil is stopped, the syndrome reoccurs. Those patients developing the syndrome most frequently have the primary lesions in the small bowel. Those patients with lesions in the rectum, stomach, or esophagus rarely develop the syndrome. This is probably related to embryonic development. Lesions in the foregut and hindgut areas develop from the so-called premature argentaffin cells. Careful attention to the blood pressure is required when performing surgery on patients having the carcinoid syndrome, for they are very unstable. Epinephrine and norepinephrine should not be administered, but Aramine or angiotensin is suitable. In the event of cardiac failure, the patient should be given digitalis and diuretics. Steroid therapy may also be necessary pre- and postoperatively in the management of such cases. Liver resection of large masses of the tumor have been performed, with temporary improvement of the carcinoid syndrome.

VIII. Carcinoid tumors may mimic other types of carcinomas, especially in their metastatic forms. In our series, a case of metastasis to the breast and the ipsilateral supraclavicular nodes was diagnosed as adenocarcinoma of the breast. Not until the patient developed the complete carcinoid syndrome was the true nature of the primary lesion evident.

Discussion

All carcinoid lesions should be looked upon favorably and attacked aggressively by surgical procedures, as long as the patient does not exhibit the carcinoid syndrome. Whenever possible, the primary lesion with the regional areas of metastasis should be removed. Frequently, the metastatic sites are quite painful, such as a lymph node in the neck or axilla, about the umbilicus, or in the bone. When possible, they should be surgically excised. If they are in the bone, X-ray therapy is the treatment of choice. In those patients with carcinoid syndrome, it may be feasible to remove as much of the tumor as possible in an attempt to lessen the effects of the syndrome; however, this must be done with caution. It should also be remembered that these patients may live for long periods of time even with metastatic disease. Therefore, when possible, aggressive surgical treatment is indicated. No matter how benign and small the lesions appear, it must be remembered that they are all potentially malignant and if not excised, will in time show evidence of their malignant potential by developing metastatic disease and possibly the carcinoid syndrome.

Ectopic Production of Adrenocorticotropic Hormone by a Bronchogenic Carcinoma

BRUCE MACKAY, M.B., Ch.B., Ph.D., F.A.C.P.,
NAGUIB A. SAMAAN, M.D., Ph.D., F.A.C.P., and
W. V. LEARY, M.D., F.A.C.P.

*Departments of Pathology and Medicine, The University of Texas
at Houston M. D. Anderson Hospital and Tumor Institute,
Houston, Texas*

In the past decade, it has become widely appreciated that conventional hormones may be produced by neoplasms of nonendocrine tissues. The literature on ectopic hormone production is burgeoning, and it is evident that a variety of functioning hormones can be elaborated by a wide range of tumors. The best known example is the association of Cushing's syndrome with bronchogenic carcinoma. Liddle *et al.* (1969) listed 104 tumors in which adrenocorticotropic hormone (ACTH) production had been demonstrated, and 50 per cent of these were carcinomas of the lung. With the increasing awareness of the existence of this entity, clinical recognition becomes more frequent. The following case report concerns a patient with an ACTH-producing bronchogenic carcinoma which was suspected on the basis of the physical examination and laboratory findings.

Case Report

A 50-year-old business executive, previously in good health, gave a four-month history of low-grade fever and substernal chest pain for which he was hospitalized elsewhere. Physical examination, electrocardiogram, and chest X-ray films were reported as being normal. Two months later, the patient noticed gradual onset of general weakness, with swelling of his lower extremities which was more pronounced at the end of the day. He received chlorothiazide and potassium chloride daily for two weeks before admission to M. D. Anderson Hospital. He had smoked one to two packs of cigarettes daily for 30 years.

On physical examination at the time of admission, his skin appeared noticeably pigmented on the exposed areas of the body, but he related this to the effect of the sun. Neither he nor his family had noticed any change in his features. Body hair distribution was normal and no lineae striae were present. The pulse was regular (80 per minute). Blood pressure was 160/100 mm. Hg while lying down and did not vary with postural change. No signs of heart failure were found. Fundus examination showed diminution of the vascular tree but no venous dilation, microaneurysms, or hemorrhages to suggest diabetic retinopathy. Results of chest examination were normal. The liver edge was two fingers below the right costal margin and was smooth and nontender. The central and peripheral nervous systems were normal. Serum sodium was 143 mEq./L; CO_2, 41 mEq./L; potassium, 1.9 mEq./L; and fasting blood sugar, 220 mg./100 ml.

Kimmelstiel-Wilson syndrome was considered. However, the absence

Fig. 1.—Lateral chest tomogram showing a mass in the anterior mediastinum.

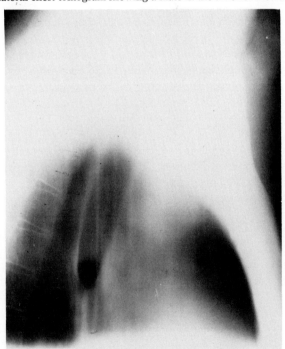

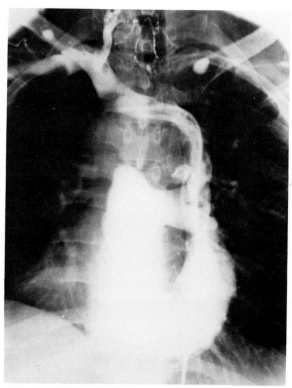

Fig. 2.—Pulmonary arteriogram showing incomplete obstruction of the left pulmonary artery.

of diabetic retinopathy, almost invariably associated with this syndrome (Epstein, 1967), the severity of the hypokalemic alkalosis, and the absence of proteinuria made this diagnosis unlikely. Therefore, the possibility of an adrenocortical carcinoma or an ACTH-producing tumor was considered. The chest X-ray films, reported as normal on two previous occasions, were carefully scrutinized. On a lateral film, a small mass in the anterior mediastinum was suspected and tomography confirmed its presence (Fig. 1). A pulmonary arteriogram revealed incomplete obstruction of blood flow through the left pulmonary artery (Fig. 2). Plasma cortisol was measured by a modified method of the protein-binding assay of Murphy (1969) and was found to be consistently elevated (130 to 140 mg./100 ml.) with no diurnal variation. The urinary 17-hydroxysteroids were measured by the Porter-Silber chromogen method and were found to be abnormally high in three basal 24-hour urine collections (73, 81, 64 mg.). Urinary 17-ketosteroids were normal. Dexamethasone in an augmented dose of 2 mg. at six-hour intervals for eight doses produced no significant change in plasma or urinary hydroxysteroid levels. Plasma ACTH was measured using a radioimmunoassay method similar to that of Landon and Greenwood (1968) and was found to be notably elevated at 3,500 pico Gm./ml. (normal 10 to 50 pico Gm./ml.). An insulin tolerance test (ITT) was performed, using twice the amount of insulin used in normal subjects in order to produce hypoglycemia (0.2 units/kg. body weight), but the patient showed no hypoglycemic response. Blood sugar was 245 at fasting, 176 at 30 minutes, 144 at 45 minutes, 130 at 60 minutes, 128 at 90 minutes, and 136 mg./100 ml. blood at 120 minutes. Growth hormone was measured during the ITT using the double antibody radioimmunoassay technique (Hunter and Greenwood, 1964; Samaan *et al.*, 1966) and showed less than 0.4 mμg./ml. serum at fasting, with no rise during the course of the ITT.

The patient's condition deteriorated rapidly with wasting of his muscle mass. He continued to have low serum potassium levels, and this was managed by Aldactone, 100 mg., and 4 Gm. potassium chloride daily, since potassium chloride alone failed to correct the hypokalemia. One month after admission to M. D. Anderson Hospital, he expired suddenly.

PATHOLOGY

At autopsy, a tumor 10 cm. in diameter was found in the left mediastinum, where it enveloped the left main bronchus and left pulmonary artery, partially constricting the artery. Multiple foci of tumor were present peripherally in both lungs. The mediastinal lymph nodes were extensively involved with metastatic tumor, and tumor nodules were present in the liver and in the vertebral bone marrow. Histologically, the tumor had the typical appearance of a small-cell, undifferentiated (oat cell) carcinoma of the lung (Fig. 3). Both adrenal glands were considerably enlarged (Fig. 4); the right weighed 30 Gm. and the left 26 Gm. Small tumor nodules were present in both glands, but the main cause of the enlargement was marked hyperplasia of the zona fasciculata (Fig. 5). The pituitary gland was not enlarged, and it appeared histologically normal.

Saline extracts of the tumor showed 4,250 pico Gm. ACTH/Gm. wet tissue as measured by radioimmunoassay. Abnormally high values were also found by bioassay. ACTH was absent in an extract from a bronchogenic carcinoma of another patient.

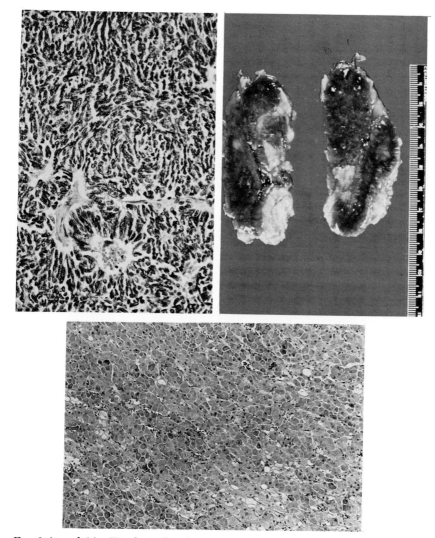

Fig. 3 (*top, left*).—Histologically, the tumor was a small-cell, undifferentiated (oat cell) carcinoma of the lung.

Fig. 4 (*top, right*).—The hemisected adrenal glands are markedly enlarged.

Fig. 5 (*bottom*).—Light micrograph showing the hyperplastic zona fasciculata of the adrenal cortex.

Discussion

Recognition of the association of Cushing's syndrome with carcinoma antedates Cushing's description. Liddle *et al.* (1969) cite a report which appeared in *The Lancet*, 1928, concerning a patient with diabetes, hirsutism, hypertension, adrenal hyperplasia, and an oat cell carcinoma of the lung, but the author of this early report did not draw the conclusion that there was a relationship between tumor and adrenal changes or endocrine symptoms. Since then, the syndrome has been described with increasing frequency. A wide variety of tumors have been implicated, but oat cell carcinoma accounts for more than 50 per cent of the reported cases. The next two most frequently mentioned tumors are thymoma and pancreatic carcinoma. The term "ectopic ACTH syndrome" was first coined by Liddle *et al.* (1963), who found ACTH-like material in nonpituitary tumors, metastatic tumors, and blood of patients whose pituitary ACTH production was subnormal.

The usual clinical picture of an ACTH-producing tumor is hypokalemia, alkalosis, edema, pigmentation, diabetes, and hypertension without the appearance of other classical features of Cushing's syndrome such as plethora, cervicodorsal fat pad, lineae striae, and osteoporosis (Liddle *et al.*, 1963). Diagnosis of the ACTH-producing tumor may be difficult if the tumor is occult and the biochemical changes are not marked. The diagnosis may be missed if the patient is given chlorothiazide as treatment for edema, in which case biochemical changes of hypokalemic alkalosis and hyperglycemia are attributed to the diuretic. Conversely, these biochemical changes after chlorothiazide administration may unmask a subclinical ACTH-producing tumor and be the first hint of the presence of such a tumor. Hypokalemic alkalosis after chlorothiazide administration also occurs in primary aldosteronism, but in this syndrome edema is absent and plasma cortisol and urinary hydroxysteroids are normal. In a patient with a pituitary tumor, adrenocortical tumor, or ectopic ACTH production, the plasma cortisol level is abnormally high and shows no diurnal variation. If the ACTH syndrome is secondary to a pituitary tumor, the pituitary fossa may be enlarged; urinary hydroxysteroids are frequently partially suppressed by an augmented dexamethasone test (Liddle, 1960), and usually the patient has plethora, lineae striae, a cervicodorsal fat pad, and osteoporosis. In the absence of these changes, the most probable diagnosis would be either adrenocortical carcinoma or ACTH-producing tumor. A high level of circulating ACTH is strong evidence of the presence of an occult ACTH-producing tumor rather than adrenocortical tumor. With adrenocortical tumors, ACTH levels are subnormal compared with the levels found in association with the ectopic ACTH-producing tumors, which produce levels far in excess of those seen with pituitary tumors (Landon and Greenwood, 1968). An intravenous pyelogram, adrenal venogram, or arteriogram may show the adrenal tumor.

In their review of hormone production by nonendocrine tumors, Liddle *et al.* (1969) list 10 different ectopic hormones. Caution with regard to the Zollinger-Ellison syndrome as an example of ectopic gastrin production has been justified by the demonstration that gastrin is produced by cells of the pancreatic islets (Lomsky, Langr, and Vortel, 1969). Nevertheless, it is apparent that many of the known hormones may be elaborated by nonendocrine tumors. The ectopic hormone may not have the physiological potency of the true hormone, and this could result from decreased efficiency of the cancer cells as they dedifferentiate. Furthermore, the ectopic hormone may not be identical to the normal hormone. Liddle and his colleagues believed, on the basis of their detailed biological, physical, chemical, and immunological tests, that the ectopic hormone was indistinguishable from the actual gland hormone, but immunologic differences between parathyroid hormone in the serum of patients with primary hyperparathyroidism and that of some patients with hypercalcemia and nonparathyroid malignant diseases have been reported (Roof, Carpenter, Fink, and Gordan, 1971).

Among attempts to explain why nonendocrine tumors should produce ectopic hormones, a theory which has aroused considerable interest is the so-called depressor-deletion hypothesis proposed by Gellhorn in 1958 which suggests that as a tumor becomes progressively less well differentiated, it loses the depressors which modify the biosynthetic mechanisms present in the multipotential primitive or embryonic cell.

A further theory was advanced more recently by Weichert (1970). Neuroendocrine cells, early in embryonic life, migrate into the mucosa of the alimentary tract, and some of these give rise to the endocrine glands. Others, Weichert suggests, can become misplaced and so find their way into the substance of nonendocrine structures that also develop as outpouchings from the gut, such as the bronchi, salivary glands, and pancreatic and biliary ducts. These widely scattered neuroendocrine cells could subsequently develop into a variety of hormone-producing tumors.

Acknowledgments

The bioassay of ACTH in the tumor tissue was performed by Doctors W. Nicholson and D. Orth of Vanderbilt Medical School, Nashville, Tennessee. The initial studies of the radioimmunoassay of ACTH were per-

212   /   *Mackay et al.*

formed using ACTH antibody given to us by Doctor John Landon of Bartholomew Hospital, London, England. The human ACTH was provided by Doctor W. Rittel of Ciba, Basel, Switzerland, and Doctor A. B. Lerner of Yale Medical School, New Haven, Connecticut.

This work was supported by American Cancer Society Grant T 558 and National Institutes of Health Central Research Grant CA 05831-10.

The Zeiss electron microscope used for these studies was purchased with the aid of a generous grant from the Kelsey-Leary Foundation.

REFERENCES

Epstein, F. H.: Functional alterations associated with diabetic nephropathy. *Diabetes Mellitus: Diagnosis and Treatment,* 2:207-210, 1967.

Gellhorn, A.: Recent studies on pathophysiologic mechanisms in human neoplastic disease. *Journal of Chronic Diseases,* 8:158-170, 1958.

Hunter, W. M., and Greenwood, F. C.: A radio-immunoelectrophoretic assay for human growth hormone. *Biochemical Journal,* 91:43-56, April 1964.

Landon, J., and Greenwood, F. C.: Homologous radioimmunoassay for plasma levels of corticotrophin in man. *The Lancet,* 1:273-276, February 1968.

Liddle, G. W.: Tests of pituitary-adrenal suppressibility in the diagnosis of Cushing's syndrome. *The Journal of Clinical Endocrinology and Metabolism,* 20: 1539-1560, December 1960.

Liddle, G. W., Island, D. P., Ney, R. L., Nicholson, W. E., and Shimizu, N.: Nonpituitary neoplasms and Cushing's syndrome. Ectopic "adrenocorticotropin" produced by nonpituitary neoplasms as a cause of Cushing's syndrome. *Archives of Internal Medicine,* 111:471-475, April 1963.

Liddle, G. W., Nicholson, W. E., Island, D. P., Orth, D. N., Abe, K., and Lowder, S. C.: Clinical and laboratory studies of ectopic humoral syndromes. *Recent Progress in Hormone Research,* 25:283-314, 1969.

Lipsett, M. B., Odell, W. D., Rosenberg, L. E., and Waldmann, T. A.: Humoral syndromes associated with nonendocrine tumors. *Annals of Internal Medicine,* 61:733-756, October 1964.

Lomsky, R., Langr, F., and Vortel, V.: Immunohistochemical demonstration of gastrin in mammalian islets of Langerhans. *Nature,* 223:618-619, 1969.

Murphy, B. E. P.: Protein binding and the assay of nonantigenic hormones. *Recent Progress in Hormone Research,* 25:563-610, 1969.

Roof, B. S., Carpenter, B., Fink, D. J., and Gordan, G. S.: Some thoughts on the nature of ectopic parathyroid hormones. *The American Journal of Medicine,* 50:686-691, 1971.

Samaan, N. A., Yen, S. C. C., Friesen, H., and Pearson, O. H.: Serum placental lactogen levels during pregnancy and in trophoblastic disease. *The Journal of Clinical Endocrinology and Metabolism,* 26:1303-1308, December 1966.

Weichert, R. F.: The neural ectodermal origin of the peptide-secreting endocrine glands. *The American Journal of Medicine,* 49:232-241, 1970.

Primary Aldosteronism: Physiology, Pathology, and Clinical Spectrum

JEROME W. CONN, M.D., Sc.D., F.A.C.P., F.A.C.S.

Department of Endocrinology and Metabolism,
University of Michigan Medical School,
Ann Arbor, Michigan

In 1954 (Conn, 1955a, 1955b), we described a fascinating new clinical syndrome which we named primary aldosteronism. The condition is produced by the presence of an aldosterone-secreting adrenocortical adenoma (rarely carcinoma), surgical removal of which results in complete reversal of the entire syndrome. The major clinical features consist of arterial hypertension (average 200/110); in the most severe cases, the hypertension is associated with hypokalemia, hypernatremia, alkalosis, and occasionally hypomagnesemia. Cortisol production is normal, but aldosterone secretion and excretion are abnormally elevated. In the severe cases, the symptomatology represents merely an expression of the biochemical abnormalities already mentioned and consists of periodic muscular weakness, episodic tetanic manifestations, nocturnal polyuria, and severe headache. Characteristically, edema is absent and hemorrhagic retinopathy with papilledema is extremely rare, although the milder forms of retinopathy are frequently observed.

From 1954 to 1964, the alerting signal for the possible presence of this syndrome was the coexistence of hypertension and hypokalemia. On this basis alone, thousands of people have been cured of hypertension, and the volume of cases detected has increased greatly with each succeeding year. Because hypokalemia had become the *sine qua non* of this syndrome, many clinics were screening their hypertensive patients by obtaining values for serum potassium. By 1960 (Laragh *et al.*, 1960), it became apparent that a large number of hypertensive patients had coexisting hypokalemia together with overproduction of aldosterone, but not all of them had primary aldosteronism. Patients with malignant hypertension and with renovascular hypertension were shown to have a newly recognized form of secondary aldosteronism (without edema) associated with hypertension. The demonstration, independently, by both Genest (1961) and Laragh (1962), that infusion of angiotensin II in man increased adrenal production of aldosterone, closed the gap in our knowledge. The renin-angiotensin-aldosterone system was thus born, and an explanation for secondary aldosteronism in ischemic renal disease became evident. But it also became clear that hypertension, hypokalemia, and overproduction of aldosterone could be produced either by an aldosterone-producing adrenal adenoma or by some forms of renal hypertension.

In 1964 (Conn, Cohen, and Rovner, 1964), we reported that in primary aldosteronism, plasma renin activity is subnormal and that in the presence of overproduction of aldosterone, this measurement could make the distinction between primary aldosteronism and those forms of secondary aldosteronism produced by renal blood flow abnormalities. In the latter group, plasma renin activity is supernormal. These observations have been confirmed repeatedly and the determination of plasma renin activity has become most useful, both in the distinction between and in the diagnosis of primary aldosteronism and renovascular hypertension. Thus, as we had indicated in 1964, if in a hypokalemic hypertensive patient with overproduction of aldosterone and normal cortisol production, plasma renin activity can be shown to be subnormal, the diagnosis of primary aldosteronism is established and renal hypertension associated with secondary aldosteronism is ruled out (exceptions are discussed below).

Detection of Primary Aldosteronism in Presence of Normal Levels of Serum Potassium

In the course of a large experience with primary aldosteronism between 1954 and 1964, it became clear that even in severely hypokalemic cases, hypertension had preceded hypokalemia by many years; still, the hypertension and the hypokalemia were corrected by removal of the adrenocortical adenoma. We concluded that a slow-growing adrenal adenoma had been present for many years, that it was the original cause of the hypertension, and that a long period of normokalemic primary aldosteronism had preceded the development of hypokalemia. We had also observed what we called "transitional cases" in which only intermittent hypokalemia occurred. Some of these cases progressed with time to a persistently hypokalemic state. We therefore set out deliberately to see if we could detect primary aldosteronism in hypertensive patients before hypokalemia became evident. Our experience with plasma renin activity determinations in the hypokalemic cases indicated that this measurement was subnormal in every proven case. Thus, we had a new exploratory tool in our search for normokalemic primary aldosteronism. If we could find a normokalemic hypertensive patient with overproduction of aldosterone, normal cortisol production, and subnormal plasma renin activity, the chances would be great that he harbored an aldosterone-producing adrenocortical adenoma. In 1965, we (Conn *et al.*, 1965) reported the first such case. This patient has now been normotensive for more than six years. His left adrenal gland contained two 5-mm. aldosterone-producing adenomas, and a unilateral adrenalectomy was performed. Preoperatively, aldosterone excretion had been four times higher than normal, cortisol production was normal, and no renin activity at all could be detected in his plasma under conditions of sodium restriction followed by four hours of upright posture—conditions which in normal people result in very high levels of plasma renin activity. After his operation, aldosterone production became subnormal precipitously and gradually returned to normal over a period of months. This phenomenon of an extremely rapid fall of aldosterone production to subnormal levels in the immediate postoperative period constitutes additional evidence that an aldosterone-producing tumor has been removed (Conn, Rovner, and Cohen, 1965), and it occurs in virtually all patients who are eventually cured by the operation. Since then, we have been able to prove the existence of normokalemic primary aldosteronism in 28 more patients. Our current figures (Conn, 1968) indicate an incidence of 8 per cent for normokalemic primary aldosteronism among hospitalized patients with essential hypertension, but a final figure for the prevalence of this disease in essential hypertension is not yet available. The laborious task of screening large numbers of hypertensive patients with aldosterone and renin determinations has limited this research. However, rapid advances have been made during the past year on methods, and we now have radioimmunoassay procedures for plasma and urinary aldosterone and for plasma angiotensin I and angiotensin II. Within a relatively short time, these tools will become available to practicing physicians so that, on a practical basis, they can screen their hypertensive patients for the possibility of primary aldosteronism.

Spectrum of Primary Aldosteronism and Its Clinical Classification

From what has already been said, primary aldosteronism can be regarded as a continuum which at one end of the scale is indistinguishable from essential hypertension (except by renin and aldosterone measurements), and at the other consists of the classical manifestations as originally described. Between these two extremes are the cases that have various degrees of intermittent hypokalemia. We now classify primary aldosteronism into three main subgroups: (1) persistently hypokalemic cases, usually the most severe cases; (2) intermittently hypokalemic cases, usually moderately severe; and (3) persistently normokalemic cases, usually the mildest cases.

There is, however, some overlapping among these groups. A given patient with intermittent hypokalemia may be periodically normokalemic or hypokalemic. This may have to do with the known variability from time to time of aldosterone secretion by such tumors, as well as with alterations in sodium and potassium intake from time to time.

The following data summarize our experience with 95 surgically explored patients, all of whom exhibited what we believe to be the most critical diagnostic criteria; namely, overproduction of aldosterone, subnormal plasma renin activity, and normal cortisol production. Of the 95 patients, 82 (86 per cent) had primary aldosteronism (tumor) and 13 (14 per cent) had bilateral hyperplasia, which we now classify as "idiopathic aldosteronism" (see under Pathological Classification below). At present, there are no critical distinguishing characteristics which can separate these cases preoperatively. (A promising approach to this problem is presented on pages 9 to 24, this volume.)

In the tumor group, aldosterone excretion ranged from 17 to 525 μg. per day. All cases with aldosterone excretion rates higher than 55 μg. per day were persistently hypokalemic. Cases with aldosterone excretion rates between 17 and 55 μg. per day fell into three groups: (1) persistently hypokalemic, (2) intermittently hypokalemic, and (3) normokalemic. In the 29 normokalemic cases, aldosterone excretion rates were between 22 and 55 μg. per day. Plasma renin activity was subnormal in all cases, whether hypokalemic or not. In the range of aldosterone excretion rates between 22 and 55 μg. per day, the degree of suppression of plasma renin activity was similar for hypokalemic and normokalemic cases. When aldosterone excretion exceeded 55 μg. per day, suppression of plasma renin activity was more intense. Those factors which allow some patients to remain normokalemic while others became hypokalemic at similar levels of aldosterone excretion and plasma renin activity are not clear. But it is likely that they involve the duration of aldosteronism, the accustomed or acquired level of potassium and sodium intake by the individual patient, and the sex of the patient.

Mention should be made now of a rare situation (Sutherland, Ruse, and Laidlaw, 1966) in which hypertension and hypokalemia coexist with overproduction of aldosterone, subnormal plasma renin activity, and normal cortisol production. In the two cases described, administration of 1 mg. of dexamethasone per day resulted in normalization of all of the abnormalities within 10 days. We have attempted this procedure in many of the cases described above but have not yet encountered one such as Laidlaw's. While the two cases described are well documented (a father and son), we conclude that this must be a very rare situation. One of these patients was explored surgically and found to have bilateral adrenocortical hyperplasia.

Pathological Classification

As stated above, it is not possible to distinguish with precision preoperatively those patients who will be found to have an adenoma from those that will show bilateral adrenocortical hyperplasia, but we (Conn et al., 1972) have recently reported suggestive progress in this area (Conn, pages 9 to 24, this volume). Both groups satisfy the preoperative criteria that we have stressed above as being diagnostic of primary aldosteronism. Our own experience with 95 cases is as follows: 82 cases (86 per cent) have been tumor cases and 13 (14 per cent) have had micronodular or macronodular hyperplasia. It is claimed that subtotal or total adrenalectomy in bilateral adrenal hyperplasia cases does not result in normalization of blood pressure, as occurs when an adenoma is removed (75 to 80 per cent). Our own experience, however, indicates that this group responds to total or subtotal adrenalectomy almost as well as do patients with primary aldosteronism whose tumors have been removed. We (Conn, Rovner, Cohen, Bookstein, et al., 1969) have reported on successful visualization of small cortical adenomas by selective adrenal venography in more than 80 per cent of cases, and Melby and colleagues (1967) have been successful in predicting the side of the tumor by measuring the aldosterone concentration of adrenal venous blood obtained by catheter from each adrenal vein. These techniques help to distinguish tumor from bilateral hyperplasia, but they are technically difficult, carry a small risk of adrenal medullary hemorrhage, and are not 100 per cent reliable. Our most recent studies (Conn et al., 1972), in which we have employed an intravenous injection of [131]I-19-iodocholesterol followed by photoscanning of both adrenal glands, suggest that it may be possible to make the preoperative distinction between those cases with bilateral hyperplasia and those with tumor (Conn, pages 9 to 24, this volume). When this can be accomplished preoperatively with certainty, we will favor surgical treatment for the tumor case and treatment with spironolactone for the hyperplasia case, pending clarification of the pathogenesis of this form of hyperplasia.

It is our current opinion that the term primary aldosteronism should presently be reserved for those cases subsequently proven to harbor an aldosterone-secreting tumor. The pathophysiology of the cases showing bilateral hyperplasia is unclear. If it should eventually be shown that it is the result of a diffuse lesion which is primary in both adrenal glands, one would be justified in classifying it as primary aldosteronism associated with bilateral hyperplasia. If, however, the bilateral hyperplasia is the result of an as yet unknown extra-adrenal stimulus for aldosterone production, the abnormality should be classified as a secondary form of aldosteronism. Since the nature of the lesion remains unknown, however, we prefer to classify this form of aldosteronism as "idiopathic" until the situation becomes clarified.

From the above discussion it should be clear that the preoperative diagnosis of bilateral hyperplasia will most likely be primary aldosteronism and that when no tumor materializes at operation it will then be classified as "idiopathic" aldosteronism with bilateral hyperplasia. Once surgical therapy has been embarked upon, it would seem wise to carry out a total or subtotal adrenalectomy when bilateral hyperplasia is found. As noted above, when preoperative diagnosis is made possible, we will consider treatment with Aldactone A to be preferable, pending clarification of the pathophysiology of the condition. Much more information is needed in the area of structure-function relationships in those cases which exhibit diffuse bilateral nodular hyperplasia.

Pathophysiology of Primary Aldosteronism

Two key points must be realized in order to understand properly the abnormal physiology involved in primary aldosteronism. First, the patient has had mild to moderate expansion of his extracellular and intravascular volume compartments, usually for several years. Second, a compensatory adjustment was made early in his disease to prevent further expansion of these spaces. This consisted of a change in renal tubular function in which proximal tubular rejection of sodium occurred (decreased proximal tubular reabsorption) and more sodium was shunted to the distal portion of the nephron. In the presence of unsuppressible aldosterone production, this increases the exchange of Na^+ for K^+ at the distal tubular ion-exchange site and initiates a period of increased urinary excretion of K^+ which may continue for many years before sufficient body K^+ is lost to produce hypokalemia. However, the major advantage is that it allows for rapid excretion of sudden salt loads which otherwise would so further overload the vascular compartment, including the heart, that acute decompensation and pulmonary edema would occur. Experimentally, this protective phenomenon has been known for many years and has been termed "renal escape" from the sodium-retaining activity of continuously administered mineralocorticoids. This latter adjustment sets up a new steady state which prevents the formation of edema and restores sodium equilibrium. The mechanism by which the hypertension is induced is not known but it too may be a response to chronic, mild overexpansion of extracellular and intravascular volumes. It has been well established that mild expansion of intravascular volume sharply diminishes the release of renal renin into the blood stream. It is clear, therefore, that when extracellular fluid volumes are expanded by excessive mineralocorticoid activity in an otherwise normal individual, a series of compensatory reactions occur which, together with the persistence of mineralocorticoid activity, lead to the clinical and biochemical picture that we recognize as primary aldosteronism.

The simplest experimental approach which would mimic the development of an aldosterone-secreting adrenocortical tumor would be the chronic daily administration of aldosterone, beginning with very tiny amounts and gradually increasing the dose over a period of years. Such information is not available, but short-term experiments of this kind have been done in man. Normal people on a fixed sodium intake, given a fixed large daily dose of aldosterone, respond in the following ways: During the first two days, urinary sodium falls sharply and total body weight increases 1 to 2 kg. By the third or fourth day, urinary sodium has returned to base line levels and weight has stabilized at the higher value, despite continuation of aldosterone injections (renal escape). The latter phenomenon is probably caused by liberation from somewhere in the body of a salt-losing hormone, sometimes referred to as "third factor." It is presumed that this hormone is responsible for the decreased proximal tubular reabsorption of sodium which occurs under conditions of intravascular volume expansion. Increased amounts of sodium are delivered to the distal tubular ion-exchange site where, under the influence of excessive amounts of aldosterone, a larger-than-normal exchange of sodium for potassium occurs, leading to increased urinary excretion of potassium. Depending upon the severity of the aldosteronism, this may quickly lead to hypokalemia, or hypokalemia may not manifest itself at all. Negative potassium balance may be so minimal that it would require many years to decrease total body potassium sufficiently to manifest hypokalemia. We (Conn, Cohen, and Rovner, unpublished data) have been able to induce in normal men our diagnostic criteria for primary aldosteronism without the induction of hypokalemia; namely, severe suppression of plasma renin activity, increased aldosterone excretion, and normal cortisol production, after five days of administration of aldosterone. Thus, it is the early volume change induced by aldosterone which is responsible for the phenomenon of low plasma renin activity; this, together with increased aldosterone production, forms the basis for our diagnostic criteria and allows us to make the diagnosis with or without hypokalemia at a particularly early stage in its development. Once chronic hypokalemia appears, the symptoms which ensue are caused wholly by potassium depletion and are no different from those of chronic potassium depletion from any other cause. These are muscular weakness or paralysis, tetany, postural hypotension, diminished renal capacity to concentrate and acidify the urine, and polyuria. Chronic potassium depletion also makes the kidneys more vulnerable to infection.

Hypertension, Decreased Plasma Renin Activity, and Normal Aldosterone Production

All investigators who have studied plasma renin activity in hypertensive patients have found a group of them falling into this category. Our figure for this group is 15 per cent, but in some studies the figure has been as high as 40 per cent (highest in black people with hypertension). We have theorized (Conn, Rovner, and Cohen, 1968) that endogenously produced sodium-retaining compounds other than aldosterone, as well as chronic ingestion of unknown compounds having a similar activity, could account for some of these cases. Ingestion of licorice is an example of an exogenous sodium retainer, and desoxycorticosterone-producing tumors and 18-hydroxy-desoxycorticosterone-producing tumors are examples of endogenously produced nonaldosterone sodium-retaining compounds. Although no one has found the precise cause of hyporeninemia in this large group of patients with essential hypertension, we believe that the hypertension in all of these situations is via the same mechanism as in aldosterone-producing tumors. In fact, in some cases an excessive end-organ response to normal quantities of aldosterone can, at least, be suggested. Until it is proved otherwise, we shall continue to assume that severely suppressed plasma renin activity in the hypertensive patient is the result of insidious, low-grade, long-term sodium retention, and we will seek to determine the causes, which, most likely, are many.

Carbohydrate Tolerance and Insulin Secretory Capacity in Primary Aldosteronism

In 1965, we (Conn, 1965) reported that more than 50 per cent of patients with primary aldosteronism exhibited a diabetic type of glucose tolerance test; in some of them this could be reversed to normal by potassium loading preoperatively, and in many of them glucose tolerance returned to normal in the postoperative period. In studying this phenomenon, we found that the plasma-insulin response to glucose loading was also diabetic in type, in that release of insulin was delayed and subnormal during the first hour after the glucose load. This too could be improved by potassium loading and, in many cases, became completely normal in the postoperative period. We suggested that an intracellular potassium deficit within the beta cells of the pancreas might account for this phenomenon, either directly or indirectly. Gorden, Sherman, and Simopoulis (1971, in press) recently reported that under conditions of potassium deficiency in man, the total insulin released into the blood stream in response to glucose is smaller than normal and is delayed. In addition, it contains a significantly higher proportion of proinsulin than is found in normal people. Proinsulin is physiologically inactive and is the precursor of the smaller molecule that we call insulin. These results confirm our suspicion that intracellular beta cell potassium is important with respect to glucose-induced pancreatic insulin release. These findings may have broad implications in the field of carbohydrate metabolism.

Summary

Primary aldosteronism is much more common among our hypertensive population than has been realized heretofore. A major limiting factor in the recognition of this disorder has been the laborious technical procedures required for the diagnosis; namely, determinations of aldosterone and plasma renin activity. As a result of those difficulties, the diagnosis of primary aldosteronism in most parts of the world has been limited to the most severe cases *i.e.*, those with chronic and persistent hypokalemia. The recent development of radioimmunoassay procedures for both of these determinations will remove part of the limitation.

The pathophysiology of primary aldosteronism has been discussed in relation to the earliest and most critical diagnostic criteria. It is likely that further study of early cases of primary aldosteronism will lead to a better understanding of the mechanism of hypertension in the large group of patients with essential hypertension who do not exhibit overproduction of aldosterone, but who do have hyporeninemia, a situation currently unexplained.

Acknowledgments

Supported in part by USPHS Grant AM 10257; USPHS Training Grant AM 05001; 5MO1-FR-4204, Division of Research Facilities and Resources.

REFERENCES

Conn, J. W.: Presidential address: 1) Painting background; 2) primary aldosteronism, a new clinical syndrome. *The Journal of Laboratory and Clinical Medicine*, 45:3-17, January 1955a.

————: Primary aldosteronism. *The Journal of Laboratory and Clinical Medicine*, 45:661-664, April 1955b.

————: Hypertension, the potassium ion and impaired carbohydrate tolerance. *The New England Journal of Medicine*, 273:1135-1143, November 18, 1965.

————: The evolution of primary aldosteronism—1954-1967. *The Harvey Lectures*, 62:257-291, 1968.

Conn, J. W., Cohen, E. L., and Rovner, D. R.: Suppression of plasma renin activity in primary aldosteronism. *The Journal of the American Medical Association*, 190:213-221, October 19, 1964.

————: Unpublished data.

Conn, J. W., Cohen, E. L., Rovner, D. R., and Nesbit, R. M.: Normokalemic primary aldosteronism: A detectable cause of curable "essential" hypertension. *The Journal of the American Medical Association*, 193:200-206, July 19, 1965.

Conn, J. W., Morita, R., Cohen, E. L., Beierwaltes, W. H., McDonald, W. J., and Herwig, K. R.: Primary aldosteronism: Photoscanning of tumors after [131]I-19-iodocholesterol. *Archives of Internal Medicine*, 129:417-425, March, 1972.

Conn, J. W., Rovner, D. R., and Cohen, E. L.: Natural history of recovery of the renin-angiotensin-aldosterone system following long term suppression by aldosterone-secreting tumors. (Abstract) *Program of the 47th Meeting of the Endocrine Society*, p. 60, June 1965.

————: Licorice-induced pseudoaldosteronism. Hypertension, hypokalemia, aldosteronopenia, and suppressed plasma renin activity. *The Journal of the American Medical Association*, 205:492-496, August 12, 1968.

Conn, J. W., Rovner, D. R., Cohen, E. L., Bookstein, J. J., Cerny, J. C., and Lucas, C. P.: Preoperative diagnosis of primary aldosteronism. *Archives of Internal Medicine*, 123:113-123, February 1969.

Genest, J.: Angiotensin, aldosterone and human arterial hypertension. *The Canadian Medical Association Journal*, 84:403-419, 1961.

Gorden, P., Sherman, B. M., and Simopoulis, A. P.: Glucose tolerance with hypokalemia: An increased proportion of circulating proinsulin-like component. *The Journal of Clinical Endocrinology and Metabolism*, 1971. (In press.)

Laragh, J. H.: Interrelationships between angiotensin, norepinephrine, epinephrine, aldosterone secretion, and electrolyte metabolism in man. *Circulation*, 25:203-211, 1962.

Laragh, J. H., Ulick, S., Januszewiza, V., Deming, Q. B., Kelly, W. G., and Lieberman, S.: Aldosterone secretion and primary and malignant hypertension. *The Journal of Clinical Investigation*, 39:1091-1106, 1960.

Melby, J. C., Spark, R. F., Dale, S. L., Egdahl, R. H., and Kahn, P. C.: Diagnosis and localization of aldosterone-producing adenomas by adrenal-vein catheterization. *The New England Journal of Medicine*, 277:1050-1056, November 16, 1967.

Sutherland, D. J. A., Ruse, J. L., and Laidlaw, J. C.: Hypertension, increased aldosterone secretion and low plasma renin activity relieved by dexamethasone. *The Canadian Medical Association Journal,* 95:1109-1119, November 26, 1966.

Adrenocortical Tumors

O. H. PEARSON, M.D.

Department of Medicine, Case Western Reserve University,
School of Medicine, Cleveland, Ohio

ADRENAL CORTICAL ADENOMAS are not uncommon findings at autopsy, but hormone-producing adrenocortical tumors diagnosed during life are rare. Aldosterone-secreting adrenal tumors are usually benign adenomas and have been discussed by Dr. Conn (see pages 213 to 223, this volume). Adrenal tumors which secrete excessive amounts of cortisol, androgens, or estrogens may be either benign or malignant but more commonly are malignant.

Adrenal cortical tumors occur in all age groups and in both sexes, although functional tumors are more frequently observed in women. With benign tumors, the endocrine disorder, either Cushing's syndrome or virilization, calls attention to the diagnosis. With malignant lesions, the presenting complaints may be related to endocrine syndromes, such as feminization, virilization, and/or Cushing's syndrome, whereas in patients without endocrine syndromes, abdominal pain or the presence of an abdominal mass may lead to the diagnosis.

The most common endocrine disorders seen in patients with adrenocortical carcinoma are Cushing's syndrome and virilization, or a combination of these two disturbances. Feminization is a less common finding. About 25 per cent of patients with malignant tumors may show no clinical evidence of endocrine disturbance. Urinary excretion of 17-ketosteroids (17-KS) and/or 17-hydroxycorticosteroids (17-OHCS) is elevated in the majority of patients with adrenal carcinoma, but the levels of steroid excretion are not well correlated with the endocrine syndrome in the patient. Thus, patients with no clinical manifestations of endocrine disturbance may nevertheless excrete large quantities of 17-KS and/or 17-OHCS in the urine. Less than 20 per cent of patients with adrenal carcinoma have normal urinary steroid excretion.

Since endocrine syndromes are a common feature in patients with adrenal carcinoma, it seems possible that the diagnosis could be established before the disease reached an advanced stage. Unfortunately, it appears that adrenal carcinoma has a low efficiency of normal steroid production, and thus the tumor mass must reach a large size before clinical manifestations of hormone excess appear. Measurement of urinary 17-KS and 17-OHCS excretion is helpful in diagnosis, since very high levels of either of these steroid determinations are suggestive of carcinoma. Failure to suppress urinary steroid excretion during administration of 8 mg. of dexamethasone in divided doses daily provides strong support for the presence of an adrenal neoplasm. The finding of a low plasma adrenocorticotropic hormone (ACTH) level in patients with Cushing's syndrome further substantiates the diagnosis of adrenal neoplasm. The finding of high levels of dehydroepiandrosterone or tetrahydro substance S in the urine may also be helpful in the diagnosis of adrenal cancer, but usually these determinations are not necessary. An ACTH stimulation test may be helpful in distinguishing between adenoma and adenocarcinoma. During intravenous ACTH administration, urinary excretion of 17-OHCS and 17-KS usually rises significantly in the presence of an adenoma, whereas there is usually no rise with adrenal carcinoma.

Excision of a functioning adrenal adenoma usually results in cure, while the rate of surgical cure in adrenal carcinoma is very low. Although the primary tumor may be resectable in about one half of the patients, this is almost invariably followed by the appearance of metastasis. Metastasis occurs most frequently in the lungs and liver and, rarely, in bone and brain. Fifty per cent of patients die within two years after the onset of symptoms. Occasionally, adrenal cancer may progress slowly, and prolonged survival may occur even in the presence of metastasis.

Treatment for adrenal neoplasms should involve surgical removal of the tumor whenever possible. Even when there is residual disease, occasional prolonged survivals may occur. In addition, removal of the major mass of tumor may result in relief of the Cushing's syndrome or virilization. Radiation therapy is usually of no benefit in adrenal cancer. The course of the disease can often be monitored by serial measurements of urinary 17-KS and/or 17-OHCS excretion.

A unique and partially effective form of chemotherapy is available for patients with adrenal cancer. Bergenstal and co-workers reported in 1959 that o,p'DDD was capable of inducing regression of metastatic adrenal cancer and inhibition of its hormonal secretion. In a subsequent report of a cooperative study (Hutter and Kayhoe, 1966), about one third of patients with metastatic adrenal cancer obtained objective tumor regression and about two thirds of the patients had significant reduction in urinary steroid excretion following o,p'DDD therapy. Despite toxicity consisting of anorexia, nausea, vomiting, diarrhea, skin rash, and mental depression, o,p'DDD has proven to be an effective agent in the management of patients with adrenal cancer. Aminoglutethamide has also been shown to suppress urinary steroid excretion in patients with adrenal cancer, but this drug appears to have little influence on the growth of the tumor.

The following case reports illustrate the course and treatment of patients with adrenal neoplasms.

CASE 1.—The first patient was 50 years of age when she presented with a large abdominal mass. A large adrenal cancer (2,880 gm.) was removed, but it was thought that residual tumor was left in the patient. She remained well for 12 years without further therapy. At that time, pulmonary and liver metastases were apparent and the tumor was nonfunctional. Treatment with o,p'DDD resulted in striking regression of the tumor which has persisted for six years. The patient is still alive but has evidence of recurrent disease in the liver. Three years after the start of o,p'DDD therapy, she developed Addison's disease which was successfully managed with replacement therapy. Five years after the treatment was started, she developed neurotoxicity consisting of somnolence, weakness, and loss of memory. This was reversed by withdrawal of therapy. She remained in remission for one year after stopping o,p'DDD, at which time recurrent disease in the liver became manifest and was refractory to o,p'DDD.

CASE 2.—The second patient developed Cushing's syndrome at age 34. A right adrenal tumor initially thought to be an adenoma was removed and the Cushing's syndrome remitted. After one year, the Cushing's syndrome returned and surgical examination revealed recurrence of tumor which was inoperable. Treatment with o,p'DDD resulted in remission of the Cushing's syndrome and one year later the recurrent tumor was removed. She remained well for two and one-half years, at which time the Cushing's syndrome recurred. At this point, the tumor was refractory to treatment with o,p'DDD, and she died of metastatic disease a year later.

CASE 3.—The third patient developed signs of virilization at one year of age and at two and one-half years a right adrenal carcinoma was removed. This was followed by transient decrease in virilization. At age four and one-half, there was a palpable mass in the abdomen which was discernible on X-ray films because of calcification. Pulmonary metastases were seen on the chest X-ray films. Treatment with o,p'DDD resulted in prompt disappearance of the pulmonary metastases and a decrease in the size of the abdominal mass. One and one-half years later the abdominal mass was removed surgically. Six months later, the abdominal mass recurred and was refractory to further treatment with o,p'DDD. She died of metastases three years after starting o,p'DDD therapy.

Three additional cases of more rapidly progressive disease failed to benefit from o,p'DDD therapy. Therapy with o,p'DDD and aminogluteth-amide produced a decrease in urinary steroids but no regression of tumor in one patient. Another patient failed to show any response to o,p'DDD therapy, either on the steroid excretion or tumor growth.

Discussion

This experience with o,p'DDD therapy in the six patients reported above is similar to that previously reported by others. Significant remissions were obtained in three patients lasting six years, three and one-half years, and two years respectively after the start of therapy. It is apparent that o,p'DDD constitutes effective chemotherapy for some patients with adrenocortical tumors.

It is also apparent that o,p'DDD may destroy normal adrenocortical tissue with sufficient time. In one patient, Addison's disease developed after three years of therapy. In another patient, autopsy revealed virtually complete destruction of the left adrenal gland after approximately three years of therapy. In a third patient, biopsy of the normal adrenal gland after one year of therapy revealed significant focal destruction of adrenocortical cells.

Toxicity associated with o,p'DDD therapy is significant, but in most cases did not preclude effective use of the drug. Gastrointestinal symptoms such as anorexia, nausea, and vomiting are the most frequent and can usually be ameliorated by brief interruptions of therapy. Severe central nervous system symptoms occurred in one of our patients after almost five years of therapy; they consisted of somnolence, weakness, and loss of memory and were associated with hyperreflexia and electroencephalographic changes suggestive of diffuse, organic brain deterioration. Fortunately, these changes appear to have been completely reversible after withdrawal of therapy.

Summary

Hormone-producing adrenocortical tumors are rare. Aldosterone-secreting tumors are usually benign, whereas those associated with Cushing's syndrome, virilization, or feminization are more commonly malignant. Hormone measurements are useful not only for diagnosis but also in monitoring the course of the disease. Surgical treatment is the initial treatment of choice and is curative with benign lesions though rarely so with malignant lesions because of the advanced stage of the disease at the time of diagnosis. Occasionally, long-term survival occurs despite the presence of metastases. A unique and partially effective chemotherapy is worthy of trial in patients with adrenocortical carcinoma despite toxicity, consisting of gastrointestinal disturbances, skin rash, and central nervous system effects. O,p'DDD may induce objective tumor regression and inhibition of hormone secretion by the tumor and in some instances is associated with long-term remissions. Other drugs, such as aminoglutethamide and metyrapone, may be useful in suppressing hormone production by the tumors but are not effective in suppressing tumor growth.

Acknowledgment

Supported by grants from the U.S.P.H.S., CA-05197-12, RR-80, and the American Cancer Society, T 461.

REFERENCES

Bergenstal, D. M., *et al.*: *Transactions of the Association of American Physicians,* 72:341, 1959.
Hutter, A. M., and Kayhoe, D. E.: Adrenal cortical carcinoma. Clinical features of 138 patients. *The American Journal of Medicine,* 41:572, 580, 1966.

The Pathology of Adrenal Cortical Carcinoma: Study of 22 Cases

MICHAEL L. IBANEZ, M.D.

Department of Anatomical Pathology, The University of Texas
at Houston M. D. Anderson Hospital and Tumor Institute,
Houston, Texas

OF 68,807 PATIENTS who have been treated for cancer at M. D. Anderson Hospital and Tumor Institute, only 22 have had a primary adrenal cortical carcinoma. This is consistent with the incidence in the large series reported (Rapaport, Goldberg, Gorden, and Hinman, 1952; Heinbecker, O'Neal, and Ackerman, 1957; Macfarlane, 1958; Lipsett, Hertz, and Ross, 1963; Hutter and Kayhoe, 1966; and Huvos, Hajdu, Brasfield, and Foote, 1970) as well as with the statistics in Cancer Registries (Griswold, Wilder, Cutler, and Pollock, 1955; Ferber, Hardy, Gerhardt, and Solomon, 1962; and Clemmesen, 1965).

Material and Methods

The hospital charts of all 22 patients with the diagnosis of adrenal cortical carcinoma were reviewed. Inclusion in this group was based upon the availability of sections of the primary tumor and metastases in ade-

---

TABLE 1.—ADRENAL CORTICAL CARCINOMA
22 Patients

		NUMBER OF PATIENTS
Functioning or Hormone-Producing Carcinomas		10*
Cushing's Syndrome	3	
Virilization	6	
Hypoglycemia	1	
Nonfunctioning Carcinomas		12†

*8 women, 2 men.
†Sex equally distributed.

231

quate numbers for evaluation. Primary tumors and metastases were compared with respect to the variability of histologic patterns and cellular morphology.

Ten of the patients had functioning carcinomas (Table 1), all of which were searched for evidence of microscopic patterns that would reflect the functional character of the carcinoma.

Analysis of Cases

AGE, SEX, AND RACE OF PATIENTS.—The ages of the 22 patients ranged from 10 to 71 years; 18 of the group being in the third, fourth, fifth, and sixth decades of life. The median age at the time of diagnosis was 44 years. Of the 22 patients, 14 were women; the ratio of men to women was 1 to 1.75. All patients were Caucasians (Table 2).

TREATMENT

Table 3 lists the surgical treatment and the type of pathologic material reviewed. The primary tumor in 19 patients was surgically excised. The three patients who had only a biopsy subsequently died, and the primary tumor was examined at autopsy.

With three exceptions, the major surgical procedures were performed outside M. D. Anderson Hospital. Postoperatively, the majority of the patients received chemotherapy, and several received radiotherapy to the site of the primary tumor.

TABLE 2.—ADRENAL CORTICAL CARCINOMA
22 Patients

AGE ON DIAGNOSIS	NUMBER OF PATIENTS	FUNCTIONING Men	FUNCTIONING Women	NONFUNCTIONING Men	NONFUNCTIONING Women
0–10	1				1
11–20	1				1
21–30	3		3		
31–40	4	1	1		2
41–50	5		3	2	
51–60	6	1	1	2	2
61–70	1			1	
71	1			1	
Total	22	2	8	6	6

Ages ranged from 10 to 71 years.
Median age on admission 45.
Median age on diagnosis 44.
Median age of onset 43 (based on 14 patients).
Ratio male to female 1 to 1.75.

TABLE 3.—ADRENAL CORTICAL CARCINOMA
22 Patients

SURGICAL TREATMENT	NUMBER OF PATIENTS
Biopsy only	3
Adrenalectomy	14°
Adrenalectomy and Nephrectomy	5

°Nephrectomy performed for recurrent disease after adre-
nalectomy in 2 patients.
Major surgical procedures performed at M. D. Anderson
Hospital on 3 of 19 patients.

PATHOLOGY

GROSS PATHOLOGIC CHARACTERISTICS OF TUMORS.—The sites of the 22 tumors were equally divided on each side of the body. The size of the
primary carcinoma removed from 15 patients was known. These were
consistently large neoplasms, the largest measuring 36 cm. in diameter.
They were round, ovoid, or lobulated, encapsulated masses of soft, yellow-
brown tumor tissue containing areas of necrosis and hemorrhage. Invasion
of the retroperitoneum was a prominent feature. Eleven of the 22 tumors
(50 per cent) had invaded the retroperitoneal soft tissues at the time of the
primary operation.

MICROSCOPIC FEATURES.—For orientation in the microscopic diagnosis
and for differentiation from adenoma, adrenal cortical carcinomas may be
divided into two groups: differentiated and pleomorphic or undifferentiated. The differentiated type is composed of polygonal cells resembling
the cells of the adrenal cortex. The neoplastic cells are arranged in more
than one cellular pattern: they may be observed in sheets (Fig. 1A), in
trabeculae (Fig. 1B), in small nests (Fig. 1C), or in a ribbon-like pattern
(Fig. 1D). The last is the least common. Primary tumors exhibiting these
patterns must be distinguished from adenoma, whereas those in metastatic
locations must be distinguished from hepatic and renal cell carcinoma.

Adrenal cortical carcinoma exhibiting the pleomorphic or undifferentiated pattern is typical of a highly malignant neoplasm. This pattern is
composed of pleomorphic cells lacking cohesion and containing bizarre
nuclei (Fig. 2). Carcinomas of this type must be distinguished from metastatic pleomorphic carcinomas.

Both pleomorphic and differentiated adrenal cortical carcinomas may be
observed in the same tumor. They were associated focally or diffusely in
variable degrees in all of the 22 tumors in this group (Fig. 3). Necrosis
(Fig. 1A) and mitotic figures are the rule in both differentiated and

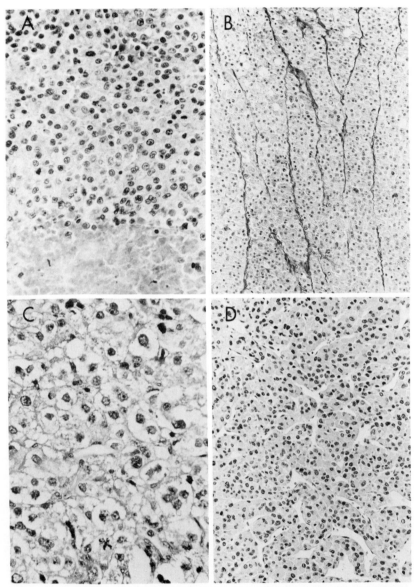

Fɪɢ. 1.—Differentiated carcinoma. *A*, diffuse or sheet pattern. Inferiorly, an area of necrosis is apparent. *B*, trabecular pattern. Here the neoplastic cells are organized in rows of more than one cell separated by fibrous septae and capillaries, although rows of single cells resembling the fascicular zone of the gland might be observed. Several

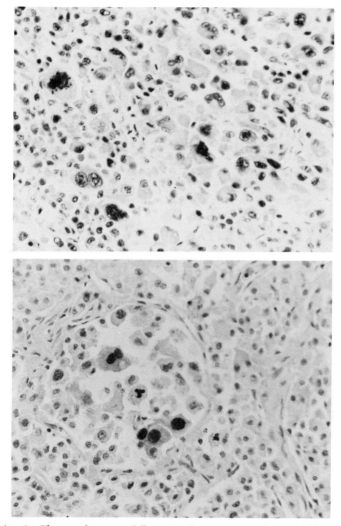

Fig. 2 (*top*).—Pleomorphic or undifferentiated pattern typical of a highly malignant tumor. The pleomorphic cells lack cellular cohesion and contain bizarre nuclei.

Fig. 3 (*bottom*).—Area of pleomorphism pattern adjacent to differentiated carcinoma. The pleomorphic cells lack cohesion. A tripolar mitosis is apparent.

---

cells in mitosis are present. *C*, small nests of vacuolated cells. A tripolar mitosis may be observed near the lower border of the picture. *D*, ribbon pattern. We have seen this pattern in scattered areas of a few tumors.

TABLE 4.—Adrenal Cortical Carcinoma
9 Autopsy Cases

Sites of Metastases	Number of Cases
Liver	7
Retroperitoneum	6
Lymph nodes	6
Lungs	5
Kidney, intestine, pancreas	2 each
Spleen, opposite adrenal, pericardium, pleura, and bone	1 each

pleomorphic adrenal cortical carcinoma. Tripolar mitosis is occasionally observed (Figs. 1C and 3).

Dissemination.—Adrenal cortical carcinoma spreads through the blood stream and lymphatic circulation to distant sites. Invasion of blood vessels at the site of the primary lesion was not a prominent feature in this group of cases. At autopsy on two subjects, the renal vein and inferior vena cava were found to have been invaded.

A combination of the clinical, radiographic, and pathologic evidence of metastases in these cases showed that the lungs, retroperitoneum, liver, and lymph nodes, in descending order, were involved most often. The sites of metastases observed at autopsy in nine patients are shown in Table 4.

Associated disease.—An occult papillary and a follicular carcinoma of the thyroid gland were discovered in one subject. Otherwise, no associated diseases were observed in this group.

Mortality

Eighteen of the 22 patients have died, 11 within two years after their operation or diagnosis; of these 11 patients, 10 died as the result of the

TABLE 5.—Adrenal Cortical Carcinoma
18 Patients—Mortality

	Number of Patients
Less than 2-year follow-up (3 had biopsy alone)	11
2 to 5-year follow-up	3
5 to 11-year follow-up	4
	18°

°14 died of disease; 2 died of other cause; 2 died, cause unknown.

tumor. The remaining seven of the 18 patients survived from two to 11 years. Four of the seven died of the carcinoma (Table 5).

Five of the 10 patients who died of the tumor within two years had functional adrenal cortical carcinoma. Also, two patients who lived from two to 11 years had functioning carcinoma.

Four of the 22 patients are still living, three of whom have evidence of disease at one, five, and six years. Two of the four had a functioning carcinoma. One patient without evidence of disease has been followed for only seven months after removal of a functioning tumor.

Discussion

Both adenomas and carcinomas, the two types of neoplastic lesions that originate in the adrenal cortex, can be functional or nonfunctional; the clinical picture depends upon the hormone produced by the tumor.

Adrenal cortical carcinomas are consistently large. At the time of diagnosis, they have usually invaded the adjacent retroperitoneal soft tissues. Invasion of the retroperitoneum was evident at operation in 11 of the 22 patients in this series.

Mitotic figures, necrosis, and cellular pleomorphism are the basis of the diagnosis of adrenal cortical carcinoma. Necrosis was observed in all of our cases in areas of well-differentiated carcinoma and also in areas with pleomorphic patterns. Mitotic figures are the rule; tripolar mitosis is occasionally observed. Invasion of blood vessels was not a prominent finding in this group.

Well-differentiated patterns of adrenal cortical carcinoma alone may be difficult to distinguish from the pattern of adenoma. The presence of necrosis and mitotic figures is unusual in adenoma. Pleomorphic nuclei appear in benign adenoma, although they are more prominent and numerous in carcinoma. Some of the problem cases may be solved only by the demonstration of invasion of the retroperitoneal soft tissues or of distant metastases.

Clinical evidence of function in an adrenal cortical tumor gives assurance of a primary lesion in the adrenal gland. Since we are dealing with a gland that frequently is the site of metastatic lesions, carcinomas should be considered nonfunctional only when the histologic criteria are strictly fulfilled. In this series, we could find no significant difference between the microscopic patterns of the functional and nonfunctional tumors, nor could we find evidence to support the suggestion of some authors that tumors with structures similar to those of the normal adrenal cortex are functional (Cahill *et al.*, 1936; Heinbecker, O'Neal, and Ackerman, 1957;

Birke *et al.*, 1959). On comparison, primary and metastatic lesions exhibited identical histologic features.

It is pointed out that metastasis to the brain is rare in adrenal cortical carcinoma, although it has been reported (Hutter and Kayhoe, 1966 and Huvos, Hajdu, Brasfield, and Foote, 1970). The brain of eight of nine patients autopsied was examined; none of the brains contained metastases.

Twelve of 19 patients who received major surgical treatment subsequently had recurrent tumor in the abdomen. A significant number of these tumors recur in the area of the primary lesion and in the retroperitoneum. In seven of the 12, the tumor recurred in the adrenal primary area.

The aggressive behavior of adrenal cortical carcinoma is portrayed by the mortality figures in this group. Fourteen of 18 patients, or 77.7 per cent, have died as the result of the disease, 10 within two years after the diagnosis.

Summary

Twenty-two cases of primary adrenal cortical carcinomas have been reviewed; 10 were functioning, while 12 were nonfunctioning tumors. Necrosis, mitotic figures, and undifferentiated patterns are helpful in establishing the diagnosis of malignant disease and in differentiation from adenoma. Functioning and nonfunctioning carcinomas exhibit a similar histologic morphology. Care should be exercised in the diagnosis of nonfunctioning carcinoma of the adrenal gland, since this structure is often the site of metastatic lesions.

The liver, retroperitoneum, lung, and lymph nodes are most often the sites of metastases. Metastasis to the brain is rare. The tumors usually recur in the retroperitoneum or at the primary site, or both.

Eighteen of the 22 patients are dead, 14 as the result of the tumor. Ten of these 14 died within two years after the diagnosis. This demonstrates the aggressive behavior of adrenal cortical carcinoma.

REFERENCES

Birke, G., Franksson, C., Gemzell, C.-A., Moberger, G., and Plantin, L.-O.: Adrenal cortical tumours. A study with special reference to possibilities of correlating histologic appearance with hormonal activity. *Acta chirurgica scandinavica*, 117:223-246, 1969.

Cahill, G. F., Loeb, R. F., Kurzrok, R., Stout, A. P., and Smith, F. M.: Adrenal cortical tumors. *Surgery, Gynecology and Obstetrics*, 62:287-313, 1936.

Clemmesen, J.: Statistical studies in the aetiology of malignant neoplasms. II. Munksgaard, Copenhagen, 1965. *Danish Cancer Registry under the National Anti-Cancer League.*

Ferber, B., Hardy, V. H., Gerhardt, P. R., and Solomon, M.: Cancer in New York State, exclusive of New York City 1941-1960. *Albany, 1962. Bureau of Cancer Control, New York State Department of Health.*

Griswold, M. H., Wilder, C. S., Cutler, S. J., and Pollock, E. S.: Cancer in Connecticut, 1935-1951. *Hartford, 1955. Connecticut State Department of Health.*

Heinbecker, P., O'Neal, L. W., and Ackerman, L. V.: Functioning and nonfunctioning adrenal cortical tumors. *Surgery, Gynecology and Obstetrics,* 105:21-33, 1957.

Hutter, A. M., and Kayhoe, D. E.: Adrenal cortical carcinoma. Clinical features of 138 patients. *The American Journal of Medicine,* 41:572-580, 1966.

Huvos, A. G., Hajdu, S. I., Brasfield, R. D., and Foote, F. W., Jr.: Adrenal cortical carcinoma. Clinicopathologic study of 34 cases. *Cancer,* 25:354-361, 1970.

Lipsett, M. B., Hertz, R., and Ross, G. T.: Clinical and pathophysiologic aspects of adrenocortical carcinoma. *The American Journal of Medicine,* 35:374-383, 1963.

Macfarlane, D. A.: Cancer of the adrenal cortex. The natural history, prognosis and treatment in a study of fifty-five cases. *Annals of the Royal College of Surgeons of England,* 23:155-186, 1958.

Rapaport, E. R., Goldberg, M. B., Gordon, G. S., and Hinman, F., Jr.: Mortality in surgically treated adrenocortical tumors. II. Reviews of cases reported for the 20 year period 1930-1949, inclusive. *Postgraduate Medicine,* 11:325-353, 1952.

Pathology of Tumors of the Adrenal Medulla

BRUCE MACKAY, M.B., Ch.B., Ph.D., AND
SIDNEY H. ROSENHEIM, M.D.

*Department of Anatomic Pathology, The University of Texas
at Houston M. D. Anderson Hospital and Tumor Institute,
Houston, Texas*

IN THIS PAPER, a brief survey of the development of the adrenal medulla and related structures is followed by a consideration of the pathology of pheochromocytoma and neuroblastoma.

Development of the Adrenal Medulla

In the three-week-old embryo, the developing central nervous system has the form of a long plate of ectoderm in which there is a longitudinal furrow, the neural groove. Cells of the neural crest first make their appearance along each side of the groove. As the sides of the neural groove approach one another and fuse, converting the developing nervous system into a tube, neural crest cells migrate dorsolaterally to form the sensory ganglia of the cranial and spinal nerves (Arey, 1965). Processes of these ganglion cells grow peripherally as the axons of the peripheral nerves, and they are accompanied by neural crest cells which form their Schwann cell sheaths.

The ganglia of the sympathetic system are formed from neural crest cells that migrate from the thoracic region of the crest about the fifth week to relocate immediately dorsolateral to the aorta where they form the sympathetic chains (Langman, 1969). Some of the sympathetic neuroblasts migrate to the anterior aspect of the aorta to form the celiac and other sympathetic ganglia. The derivation of the parasympathetic ganglia which are formed along sensory cranial nerves is less well understood (Langman, 1969).

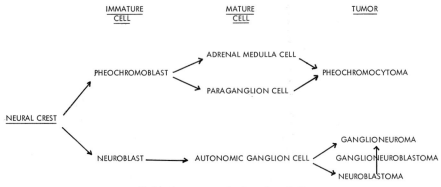

Fɪɢ. 1.—Cellular derivation of adrenal medullary tumors.

A secondary migration of neural crest cells occurs during the seventh week, and these cells differ from neuroblasts in that they develop an affinity for chromium salts, hence their designation as pheochromoblasts. Groups of these cells invade the medial aspect of the developing adrenal cortex, which is of mesodermal origin, and form the adrenal medulla (Hervonen, 1971). Others form the para-aortic bodies (of Zückerkandl), paired structures on each side of the abdominal aorta close to its bifurcation, and small clusters of pheochromocytes are found at other levels in the paravertebral region. Neuroblasts also migrate into the developing adrenal medulla where they differentiate into ganglion cells (Hervonen, 1971).

The two lines of cells of neural crest origin, and the tumors that arise from them, are summarized in Figure 1.

Pheochromocytoma

Pheochromocytoma is a tumor of pheochromocytes and it may therefore occur at any site where these cells are found. Approximately 90 per cent of these tumors are located within the adrenal gland, and the majority of the extra-adrenal tumors are related to the para-aortic bodies (Evans, 1966). The tumor has been described in a wide variety of locations, however, including the scrotum (into which the pheochromocytes are drawn by the descending testis), urinary bladder, mediastinum, and the cervical sympathetic chain.

Pheochromocytoma is a relatively rare tumor. It occurs most frequently in the third through the sixth decades, but juvenile patients have been reported (Stackpole, Melicow, and Uson, 1963). In adults, the sexes are equally affected, but pheochromocytomas occur more frequently in boys than girls (Stackpole, Melicow, and Uson, 1963). The adrenal tumors are bilateral in 10 per cent of patients, but this figure rises to 40 per cent in familial cases and to 70 per cent in cases of Sipple's syndrome (Catalona, Engelman, Ketcham, and Hammond, 1971), in which the pheochromocytoma coexists with medullary carcinoma of the thyroid and parathyroid adenoma. Simultaneous intra- and extra-adrenal pheochromocytomas may occur.

The tumors are typically encapsulated and vary tremendously in size. Pharmacologically active tumors measuring 1 cm. in diameter have been reported (Russell and Rubenstein, 1971), and at the other extreme Sherwin described a tumor that weighed 2,200 Gm. (Sherwin, 1959). The cut surface is generally dark grey to dark red, and while the appearance may be uniform, zones of hemorrhage and necrosis and cyst formation are generally present.

The pheochromocytoma is "chromaffin positive," a property reflecting the affinity of its cells for chromium salts. The reaction is not specific, but it may be of some assistance in the diagnosis of a tumor where the histological appearance is not diagnostic. The reaction depends on the oxidation of the catecholamines present within the tumor cells, and in fact is not necessarily dependent on chromium salts since certain other oxidizing agents will also give positive results (Sherwin and Rosen, 1965). However, Zenker's fixative solution, available in most pathology laboratories, provides a convenient reagent for the performance of the chromaffin reaction. Fresh tissue must be used, since catecholamines react with formalin and may not be detectable even by chemical analysis after fixation (Walters, 1969). A satisfactory procedure is to place a thin slice of the tumor on a glass slide and to apply to the cut surface a few drops of Zenker's solution from which the acetic acid has been omitted. As described in the AFIP Staining Manual, the composition of the fluid is as follows:

distilled water	100 ml.
mercuric chloride	5 Gm.
potassium dichromate	2.5 Gm.
sodium sulfate	1 Gm.

The pH of the solution should be between 5.0 and 6.0 (Kennedy, Symington, and Woodger, 1961). A positive result is indicated by the tumor surface becoming a deep chocolate brown within 30 minutes. The catecholamines are oxidized by the dichromate to give the brown reaction product. Pheochromocytomas which produce only norepinephrine may give a weak reaction, and the reaction product may then be difficult to recognize in the presence of the Zenker's solution. In this situation, 10 per cent potassium iodide, a colorless solution which oxidizes norepinephrine, may be applied to the cut surface of the tumor. It will become deep brown within 30 minutes if the reaction is positive (Sherwin and Rosen, 1965).

The microscopic pattern of a pheochromocytoma can vary, but sections typically contain nests of cells separated by thin connective tissue septae (Fig. 2A). Numerous sinusoids and thin-walled veins are present. Diffuse sheets of cells, and occasionally a pseudopapillary arrangement, may be seen. The tumor cells are usually polyhedral or spherical, and tend to be

Fig. 2.—Pheochromocytoma. A, light micrograph showing nests of tumor cells encircled by partitions of connective tissue containing blood vessels. Very little pleomorphism is seen. Hematoxylin and eosin. × 250. B, light micrograph of a number of cells from a pheochromocytoma processed for electron microscopy. Intracytoplasmic granules are evident in this Epon-embedded section. Methylene blue. × 400.

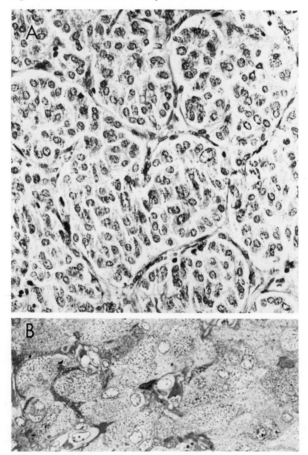

larger than those of the normal adrenal medulla. The cytoplasm is often lightly basophilic and finely granular. This granular character becomes readily apparent in sections of tissue prepared for electron microscopic study and viewed with the light microscope after staining with methylene blue (Fig. 2B). The nuclei of the tumor cells are typically spherical, central, and regular in appearance. However, cellular and nuclear pleomorphism does occur and is not a reliable criterion of malignancy since it is frequently seen in benign tumors. Likewise, capsular invasion and vascular penetration, while they may occasion suspicion of an aggressive disposition, are not proof of malignancy (Evans, 1966; Russell and Rubenstein, 1971). The only way to establish the diagnosis of malignant pheochromocytoma is to demonstrate unequivocal metastases in sites at which chromaffin tissue does not normally occur, such as lymph nodes and liver. Since pheochromocytomas may be multicentric, the surgeon and the pathologist must be cautious in assessing the significance of multiple tumors, and an awareness of the normal distribution of chromaffin tissue can be helpful. The incidence of malignancy is not greater than 10 per cent (Symington and Goodall, 1953).

Electron microscopic studies (Tannenbaum, 1970; Cornog *et al.*, 1970; Yokoyama and Takayasu, 1969; Misugi, Misugi, and Newton, 1968) have shown that the fine structural features of pheochromocytoma cells are similar to those of normal adrenal medulla. The tumor cells may possess short peripheral processes (Fig. 3A), but these appear to be unusual features. Many catecholamine granules are present within the cytoplasm, and these appear in electron micrographs as approximately spherical electron-dense bodies surrounded by a limiting membrane. In contrast, cells of the adrenal cortex and its tumors do not possess these secretory granules.

Morphological differences have been described between epinephrine and norepinephrine granules in the normal adrenal medulla (Coupland and Hopwood, 1966; Kadin and Bensch, 1971). Mature norepinephrine granules possess a uniform electron density and are often eccentrically positioned within the limiting membrane. Epinephrine granules are larger, less electron dense, and have a finely granular character. In the normal human adrenal medulla, chemical analysis shows that norepinephrine represents from 5 to 15 per cent of the total catecholamines (Blaschko *et al.*, 1968). Analysis of pheochromocytomas has shown the reverse: most tumors contain a predominance of norepinephrine (Blaschko *et al.*, 1968; Tannenbaum, 1970). Tannenbaum (1970), in his review of the fine structural features of adrenal medullary tumors, observed that 12 of 14 tumors in his series contained a predominance of norepinephrine by chemical analysis, and the great majority of the cells in these tumors possessed nor-

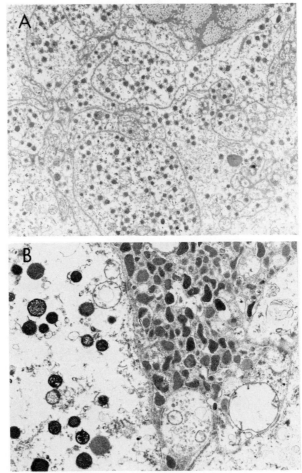

FIG. 3.—Pheochromocytoma. *A*, electron micrograph of an area removed from the adrenal gland of a 26-year-old female patient who also had a solid (medullary) carcinoma of the thyroid. There was a family history of both tumors. Many transversely sectioned cell processes can be seen, containing electron-dense secretory granules. × 7,000. *B*, electron micrograph of parts of two pheochromocytoma cells with an obvious difference in numbers of secretory granules. A nerve ending is present on the periphery of the cell containing many granules and small synaptic vesicles are seen within the nerve. The clear circle to the right of the nerve ending is a distended mitochondrion. × 10,000.

epinephrine granules. Our own observations on the fine structure of pheochromocytomas suggest that while variations in the number and appearance of the granules may be striking from one cell to another (Fig. 3), sharp distinctions between the two types of granules may be less readily apparent than in the normal human adrenal medulla. Nerve endings containing synaptic vesicles are present on the cells of the normal adrenal medulla, but are rarely detected on pheochromocytoma cells (Fig. 3B).

Neuroblastoma

Neuroblastoma is a tumor of neuroblasts, the undifferentiated precursors of cells of the peripheral nervous system. It is a highly malignant tumor with peak incidence in the first two years of life. In a recent series, 21 per cent of the patients were under one year of age, and 83 per cent were under four years of age (Stella, Schweisguth, and Schlienger, 1970). Neuroblastoma is infrequent in adolescents and rare in adults. The sexes are affected approximately equally.

Approximately two thirds of all neuroblastomas arise in the retroperitoneal region, the majority within the adrenal glands, although the primary site may be impossible to determine in the presence of extensive retroperitoneal disease. Extra-abdominal sites include the mediastinum, pelvis, and neck region. Usually (Russell and Rubenstein, 1971; Stella, Schweisguth, and Schlienger, 1970), the tumor is unilateral. Metastatic disease frequently is present when the patient is first seen: lymph nodes, bone, and liver are the sites most likely to be involved (Stella, Schweisguth, and Schlienger, 1970). Grossly, neuroblastomas are soft, friable tumors which appear to be encapsulated. The cut surface is dark red to dark gray, and zones of hemorrhage and necrosis are characteristic. Focal calcification may be present. Histologically (Fig. 4), neuroblasts resemble small lymphocytes, being small round cells with hyperchromatic nuclei and scanty cytoplasm. As the differentiation of the tumor increases, the nuclear staining becomes less dense and the cells are larger with more obvious cytoplasm. Rosette formation, a circle of tumor cells surrounding a small central tangle of neurofibrils, is an inconstant finding, and attempts to demonstrate rosettes by silver impregnation techniques are often disappointing (Russell and Rubenstein, 1971). The presence of well-differentiated ganglion cells indicates that the tumor is undergoing maturation.

Electron microscopic studies of neuroblastomas have shown that the fine structural appearance of the tumor cells varies to some degree with the differentiation of the tumor (Misugi, Misugi, and Newton, 1968). The better differentiated tumor cell is roughly spherical with a centrally placed

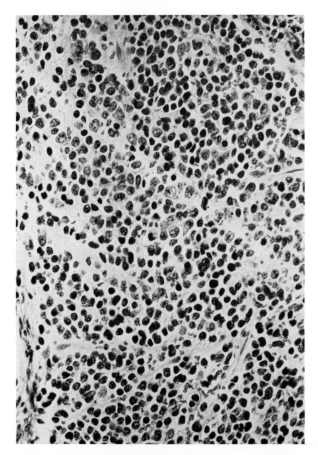

FIG. 4.—Light micrograph of a mediastinal neuroblastoma removed from an 11-year-old boy. The tumor cells resemble poorly differentiated lymphocytes. Hematoxylin and eosin. × 250.

nucleus which usually has a regular, circular profile. The cell membranes of adjacent cells are typically closely apposed (Fig. 5) and occasional small thickenings of the membranes are present. It is tempting to suggest that these structures are poorly developed desmosomes, but we have never seen intermediate lines or associated bundles of tonofilaments to justify this assertion. The cytoplasmic organelles are not remarkable. Mitochondria are not particularly numerous, and the endoplasmic reticulum tends to be limited to scattered, rough-surfaced cisternae (Tannenbaum 1970; Misugi, Misugi, and Newton, 1968). A characteristic finding is the presence of variable numbers of secretory granules (Fig. 5) which are smaller than those found in pheochromocytoma cells but which possess the same basic structure, comprising a spherical electron-dense core intimately surrounded by a limiting membrane (Misugi, Misugi, and Newton, 1968). Slender dendritic processes are present at the periphery of the cells, and these also contain secretory granules. Neuroblastoma cell processes may also contain longitudinally oriented microtubules (Fig. 5), although these are not as numerous as in the processes of ganglioneuroma cells. Synaptic-like structures have been reported by different observers (Tannenbaum, 1970; Kadin and Bensch, 1971; Yokoyama and Takayasu, 1969; Misugi, Misugi, and Newton, 1968). In the poorly differentiated neuroblastoma cell, cytoplasmic processes are poorly developed and the cells may contain only occasional secretory granules. The secretory granules in neuroblastoma cells represent stored catecholamines, and the diagnosis often can be confirmed biochemically by quantitating urinary excretion of catecholamine metabolites (Kaser, 1966; Gitlow *et al.*, 1970). Patients with neuroblastoma usually have elevated levels of more than one urinary catabolite (Gitlow *et al.*, 1970). The determination of homovanillic acid also is of value in the differential diagnosis of neural crest tumors because the excretion of this metabolite almost always is normal in patients with benign pheochromocytoma and is elevated in patients with neuroblastoma (Walters, 1969; Kaser, 1966; Gitlow, Mendlowitz, and Bertani, 1970).

The pathological diagnosis of neuroblastoma frequently is difficult. The tumor metastasizes rapidly and extensively and a metastatic focus often is the first indication that a neoplasm is present. A poorly differentiated neuroblastoma may be difficult to distinguish from other tumors composed of small lymphocyte-like cells, and the differential diagnosis must include lymphoma, Ewing's sarcoma, and embryonal rhabdomyosarcoma. Many lesions diagnosed as Ewing's tumor of bone are, in fact, metastases from a neuroblastoma (Symington, 1967). Clinical or radiological localization of the primary tumor also can be difficult, particularly when the tumor is outside the adrenal gland. In these situations, electron microscopic study may prove valuable. The characteristic fine structural appearance of neuroblastoma cells readily distinguishes them from the other tumors which neuroblastoma may resemble at the light microscopic level (Friedman and Hanaoka, 1971). In disseminated neuroblastoma, no metastatic focus may be accessible for biopsy, but tumor cells frequently are present in the bone marrow and can be seen in smears of the marrow aspirate. The diagnosis then may be established by electron microscopy. The technical aspects of processing this specimen are important if well-preserved tumor cells are to be obtained, but with careful techniques, diagnosis is possible. Even the poorly differentiated neuroblastoma cells usually contain at least a few

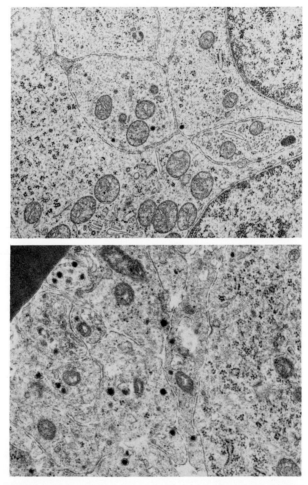

Fig. 5 (*top*).—Electron micrograph of a metastatic neuroblastoma in the scrotal sac of a 3-year-old boy. The primary tumor in the adrenal gland had been previously excised. Parts of the nuclei of two tumor cells are visible with portions of the cytoplasm of the two cells, and three cell processes are present between the cells. The membranes of cells and processes are intimately apposed. Occasional small electron-dense secretory granules are seen and in the process on the right of the illustration many slender microtubules are present in cross section. × 13,000.

Fig. 6. (*bottom*).—A 6-year-old girl was referred with the diagnosis of acute leukemia. Electron microscopy of a bone marrow aspirate revealed tumor cells having numerous slender processes in which secretory granules were present. The diagnosis of neuroblastoma was confirmed at autopsy. × 20,000.

catecholamine granules. Electron microscopic study of the bone marrow may provide the diagnosis and avoid the time, expense, and inconvenience of more complex diagnostic procedures, thereby permitting earlier initiation of therapy than would otherwise be possible. The electron micrograph in Figure 6 is of a bone marrow aspirate from a six-year-old girl referred to M. D. Anderson Hospital with the diagnosis of acute leukemia, based on abnormal cells present in her bone marrow. The tumor cells possessed many dendritic processes, and catecholamine granules were readily demonstrated, establishing the diagnosis of neuroblastoma.

Several unusual aspects of the biology of neuroblastoma merit comments. Where the neuroblastoma has not metastasized, a child less than two years old will have a better prognosis than an older child (Sutow *et al.*, 1970). The five-year survival rate in the younger age group is 72 per cent compared to 12 per cent for the older children. Neuroblastomas may regress spontaneously. This occurs primarily in children under six months of age (Bolande, 1971). The finding of a much higher incidence of *in situ* adrenal neuroblastoma in autopsied infants (1 in 39 to 1 in 500) compared with the over-all incidence of neuroblastoma (1 in 10,000) suggests that these *in situ* tumors normally regress during the first few months of life (Bolande, 1971; Guin, Gilbert, and Jones, 1969). Some neuroblastomas undergo maturation to ganglioneuroma. Two well-documented cases of neuroblastoma in infants of 7 months and 18 months were followed for 20 years and 46 years, respectively, during which periods the tumors matured to ganglioneuromas (Fox, Davidson, and Thomas, 1959). Another patient was born with approximately 40 subcutaneous masses of neuroblastoma which were diagnosed by surgical biopsy. Treatment was not undertaken but growth and development proceeded normally. At ages five and eight, biopsy specimens of lesions had the histological appearance of ganglioneuromas, and the patient was alive at age 14 with radiologic evidence of calcification in the liver, left adrenal, and retroperitoneal lymph node areas (Griffin and Bolande, 1969). A further case of maturation of a neuroblastoma is described by Haber and Bennington (1963).

Ganglioneuroma, a benign tumor derived from neuroblasts, occurs more frequently than neuroblastoma and is found in older patients. Ganglioneuromas usually occur in the posterior mediastinum but also may be found in the retroperitoneum, mesentery, and gastrointestinal tract. The tumors are slow growing and frequently do not produce clinical symptoms. A mass may be discovered during a routine physical examination or on X-ray films obtained for other purposes. Grossly, the tumor is encapsulated and firm in consistency. The tumor may be large, and attachment to the sympathetic chain may be evident. The cut surface is grayish-white and a whorled pattern may be apparent. Myxomatous change and calcification can occur.

The light microscopic appearance of the ganglioneuroma is quite characteristic (Fig. 7A). Mature ganglion cells, solitary and in small groups, are present amid bundles of nerve fibers and scattered collagen. Degenerative changes may be seen in the ganglion cells. Satellite cells are usually

FIG. 7.–Ganglioneuroma. *A*, light micrograph of a ganglioneuroma removed from the retroperitoneal region of a 10-year-old girl. Mature nerve cells are present amid bundles of nerve fibers. Hematoxylin and eosin. × 250. *B*, electron micrograph of a ganglioneuroma from the retroperitoneal region of a 7-year-old girl, showing unsheathed nerve fibers separated by zones of collagen fibrils. Longitudinally oriented microtubules are present within the nerve fibers, together with occasional catecholamine granules. × 13,000.

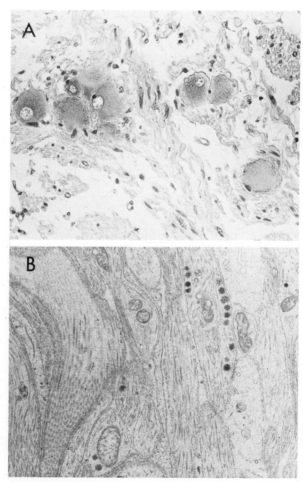

sparse. Electron microscopy (Fig. 7B) demonstrates that the nerve fibers are for the most part unmyelinated. However, myelin sheaths occasionally do occur and are often morphologically distorted. Some axons do not possess a Schwann cell sheath, and in these the basal lamina is usually prominent. Longitudinally oriented microtubules and groups of secretory granules are present within the axoplasm. Synaptic structures may be seen where a nerve fiber contacts the membrane of a ganglion cell.

The term ganglioneuroblastoma connotes a tumor which possesses histological features of both neuroblastoma and ganglioneuroma. The tumor is a neuroblastoma which is undergoing maturation, but it may metastasize, and it is therefore advisable to section many areas of an apparent ganglioneuroma before concluding that the tumor is benign.

Tumors of the carotid body and other branchial glomera, the so-called nonchromaffin paragangliomas, are composed of nests of tumor cells (Zellballen) surrounded by connective tissue septae containing blood vessels. With the electron microscope, the cells of these tumors are seen to contain membrane-bound granules similar to those in adrenal medullary cells. Histologically they thus resemble pheochromocytomas. Occasionally, a tumor occurring in one of these bodies is functional and gives a positive chromaffin reaction; as Symington (1953) points out, there is no good reason for not calling such a tumor a pheochromocytoma. Most tumors of the chemoreceptor organs are, however, chromaffin negative, and presumably this reflects their origin from the chief cells of the chemoreceptor organ rather than from pheochromocytes.

REFERENCES

Arey, L. B.: *Developmental Anatomy: A Textbook and Laboratory Manual of Embryology.* 7th edition. Philadelphia, Pennsylvania, W. B. Saunders Co., 1965, 695 pp.

Blaschko, H., Jerrome, D. W., Robb-Smith, A. H. T., Smith, A. D., and Winkler, H.: Biochemical and morphological studies on catecholamine storage in human phaeochromocytoma. *Clinical Science*, 34:453-465, 1968.

Bolande, R. P.: Benignity of neonatal tumors and concept of cancer repression in early life. *American Journal of Diseases of Children*, 122:12-14, July 1971.

Catalona, W. J., Engelman, K., Ketcham, A. S., and Hammond, W. G.: Familial medullary thyroid carcinoma, pheochromocytoma, and parathyroid adenoma (Sipple's syndrome): Study of a kindred. *Cancer*, 28:1245-1254, November 1971.

Cornog, J. L., Wilkinson, J. H., Arvan, D. A., Freed, R. M., Sellers, A. M., and Barker, C.: Extra-adrenal pheochromocytoma: Some electron microscopic and biochemical studies. *The American Journal of Medicine*, 48:654-660, May 1970.

Coupland, R. E., and Hopwood, D.: Mechanism of a histochemical reaction differentiating between adrenaline- and noradrenaline-storing cells in the electron microscope. *Nature*, 209:590-591, February 1966.

Evans, R. W.: *Histological Appearance of Tumours; With a Consideration of Their Histogenesis and Certain Aspects of Their Clinical Features and Behaviour.* 2nd edition. Edinburgh, Scotland, Livingstone, 1966, 1255 pp.

Fox, F., Davidson, J., and Thomas, L. B.: Maturation of sympathicoblastoma into ganglioneuroma: Report of 2 patients with 20- and 46-year survivals respectively. *Cancer*, 12:108-116, January-February 1959.

Friedman, H., and Hanaoka, H.: Round-cell sarcomas of bone. *The Journal of Bone and Joint Surgery*, 53-A:1118-1136, September 1971.

Gitlow, S. E., Mendlowitz, M., and Bertani, L. M.: The biochemical techniques for detecting and establishing the presence of a pheochromocytoma. *The American Journal of Cardiology*, 26:270-279, September 1970.

Gitlow, S. E., Bertani, L. M., Rausen, A., Gribetz, D., and Dziedzic, S. W.: Diagnosis of neuroblastoma by qualitative and quantitative determination of catecholamine metabolites in urine. *Cancer*, 25:1377-1383, June 1970.

Griffin, M. E., and Bolande, R. P.: Familial neuroblastoma with regression and maturation to ganglioineurofibroma. *Pediatrics*, 43:377-382, March 1969.

Guin, G. H., Gilbert, E. F., and Jones, B.: Incidental neuroblastoma in infants. *The American Journal of Clinical Pathology*, 51:126-136, January 1969.

Haber, S. L., and Bennington, J. L.: Maturation of congenital extra-adrenal neuroblastoma. *Archives of Pathology*, 76:121-125, August 1963.

Hervonen, A.: Development of catecholamine-storing cells in human fetal paraganglia and adrenal medulla: A histochemical and electron microscopical study. *Acta Physiologica Scandinavica*, Suppl. 368, Helsinki, 1971, 94 pp.

Kadin, M. E., and Bensch, K. G.: Comparison of pheochromocytes with ganglion cells and neuroblasts grown in vitro. An electron microscopic and histochemical study. *Cancer*, 27:1148-1160, May 1971.

Kaser, H.: Catecholamine-producing neural tumors other than pheochromocytoma. *Pharmacological Reviews*, 18:659-665, 1966.

Kennedy, J. S., Symington, T., and Woodger, B. A.: Chemical and histochemical observations in benign and malignant phaeochromocytoma. *The Journal of Pathology and Bacteriology*, 81:409-418, 1961.

Langman, J.: *Medical Embryology*. 2nd edition. Baltimore, Maryland, The Williams and Wilkins Co., 1969, 386 pp.

Luna, L. G., Ed.: *Manual of Histologic Staining Methods of the Armed Forces Institute of Pathology*. 3rd edition. New York, New York, Blakiston Division, McGraw-Hill Book Co., 1968, p. 4.

Misugi, K., Misugi, N., and Newton, W. A., Jr.: Fine structural study of neuroblastoma, ganglioneuroblastoma, and pheochromocytoma. *Archives of Pathology*, 86:160-170, August 1968.

Russell, D. S., and Rubenstein, L. J.: *Pathology of Tumours of the Nervous System*. 3rd edition. Baltimore, Maryland, The Williams and Wilkins Co., 1971, 429 pp.

Sherwin, R. P.: Histopathology of pheochromocytoma. *Cancer*, 12:861-877, September-October 1959.

Sherwin, R. P., and Rosen, V. J.: New aspects of the chromoreactions for the diagnosis of pheochromocytoma. *The American Journal of Clinical Pathology*, 43:200-206, March 1965.

Stackpole, R. H., Melicow, M. M., and Uson, A. C.: Pheochromocytoma in children: Report of 9 cases and review of the first 100 published cases with follow-up studies. *The Journal of Pediatrics*, 63:315-330, August 1963.

Stella, J. G., Schweisguth, O., and Schlienger, M.: Neuroblastoma: A study of 144 cases treated in the Institut Gustave-Roussy over a period of 7 years. *The American Journal of Roentgenology, Radium Therapy and Nuclear Medicine*, 108:324-332, February 1970.

Sutow, W. W., Gehan, E. A., Heyn, R. M., Kung, F. H., Miller, R. W., Murphy, M. L., and Traggis, D. G.: Comparison of survival curves, 1956 versus 1962, in children with Wilm's tumor and neuroblastoma. *Pediatrics*, 45:800-811, May 1970.

Symington, T.: Adrenal Gland. In Robbins, S. L.: *Pathology*. 3rd edition. Philadelphia, Pennsylvania, W. B. Saunders Co., 1967, pp. 1219-1247.

Symington, T., and Goodall, A. L.: Studies in pheochromocytoma; I. Pathological aspects. *Glasgow Medical Journal*, 34:75-96, 1953.

Tannenbaum, M.: Ultrastructural pathology of adrenal medullary tumors. In Sommers, S. C., Ed.: *Pathology Annual*. New York, New York, Appleton-Century-Crofts, 1970, pp. 145-171.

Walters, G.: Secretory characteristics of phaeochromocytoma and related tumors. Their diagnostic and clinical significance. *Annals of the Royal College of Surgeons of England*, 45:150-161, 1969.

Yokoyama, M., and Takayasu, H.: An electron microscopic study of the human adrenal medulla and pheochromocytoma. *Urologia Internationalis*, 24:79-95, 1969.

Polyglandular Disease and Pancreatic Islet Cell Cancer

ROBERT C. HICKEY, M.D.

Department of Surgery, The University of Texas at Houston
M. D. Anderson Hospital and Tumor Institute,
Houston, Texas

DURING THE PAST TWO DECADES, considerable interest has centered around multiple endocrine adenomatosis (MEA) as being a group of syndromes, variously identified with descriptive adjectives or names. The polyglandular disease(s) focuses on those glands of ectodermal and endodermal origins which produce peptide substances or hormones; those glands which arise from the nephrogenic ridge, i.e., testes, ovaries, and adrenal cortex, are generally excluded, and also they are influenced by trophic discharges from the other glands.

The collective nosologic entity of anterior pituitary, parathyroid, and pancreatic adenomas has been well recognized for several decades as an individual patient entity, even though its occurrence is rare. The familial disease aspect was described by Wermer (1954) and Moldawer, Nardi, and Raker (1954) as being a pattern of anterior pituitary, parathyroid, and islet cell pancreatic tumors. Wermer described the dominant autosomal gene inheritance with a high degree of penetrance in his description of a father and four of nine offspring afflicted with MEA.

The expression of the genetic defect appears to be variable, since there were five different endocrine tumor combinations in the kindred reported by Steiner, Goodman, and Powers (1968). These genealogic data, traced for seven generations, showed that endocrine neoplasia is inherited as an autosomal dominant gene with high penetrance. Karbach and Galindo (1970) described a Mexican-American family in which pancreatic nonbeta cancers, insulinomas, and parathyroid adenoma occurred. It must be recognized, however, that multiple endocrine disease is not familial in all or even most instances.

The polyglandular disease is highly variable. Attention does, however, focus on the syndrome of medullary cancer of the thyroid with pheochromocytomas, neurofibromatosis, and parathyroid adenoma, and on the mosaic identified as Wermer's syndrome (familial or not), which consists of pancreatic islet cell adenoma, parathyroid adenoma, and pituitary adenoma. To this latter is added, in the minds of many, a syndrome linked to the names of two American surgeons. This syndrome, identified with non-beta cell pancreatic tumors, gastric hypersecretion and hyperacidity, and severe peptic ulcer diathesis was described in detail initially in two cases reported by Zollinger and Ellison (1955), and it now bears their names. In the Milwaukee, Wisconsin, registry on the Zollinger-Ellison (Z-E) syndrome (Wilson, personal communication), approximately 1,000 patients with Z-E had been recorded by late 1971.

In an earlier report from the Ellison and Wilson registry, approximately 25 per cent of patients had MEA (Ellison and Wilson, 1964). Way, Goldman, and Dunphy (1968) reported that 12 of their 25 patients (48 per cent) had MEA; the authors commented that autopsy augmented this identification, and the great overlap necessitated a clinical investigation for pituitary, parathyroid, pancreatic, adrenal, thyroid, and carcinoid disease in all patients who appeared to have one facet of the syndrome.

Clinical Data

Stimulated by the background of interest in multiple endocrine disease, a retrospective review was done of all patients with islet cell carcinoma seen as inpatients or in consultation at The University of Texas M. D. Anderson Hospital and Tumor Institute from 1946 and 1970 (14 patients). All had a recent histologic review and confirmation with light microscopic techniques by Drs. William Russell and Serge Masse. Histological differentiation between glucagon-producing, gastrin-producing, insulin-producing, and noninsulin-producing islet cells, particularly when the tissue is neoplastic, is not possible. The tumors were scattered throughout the pan-

TABLE 1.—PANCREATIC ISLET CELL CANCER

Total:	14 patients, age 35 to 72 years	
Sex:	F. 5	M. 9
Hormonal Syndrome:	$\bar{s}$ 8	$\bar{c}$ 6
Average Age:	48 yrs.	53 yrs.

TABLE 2.—POLYGLANDULAR DISEASE AND PANCREATIC ISLET CELL CANCER
(14 PATIENTS) AT M. D. ANDERSON HOSPITAL

MAIN SYMPTOMS	No.
Pancreatic Related	7
Peptic Ulcer only	1
Diarrhea only	1
Peptic Ulcer and Diarrhea	1
Incidental	4
Multiple Endocrine Adenopathy	(0)
Other Cancer(s)	(4)

creas and had no location pattern. All seemed to develop from a single focus.

Of the 14 patients, 12 were Caucasian, 1 Latin American, and 1 Negro. The average age of the entire group was 51 years, the range in years being 35 to 72. There were nine men and five women. With respect to hormonal effects, six patients showed clinical activity and eight did not. In brief, eight patients had nonfunctioning islet cell cancers, one patient had preponderantly severe diarrhea, four patients had predominantly acid-peptic disease, and one had a measure of concomitant diarrhea or peptic ulcer disease (Tables 1 and 2). There was no evidence of MEA in the entire group, although one Hebrew patient had moderately severe diabetes mellitus but also had a familial history of diabetes mellitus. One patient had undescended testicles and hyperestrogenism. Four patients had other cancers, one of which was of thyroid origin. This latter merits further comment.

ISLET CELL CARCINOMAS OF THE PANCREAS, FUNCTIONING TUMORS

There were six patients, one woman and five men, with functioning islet-cell carcinomas of the pancreas. One, a white man aged 52, had a 15-year survival after metastasis to the liver was identified at time of posterior gastroenterostomy (February 1950). Two years before, symptoms of duodenal ulcer and diarrhea had begun. Total gastrectomy was done in April 1963, but he died 31 months later from liver replacement by cancer.

The total gastrectomy was the fourth surgical attempt to control the ulcer diathesis. The patient did well (31 months), but no definite tumor regression was noted. Total survival was 17 years, during 15 of which he had known liver metastases.

A second white man, aged 70, was found to have a hard, indurated, and fixed pancreas at time of partial colectomy for adenocarcinoma of the sigmoid colon (October 1968). Biopsy was not done. At M. D. Anderson Hospital, a celiac arteriogram made in February 1970 showed a pancreatic lesion with metastasis to the liver. Exploratory laparotomy and biopsy of the pancreas was done; diagnosis was islet cell carcinoma, which was treated with 5-fluorouracil (5-FU). He also had hypersecretion, prepyloric ulcer, and gastritis, which were managed medically. He died at home at age 75 of emaciation.

In this case, pancreatic cancer was diagnosed clinically two years before any peptic ulcer manifestations. The ulcer was controlled medically.

A white man aged 58 with fulminant Z-E triad, survived five months. The cause of death was exsanguination after total gastrectomy from an existing peptic ulcer erosion into an unligated pancreatic-duodenal artery. He had 89 mEq./L. free HCl and 108 mEq./L. total HCl and a 12-hour gastric juice volume of 1,640 ml.

A 38-year-old white woman was admitted in 1963 for left thyroid lobectomy for follicular carcinoma after supraclavicular lymph node biopsy. The specimen was interpreted as metastatic, poorly differentiated carcinoma "of the thyroid." An inoperable abdominal mass was found in 1967; biopsy indicated islet cell carcinoma of the pancreas. Histologic review of the supraclavicular biopsy done in 1963 indicated that this specimen was also islet cell cancer. After a five-year survival, she died in 1968 from massive neoplastic disease and duodenal ulcer hemorrhage.

This patient had two separate cancers. The islet cell pancreatic metastasis attracted attention to the thyroid and an incidental follicular thyroid cancer with metastases was found. Acid peptic disease was not present clinically for five years although islet cell cancer existed. Multiple endocrine cancers were present.

A Negro man aged 60 was admitted in August 1970 and is currently being seen in the clinic. His father had gynecomastia and died of diabetes mellitus; two brothers suffer from gynecomastia. The patient has undescended testicles, proved hyperestrogenism, severe diarrhea, and a medically controlled peptic ulcer.

On 5-FU therapy, this patient has had decreased gastric acidity from maximum acid output (MAO) level of 73 mEq./L. to 3 mEq./L. and no appreciable change in diarrhea. With relative anacidity, gastrin level is 948 picogm./ml. by radioimmunoassay.

A 42-year-old white man with a functioning malignant pancreatic islet cell tumor, had medically controllable peptic ulcer and diarrhea for four months before first laparotomy. At the initial laparotomy, histologic diagnosis was reticulum cell sarcoma, but the clinical course of disease suggested pancreatic cancer. More tissue was obtained at M. D. Anderson Hospital and a diagnosis of islet cell carcinoma was made.

This patient had both peptic ulcer disease and diarrhea of four months' duration. These conditions prompted the original laparotomy and were the first symptoms leading to diagnosis. The ulcer is medically controlled. Histological interpretation in such a case may be confusing and difficult. The patient's clinical course has declined rapidly over the last 18 months.

Islet Cell Carcinomas of the Pancreas, Nonfunctioning Tumors

A white woman, 57, had an 11-month survival after discovery of pancreatic islet cell cancer with biliary obstruction from cancerous nodes and huge liver metastases. She showed no appreciable response to drug therapy.

A Latin American woman aged 49 is now 19 years after resection of pancreatic body and tail because of islet cell carcinoma of the pancreas. Although she had bled massively preoperatively because of carcinomatous extension causing splenic vein occlusion and portal hypertension and had multiple postoperative infections, she is living and well (Fig. 1).

Localized islet cell cancer was an incidental finding at autopsy in a 40-year-old white man who showed no symptoms of this cancer. Death was from advanced malignant melanoma. Melanomatous erosion into the duodenum was the immediate cause of death, with bleeding and peritonitis. There was no known hormonal disease.

A white man aged 58 was treated by 5,000 rads ^{60}Co after a laparotomy diagnosis of a nonresectable body lesion. He had a history of duodenal ulcer for 14 years before admission but the ulcer was asymptomatic during this illness. Adenoma (microscopic) of the thyroid was found at autopsy. The patient had clinical response to ^{60}Co and later to 5-FU, but no lasting response to other chemotherapeutic drugs was obtained. Total survival was two years.

A white man aged 46 experienced a 10-year survival after diagnosis of proved islet cell carcinoma of the pancreas with metastasis to liver. Biliary and later gastric bypass procedures were done. There was a suggestion of clinical metastasis to bones or of parathyroid adenoma, but adenoma was not described at autopsy. His mother had diabetes mellitus, as did this man.

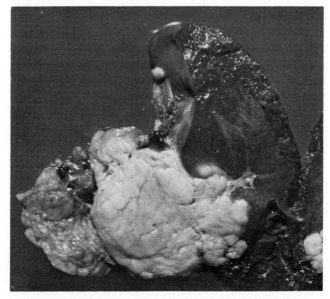

Fɪɢ. 1.—Resected islet cell tumor specimen from a 49-year-old patient who had splenic vein hypertension due to cancer invasion. The patient was in urgent condition when operated on, and is living 19 years later.

This patient may have been benefited by maintaining 5-FU therapy. He developed fluffy calcified liver metastasis. Ultimately he died because of the cancer, with acute bacterial endocarditis as the terminal event.

A white man aged 59 had four months of premonitory symptoms and a four-month survival after islet cell carcinoma in the tail of the pancreas with liver involvement was found at laparotomy. His disease was fulminant, and he tolerated chemotherapy poorly. His total survival period was eight months.

A 35-year-old white woman was admitted in 1966 after diagnosis and resection of islet cell carcinoma, metastatic to nine of 24 regional lymph nodes. She underwent, as the only therapy, subtotal distal resection of pancreas, splenectomy, and regional adenectomy. When last seen in December 1971, she was well and had survived five years with nodal spread of disease.

A white woman aged 54 had a four-year survival. She had had a pancreatic (neck) mass resected elsewhere in 1965, and was thought free of all gross cancer. At laparotomy for vascular disease in June of 1966, peritoneal implants and a liver hilar neoplastic mass were found. 5-FU therapy was begun and at next laparotomy done October 1967, no tumor was found. Although she eventually died of cancer, her response to 5-FU was favorable.

Discussion

During the same time period at this institution there were 14 patients with islet cell cancer of the pancreas and 344 patients with adenocarcinoma of the pancreas and two patients with benign insulinomas. The 14 patients presented, for the main part, because of abdominal distress or pain which was related to the pancreas. The differential diagnosis depended on physical examinations, with pancreatic pseudocyst, other alimentary tract cancer, and abdominal great-vessel arterial aneurysm, an acid-peptic entity, and, of course, other pancreatic disease being possible diagnoses. Contrary to the experiences of others, arterial contrast radiography was of great diagnostic aid when it was employed; admittedly, however, most patients had advanced disease. Two patients with slowly growing disease developed fluffy calcified metastases in the liver; these were not related to calcium metabolic disturbance. These findings and those of gastrointestinal radiography, which are diagnostic, will be described by Dodd (see pages 283 to 295, this volume). In the true Zollinger-Ellison syndrome, he noted hypersecretion, large gastric folds, peptic ulceration (usually duodenal), dilated descending limb of duodenum, edema, barium dilution, sprue-like small bowel pattern, and possible rapid propulsion through the bowel. The other findings were those of pancreatic cancer.

Longevity has been encouraging for the main part (Figs. 2 and 3), but the clinical course is unpredictable; a rampant course is a possibility. In general, life expectancy is considerably better than with ductal pancreatic cancer. Biologically, this tumor tends to spread to regional nodes and to the liver; pulmonary spread was not observed. As noted, a long life is still a possibility with liver involvement. Cervical lymph node spread occurred on only one occasion.

If resection is possible, this offers the patient the best chance for therapeutic benefit. It is difficult to assess the efficiency of anticancer drugs, but they seemingly are of some benefit. In one patient with known abdominal carcinomatosis, complete clearing occurred after one year of continuous maintenance therapy with 5-FU, as determined at the time of an unrelated abdominal celiotomy. Another patient in whom the presenting complaint was diarrhea had proved reduction of gastric acid secretion after 5-FU therapy.

In the single opportunity for observation after total gastrectomy, spon-

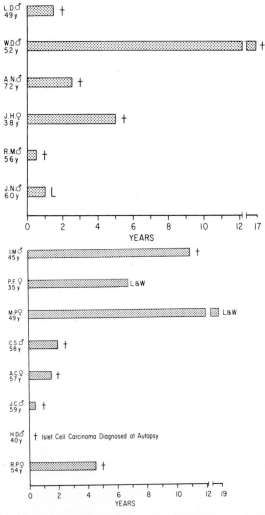

FIG. 2 (*top*).—Islet cell carcinomas of the pancreas—functioning. (Length of survival after initial diagnosis). † dead; L living.

FIG. 3 (*bottom*). Islet cell carcinomas of the pancreas—nonfunctioning. (Length of survival after initial diagnosis). † dead; L & W, living and well.

taneous remission of a pancreatic islet cell cancer as described by Friesen (1968) was not discerned in the 31 months after the total gastrectomy. Melnyk, Krippaehne, Benson, and Dunphy (1965) described symptomatic regression as a biological change after only lymph node biopsy for some 20 months with no specific change in the cancer. This phenomenon also was not observed.

The proved stimulants to gastric secretion are histamine, acetylcholine, and gastrin. These physiological substances cause the functioning gastric parietal cell mass to change pH from 7.4, that of the serum, to pH 1.0, that of pure gastric juice. The observations of Zollinger and Ellison and Gregory and Tracy (1960) in identifying gastrin as the tumor agent emphasize that cancer tissue can be very active biologically, beyond the effects of the cancer from local or metastatic growth phenomena.

We have accepted as hormonal activity some new symptomatic alimentary tract changes associated with the presence of the tumor: (1) onset of ulcer pain and diarrhea; (2) Z-E triad of tumor hypersecretion, severe peptic ulcer disease, and proved marked hyperacidity; (3) duodenal ulcer diathesis with exsanguination; (4) radiographic proof of a new peptic ulcer, hypersecretion, and gastritis; and (5) diarrhea involving 10 to 16 movements daily with variable acidity. We would interpolate that five tumors secreted gastrin, one gastrin and a possible diarrheal substance, and the other predominantly a possible diarrheal substance only.

This group of patients had no evidence of observed hypercalcemia, so the augmentative effects of hypercalcemia on the ulcer diathesis, gastric hypersecretion, or diarrhea were not subject to observation. Passaro, Basso, Sanchez, and Gordon (1970) had noted after calcium infusion that gastric acidity equals that of Histolog stimulation.

Another significant observation relates to a report by Passaro of two patients, treated by operation for acid-peptic disease, in whom the islet cell carcinoma was visualized as small with "incidental" metastases existing in the liver; the acid secretion increased notably to true Z-E level in each patient by 30 months. In two of our patients, the observations of Passaro were repeated; namely, for two to five years with known cancer there was no disturbance of gastrointestinal function, and then a severe ulcer diathesis developed with the Z-E syndrome. Our 60-year-old Negro patient with extreme diarrhea had a notable fluctuation of the gastric acidity, but an additional variable was the maintenance 5-FU therapy. The severity of his potential acid-peptic disease was relatively less and could be easily controlled by symptomatic care. His serum gastrin levels measured in the laboratory of Dr. Paul Jordan were above normal, 948 pico Gm./ml. serum at a time of relative anacidity and severe disabling diarrhea.

One 42-year-old man had a histological interpretation that resulted in the diagnosis of reticulum cell sarcoma at an initial laparotomy. Later, the clinical manifestations of the patient's disease at M. D. Anderson Hospital were those of pancreatic cancer, and with the examination of more tissue, the diagnosis of pancreatic islet cell cancer was made. In another patient, the true nature was not identified in the first manifestation of disease until five years after an involved lymph node had appeared in the supraclavicular area. This was thought to be follicular thyroid cancer, and such a disease was discovered upon thyroid exploration, but the original node was judged to contain islet cell cancerous deposits in later studies when the pancreatic islet tumor was uncovered five years later and at which time the Z-E diathesis developed. This served especially to reemphasize the problem of using light microscopic techniques. In no instance was it possible with this instrument to anticipate histologically the presence or absence of Z-E hormonal activity.

The problem of multiple endocrine adenomatosis merits further mention. While no MEA was discovered, one patient did have two endocrine cancers: thyroid cancer and pancreatic islet cell cancer. A benign thyroid nodule was present also in one patient in addition to the islet cell cancer, but such a finding probably lacks correlative significance.

In Macdonald's (1960) El Paso study, multiple cancers with cancer of the thyroid occurred in 1 of 87 instances within a population of 200,000. The other primary cancer was not listed. Wyse, Hill, Ibanez, and Clark (1969) studied 635 thyroid cancer patients at risk and found 65 (10.2 per cent) to have second primaries. There were a total of six endocrine tumors including that of this patient; these included adrenal cortical cancer (1), embryonal cell testicular cancer (1), adenocarcinoma ovary (1), and malignant pheochromocytoma (with medullary thyroid cancer) (2), plus two parathyroid adenomas.

A special significance to the association in the patient included herein does not seem warranted.

Summary

1. Fourteen patients with islet cell carcinoma of the pancreas were reviewed retrospectively. Of these, probably six patients had evidence of tumor hormonal activity which disturbed alimentary tract function, *i.e.*, caused diarrhea and/or acid-peptic disease.

2. The intensity of this response and the measures necessary to control the effects on the end-organ varied.

3. The tumor hormonal activity may not cause effects, even in the pres-

ence of cancer, for protracted periods. Two instances are presented where the tumor was present for two and five years before other digestive tract disturbances occurred.

4. Other pertinent observations may be presented. In this group of patients there was no proved evidence of MEA, although one patient had two endocrine cancers, follicular thyroid cancer, and islet cell cancer. A prior study with thyroid as the primary study lesion had been done here and in that review no MEA was discovered.

5. The histological interpretations of tissue can be misleading as proved in two instances with islet cell cancer.

6. The clinical biological course of the cancer may be fulminant, progressing from first symptom to death in eight months, or it may be less severe, extending over 19 years and up to 15 years in the presence of liver metastatic disease.

7. Radical extirpation therapy for local and regionally localized disease offers the best therapeutic chance for cure.

Acknowledgments

Appreciation is expressed to William O. Russell, M.D., Head and Professor of Anatomical Pathology, and Serge Masse, M.D., Fellow in Anatomical Pathology, for reconfirming the histological data; also, to Robert Nelson, M.D., Professor of Medicine, and Richard G. Martin, M.D., Professor of Surgery, for clinical data; Miss Eleanor Macdonald and staff, Department of Epidemiology, gave invaluable assistance. All the aforementioned are of The University of Texas at Houston M. D. Anderson Hospital and Tumor Institute. Also, appreciation is expressed to E. K. Sanders, M.D., and Henry Holle, M.D., both of Houston, who supplied data on individual patients.

REFERENCES

Ellison, E. H., and Wilson, S. D.: The Zollinger-Ellison Syndrome: Re-appraisal and evaluation of 260 registered cases. *Annals of Surgery*, 160:512-530, July-December, 1964.

Friesen, S. R.: A gastric factor in the pathogenesis of the Zollinger-Ellison Syndrome. *Annals of Surgery*, 168:483-501, 1968.

Gregory, R. A., Tracy, H. J., French, J. M., and Sircus, W.: Extraction of a gastrin-like substance from a pancreatic tumor in a case of Zollinger-Ellison Syndrome. *The Lancet*, 1:1045-1048, January-June, 1960.

Karbach, H. E., Jr., and Galindo, D. L.: Familial endocrine adenomatosis. *Texas Medicine*, 66:54-63, 1970.

Macdonald, E. J.: Occurrence of multiple primary cancers in a population of 200,000. *Unio Internationalis Contra Cancrum* (ACTA), 16:1702-1710, 1960.

Melnyk, C. S., Krippaehne, W. W., Benson, J. A., Jr., and Dunphy, J. E.: Spontaneous remission of Zollinger-Ellison Syndrome. *Archives of Internal Medicine*, 115:42-47, January 1965.

Moldawer, M. P., Nardi, G. L., and Raker, J. W.: Concomitance of multiple adenomas of the parathyroids and pancreatic islets with tumor of the pituitary: A syndrome with familial incidence. *The American Journal of the Medical Sciences*, 228:190-206, 1954.

Passaro, E., Jr., Basso, N., Sanchez, R. E., and Gordon, H. E.: Newer studies in the Zollinger-Ellison Syndrome. *The American Journal of Surgery*, 120:138-143, August 1970.

Steiner, A. L., Goodman, A. D., and Powers, S. R.: Study of a kindred with pheochromocytoma, medullary thyroid carcinoma, hyperparathyroidism and Cushing's Disease: Multiple endocrine neoplasia, type 2. *Medicine*, 47:371-409, 1968.

Way, L., Goldman, L., and Dunphy, J. E.: Zollinger-Ellison syndrome. An analysis of twenty-five cases. *The American Journal of Surgery*, 116:293-304, August 1968.

Wermer, P.: Genetic aspects of adenomatosis of endocrine glands. *The American Journal of Medicine*, 16:363-371, 1954.

Wilson, S. D.: Personal Communication.

Wyse, E. P., Hill, C. S., Ibanez, M. L., and Clark, R. L.: Other malignant neoplasms associated with carcinoma of the thyroid: Thyroid carcinoma multiplex. *Cancer*, 24:701-708, 1969.

Zollinger, R. M., and Ellison, E. H.: Primary peptic ulcerations of the jejunum associated with islet cell tumors of the pancreas. *Annals of Surgery*, 142:709-728, October 1955.

GENERAL REFERENCES

Ballard, H. S., Frame, B., and Hartsock, R. J.: Familial multiple endocrine adenoma-peptic ulcer complex. *Medicine*, 43:481-516, 1964.

Cushman, P., Jr.: Familial endocrine tumors. Report of two unrelated kindred affected with pheochromocytomas, one also with multiple thyroid carcinomas. *The American Journal of Medicine*, 32:352-360, 1962.

Finegold, M. J., and Haddad, J. R.: Multiple endocrine tumors. Report of an unusual triad in a family. *Archives of Pathology*, 76:449-455, 1963.

Hazard, J. B., Hawk, W. A., and Crile, G., Jr.: Medullary (solid) carcinoma of the thyroid—a clinicopathologic entity. *The Journal of Clinical Endocrinology and Metabolism*, 19:152-161, 1959.

Schulte, W. J., Hensley, G., Garancis, J. C., Wilson, S. D., and Ellison, E. H.: Zollinger-Ellison Syndrome: Clinical and histopathologic manifestations. *The American Journal of Surgery*, 117:866-875, June 1969.

Carcinoid Islet Cell Tumors of the Duodenum

PAUL H. JORDAN, JR., M.D.

*Department of Surgery, Baylor College of Medicine, and
the Veterans Administration Hospital, Houston, Texas*

IN 1952, Forty and Barrett described a patient who had hypersecretion of gastric juice, fulminating ulcer diathesis, and an islet cell tumor of the pancreas. Because of the tumor's histology, it was thought, but not documented, that the hypersecretion occurred in response to hypoglycemia caused by hyperinsulinism. In reality, this may have been the first described ulcerogenic tumor of the pancreas. Zollinger and Ellison (1955) later described a syndrome of peptic ulcer disease that developed in response to a gastric secretagogue that developed from islet cell tumors of the pancreas. The recognition (Gregory, Tracy, French, and Sircus, 1960) that the secretagogue from this type of tumor was gastrin and the increased availability of McGuigan's (1968) radioimmunoassay for its determination increased physicians' awareness of this entity and their ability to diagnose patients with this syndrome.

Islet cell tumors are not confined to the pancreas. While the first islet cell tumor of the duodenum was reported in 1928 (Stewart and Hartfall), the first functioning islet cell tumor of the duodenum associated with the Zollinger-Ellison syndrome was described in 1956 (Porter and Frantz). Since that time, a number of patients with islet cell tumors of the duodenum associated with ulcer disease have been reported. Oberhelman and Nelsen (1964) reported nine patients, and Weichert *et al.* (1971) reported 13 patients with the Zollinger-Ellison syndrome in which the gastrin-producing tumors were in the duodenum rather than the pancreas. In a search of the literature, Zollinger (Weichert *et al.*, 1971, discussion by Zollinger) found that of 650 ulcerogenic tumors reported, 82 were located in the duodenum.

This paper reports on seven patients with severe ulcer diathesis whose cases are summarized in Table 1. Five of these patients represent new

TABLE 1.—Seven Patients with Virulent Peptic Ulcer Disease

Case	Duodenal Tumor	Islet-Cell Hyperplasia	Metastasis	Operations	Follow-up
1. H. D.	+ First op.	?	1 Lymph node at second op.	1. V – A – BII 2. Resection of marginal ulcer	Living and well 7 years after first and 2 years after second operation
2. E. P.	+ Third op.	–	0	1. V – SGR 2. Thoracic vagotomy 3. Re-resection	Living and well 3 years after third operation
3. H. K.	+ Third op.	–	0	1. SGR 2. SGR 3. V – Resection of marginal ulcer	Living and well 1 year after third operation
4. An. J.	+ First op.	+	1 Lymph node at first op.	1. Near total gastric resection	Living and well 1 year
5. Ar. J.	+ Autopsy	+	1 Lymph node at autopsy	1. V + P → GE 2. SGR + BII 3. SGR	Died 20 months after first operation
6. A. F.	0	+	0	1. V – A – BII 2. Thoracic vagotomy Total gastrectomy 3. Distal pancreatectomy	Died 12 months after first operation
7. W. H.	0	+	0	1. V – A – BII 2. Re-resection 3. Re-resection	Died 9 years after third operation

Abbreviations: V = Vagotomy; A = Antrectomy; BII = Billroth II anastomosis; SGR = Subtotal gastric resection; GE = Gastroenterostomy.
+ Present.
0 Not found.
– Not looked for.

cases of islet cell tumors of the duodenum. Tumors were not found in the other two; instead, each had notable hyperplasia of the pancreatic islets of Langerhans. The high incidence of islet cell hyperplasia in patients with islet cell tumors of the duodenum suggests that the tumors may have been present in these two patients as well but were unrecognized because of their small size.

Case Reports

CASE 1.—H. D. was 60 years old when he was admitted for epigastric pain and hematemesis which required the administration of eight units of blood. He had had an ulcer history of several years' duration. At operation, a vagotomy, gastric resection, and a Billroth I anastomosis were performed. The specimen contained a small tumor, originally called a carcinoid tumor and subsequently identified as an islet cell tumor of the duodenum. The gastroduodenostomy failed to function, and a gastrojejunostomy was performed. Five years later, he returned with epigastric pain and melena. A marginal ulcer was identified at the gastrojejunostomy. At operation, the jejunum containing the ulcer was resected, the stomach closed, and a jejunojejunostomy performed. The gastroduodenostomy was adequately patent. A lymph node removed from the area of the gastroduodenostomy contained a tumor similar to the original tumor removed five years previously. No other positive lymph nodes were identified. A biopsy of the pancreas did not reveal unequivocal evidence of islet cell hyperplasia. The patient has gone two years without further ulcer symptoms. His serum gastrin level ranges from 70 to 90 pico Gm., and he is achlorhydric.

Comment.—This patient is asymptomatic, has a normal serum gastrin level, and is achlorhydric after having been initially treated by hemigastrectomy and vagotomy seven years ago. The patient has had one episode of recurrent ulcer during this interval which was treated by resection of the ulcer and removal of a lymph node containing metastatic islet cell tumor.

The events in this patient's case suggest that the residual islet cell tumor, during the interval between operations, was exceedingly slow-growing but had the potential to stimulate secretion when the tumor mass obtained sufficient size. Presently, the normal serum gastrin level and the gastric achlorhydria are objective evidence that insufficient tumor, if any, is present to exert an effect on gastric secretion. Although this patient has had one recurrent ulcer, he would not have had the benefit of his gastric reservoir for seven years had total gastrectomy been performed as the initial operation. Whether tumor will subsequently recur cannot be predicted. Our ability to monitor the serum gastrin level should permit us to antici-

pate and take measures to avoid future complications from gastric hypersecretion.

CASE 2.—E. P. was a 48-year-old man who had undergone vagotomy,
hemigastrectomy, and a Billroth II anastomosis for a duodenal ulcer
known to have existed for one year. Two years later, he began to complain
of episodic epigastric pain and vomiting. Four years after operation, he
was thought to have a marginal ulcer and was treated by transthoracic
vagotomy. The pain was unrelieved by operation. Roentgenograms showed
a persistent marginal ulcer, and he was reoperated on one month later. An
abdominal vagotomy, repeat gastric resection, and a Billroth II anastomosis were performed. A tumor, 1 cm. in greatest diameter, was palpated in
the wall of the duodenum and removed by a wedge resection. The tumor
was initially called a carcinoid, but in considering the clinical history, the
diagnosis was changed to islet cell tumor. He was asymptomatic three
years after the last operation. His serum gastrin level is normal and he is
achlorhydric.

Comment.—The islet cell tumor may have been too small to recognize at
the first operation. Apparently, four years were required for the tumor to
achieve sufficient size and functioning capacity to stimulate the remaining
parietal cells sufficiently to cause a recurrent ulcer. It is unknown whether
islet cell hyperplasia occurred in this patient because biopsy of the pancreas was not done.

This patient, like the first, has had the benefit of retaining his gastric
reservoir for two years since the islet cell tumor in the wall of the duodenum was discovered. If his serum gastrin level and/or his gastric secretion
becomes significantly elevated, the patient will be considered for reexplo-
ration without waiting for signs of recurrent ulcer. The results of this case
appear to support the contention of Oberhelman and Nelsen (1964) that
local excision of the tumor, particularly if it is in the duodenal wall, will
cure these patients if metastases are not present.

CASE 3.—H. K. was a 61-year-old woman who had had a subtotal gastric
resection for duodenal ulcer five years previously. Another resection and a
Billroth II anastomosis were performed for marginal ulcer ten days after
the first operation. Three years later, she developed left upper quadrant
pain which became gradually worse. The pain woke her at night and was
relieved by drinking milk. Roentgenograms suggested marginal ulcer. In
spite of having a very small gastric pouch, she produced 1.5 to 3.5 mEq. of
acid per hour basally. Her serum gastrin level was 1,175 pico Gm./ml.
which was significantly elevated. She was operated on for a marginal ulcer
secondary to a Zollinger-Ellison tumor or retained antrum. She had a large
marginal ulcer, but no evidence of a Zollinger-Ellison tumor was apparent

grossly. The duodenal stump was resected because it appeared to be retained antrum. Frozen-section examination failed to demonstrate any antral mucosa but, instead, a small islet cell tumor 0.6 cm. in size was found lying beneath the mucosa. A vagotomy, resection of the ulcer, leaving about 15 per cent of her stomach, and a Billroth II anastomosis were performed. Postoperatively, the patient did well. She became achlorhydric, and her serum gastrin level fell to normal.

Comment.—The marked secretory capacity of even a small tumor such as this patient had is demonstrated by the fall in the serum gastrin level to normal and the occurrence of achlorhydria, even though very little stomach was removed at the last operation. The finding of the tumor in this patient was fortuitous and occurred only because the duodenal stump appeared to be antrum and was resected. Because Oberhelman, Nelsen, Johnson, and Dragstedt (1961) had the identical experience in two patients, they came to the conclusion with which we now agree: that the duodenal stump should be reexcised to the vicinity of the ampulla of Vater if a tumor is suspected but cannot be found. A biopsy of the pancreas for islet cell hyperplasia was not done in this case. We now believe that this may be sufficiently indicative of the presence of tumor that it should become a routine part of an operation in which an islet cell tumor is suspected.

CASE 4.—An. J. was a 43-year-old man who had had diarrhea, weight loss, and epigastric symptoms suggestive of duodenal ulcer for six months. The patient was a hypersecretor, producing 32 mEq. of acid per hour basally and 51 mEq. per hour after Histalog stimulation. The dry weight of his stool was 20 per cent fat. Roentgenograms suggested a duodenal ulcer. On exploration, the patient appeared to have a healed duodenal ulcer. After an exhaustive search, one lymph node in the area of the celiac axis was found to contain carcinoid islet cell tumor. Resection of the stomach was begun and on transecting the duodenum, a small carcinoid islet cell tumor lying beneath the mucosa of the first portion of the duodenum was noted. A bilateral vagotomy and a nearly total gastrectomy, leaving about 10 per cent of the stomach, were performed. The patient was asymptomatic one year after operation, and his diarrhea had not returned. His serum gastrin level remains elevated, but his basal secretion is achlorhydric.

Comment.—Although this patient showed no evidence of active peptic ulcer at operation, he did have extreme hypersecretion which accounted for his steatorrhea and which was relieved by the operation. He had a duodenal carcinoid islet cell tumor, with metastasis to one lymph node, as well as pancreatic islet cell hyperplasia. Because it was not known whether residual tumor remained, a nearly total gastrectomy was performed. A less radical operation was not done for fear of causing an ulcer, as had occurred in a similar patient reported by Petersen, Myren, and Liavåg (1969). If the patient had had evidence of an active ulcer, a total gastrectomy would have been performed.

The serum gastrin level has remained elevated since operation. It may be that the source of this elevated gastrin level is either residual islet cell tumor or the hyperplastic islet cells of the pancreas. The absence of acid in the basal secretion suggests that the functional capacity of the gastrin produced is inadequate to stimulate the few remaining parietal cells. By monitoring these two parameters, serum gastrin and basal acid secretion, we expect to anticipate any ulcer complications that might occur from rising gastrin concentrations.

CASE 5.—Ar. J. was a 39-year-old man whose first episode of hematemesis occurred on the day of admission. He had had a four-week history of anorexia and epigastric pain and was in shock. At operation, he had a posterior, penetrating, bleeding duodenal ulcer. The ulcer was oversewn and a pyloroplasty and vagotomy were performed. Because the stomach did not empty properly, a gastrojejunostomy was performed. Following this, his postoperative course was uneventful.

Three weeks after operation, the patient began to have left upper quadrant pain. He was operated on again eight months later, and a large marginal ulcer was found at the gastrojejunostomy. Gastric resection and a Billroth II anastomosis were performed. A large vagal trunk was found and resected.

One year later, a perforation from a marginal ulcer developed. Evidence of a Zollinger-Ellison tumor was sought, including a careful inspection of the duodenum. None was found. Because of the degree of abdominal contamination, total gastrectomy was not done. The gastrojejunostomy was resected and a new anastomosis performed. The patient had a severe septic course and expired.

At autopsy, a tumor measuring 1 cm. in diameter was found lying beneath the mucosa in the second portion of the duodenum. One lymph node in the area of the head of the pancreas contained metastatic disease. The pancreas showed notable islet cell hyperplasia.

Comment.—The fact that an obvious tumor with a metastasis to a large lymph node was readily apparent at the autopsy, but not appreciated at operation, indicates the difficulty in recognizing the presence of a tumor and the great caution that one must utilize in the careful inspection of the duodenum if such lesions are not to be overlooked. Surgical biopsy of the pancreas revealed significant pancreatic islet cell hyperplasia. Subsequent studies showed that the gastrin content of the tumor was 4,000, the metastatic lymph node was 2,952 and the pancreas was 1,150 pico Gm. per gram of wet weight, indicating that the tumor, as well as the pancreas, was contributing to the elevated serum gastrin level. The serum gastrin results were not available for several days after operation, since the patient had a perforated ulcer and had undergone an emergency operation. In the future, the presence of pancreatic islet cell hyperplasia will be sufficient warning that the patient's ulcer diathesis is virulent, probably requiring total gastrectomy if an obvious cause for recurrent ulcer is not found.

CASE 6.—A. F., a 44-year-old patient, was found to have massive upper gastrointestinal bleeding while being evaluated for right upper quadrant pain of one week's duration. Vagotomy, hemigastrectomy, and a Billroth II anastomosis were performed as emergency procedures for a bleeding duodenal ulcer. He continued to have midepigastric pain and was readmitted for gastrointestinal bleeding five months after operation. The results of the Hollander test were positive. Transthoracic vagotomy was performed for suspected marginal ulcer. His symptoms subsided and results of the Hollander test were now negative. Epigastric pain and frequent episodes of melena began seven months later. Gastroscopy revealed one gastric ulcer and one jejunal ulcer. He was operated on again, and a total gastrectomy was performed after biopsy of the duodenal stump revealed no retained antrum or duodenal tumor, and resection of body and tail of the pancreas revealed no pancreatic tumor. The esophagojejunal anastomosis failed and the patient developed severe sepsis from which he did not recover. Permission for an autopsy was not granted.

Comment.—A total gastric resection in the absence of a known Zollinger-Ellison tumor was performed because of the patient's virulent ulcer diathesis. Since a functioning islet cell tumor may be so small as to be undetectable by visual inspection or palpation, we have no assurance that this patient did not have such a tumor. Conversely, we do know that he had definite hyperplasia of the islet cells of the pancreas. Whether the ulcerogenic syndrome was the result of islet cell hyperplasia in the absence of a tumor, as suggested by Zollinger *et al.* (1962), or whether the islet cell hyperplasia was merely indicative of the presence of an islet cell tumor of the duodenum which was not recognized, is unclear.

CASE 7.—W. H. was a 55-year-old man with a long history of duodenal ulcer who had undergone vagotomy, gastrectomy, and a Billroth II anastomosis nine years previously. He continued to use aspirin and alcohol and had recurrent episodes of hematemesis and melena. A marginal ulcer was detected by gastroscopy. At operation, a marginal ulcer was found at the gastrojejunostomy. Another resection was performed and on the sixth postoperative day, the patient experienced hematemesis and melena. He received a transfusion and made a satisfactory recovery. He returned in one month because of further severe upper gastrointestinal bleeding. He was reexplored, and further resection was performed for a marginal ulcer. The duodenal stump was biopsied and showed no evidence of retained antrum or duodenal tumor. The patient developed severe sepsis and died after a prolonged hospital course. Autopsy revealed recurrent marginal ulcer, adrenocortical hyperplasia, pancreatic islet cell hyperplasia, and parathyroid hyperplasia. No duodenal or pancreatic tumors were found at autopsy, but it is not known how carefully these were sought.

Comment.—This patient had a virulent peptic ulcer diathesis, and total gastrectomy should have been performed when reoperation was required six days after his second gastric resection, even though a Zollinger-Ellison tumor was not found. This patient was similar to the patient described in case 6, and it is not known for certain whether this patient had no tumor or whether it was overlooked because of its small size. Thus, it is not possible to determine whether the pancreatic islet cell hyperplasia was merely the reflection that a carcinoid islet cell tumor was present or whether the hyperplastic pancreatic islet cells had the inherent capacity to initiate gastric hypersecretion.

Discussion

PATHOLOGY

The duodenal tumors reported in this paper were small, none being larger than 1 cm. in dimension. This experience is similar to that reported by others. All tumors were located in the submucosa of the first and second portions of duodenum. The tumors were circumscribed, but nonencapsulated. The cells were small, uniform in size, and arranged in nests and ribbons. They sometimes permeated the mucosa and muscularis mucosa, but mitotic figures were absent. There was no evidence of pancreatic acinar tissue in the tumors. Most of these tumors were diagnosed initially as carcinoid tumors on the basis of light microscopy. The tumors did not take the silver stain, and on the basis of the clinical history, the diagnoses were changed to islet cell tumor, which is indistinguishable from carcinoid tumor by light microscopy. Subsequent electron microscopic study (by Dr. Ferenc Gyorkey) demonstrated that the granules within the tumor cells resembled those seen in alpha cells of the islets of Langerhans. This provided supporting evidence that these tumors were indeed islet cell tumors. In two patients (CASES 3 and 4), we made the preoperative diagnoses of gastrin-producing tumors on the basis of elevated serum gastrin levels. When frozen sections of the tumors from these patients revealed the carcinoid islet cell characterization, it was recognized immediately, on the basis of their biological behavior, that they represented islet cell and not carcinoid tumors.

EMBRYOLOGY

There is evidence to suggest that primitive precursor cells migrate from the neural crest to form the chromaffin system and also diffusely populate the mucosa of the foregut (Weichert, Reed, and Creech, 1967). These enterochromaffin cells are incorporated in the nonendocrine derivatives of the foregut such as the bronchi, stomach, bile ducts, and pancreatic ducts. They also migrate with the primordial buds of the endocrine glands that form the thyroid, parathyroid, thymus, ultimobranchial bodies, and pancreas. Because of their multipotentiality, these cells produce on maturation the hormones appropriate for the various endocrine glands. In the case of endocrine tumors, these cells may produce hormones that are both appropriate and inappropriate for a particular gland. The pluripotential precursor cells of neural ectodermal origin also provide an explanation for the secretion of peptide hormones by tumors of nonendocrine derivatives of the foregut such as the oat cell carcinoma of the lung. Such a hypothesis aids in an understanding of how tumors which appear histologically similar can originate in such diverse organs and can produce such a wide variety of hormones which cannot be completely predicted by the location of the tumor. Thus, the small lesions within the duodenum that histologically resemble both carcinoid and islet cell tumors can produce a variety of clinical conditions, depending on the peptide they produce. One of the most frequent syndromes for which this tumor is accountable is the Zollinger-Ellison syndrome.

MULTIPLE ENDOCRINE ADENOMATOSIS AND DUODENAL CARCINOID ISLET CELL TUMORS

The hypothesis that the endocrine organs arising from the foregut depend on a common precursor cell from the neural crest for the production of hormones has been helpful in understanding the syndrome of multiple endocrine adenomatosis. The syndrome can be considered as a familial dysplasia of this neural-ectodermal cell system (Weichert, 1970). Nearly 30 per cent of patients with islet cell tumors of the pancreas demonstrate a multiglandular involvement. In the series of Oberhelman and Nelsen (1964) of islet cell tumors of the duodenum, only one of nine patients had an associated endocrine dysfunction, and it was limited to the parathyroid glands. Hyperplasia of the pancreatic islets was also reported in their first six patients (Oberhelman, Nelsen, Johnson, and Dragstedt, 1961); however, the functional significance of this finding was not determined. In the report by Weichert *et al.* (1971), multiple endocrine adenopathy occurred in 31 per cent of 13 patients. No mention was made of pancreatic islet cell hyperplasia. In our series, one patient had hyperplasia of the parathyroids, but this caused no abnormality in the serum calcium level. Four of seven patients were known to have pancreatic islet cell hyperplasia. This was absent in one patient and not looked for in the other two patients.

Pancreatic Islet Cell Hyperplasia and Duodenal Islet Cell Tumors

Zollinger *et al.* (1962) suggested that pancreatic islet cell hyperplasia may be associated with the ulcerogenic syndrome in the absence of tumor. Oberhelman and Nelsen (1964) did not accept this concept because gastric hypersecretion decreased after excision of duodenal tumors in patients that also had pancreatic islet cell hyperplasia. In our experience, two patients (cases 6 and 7) with a virulent ulcer diathesis had pancreatic islet cell hyperplasia. An islet cell tumor could not be demonstrated although a diligent search was made at operation in both cases and at autopsy in one of the cases. Since these tumors are so small, it is entirely possible that they were overlooked. However, the absence of tumor in these patients suggests that while the presence of pancreatic islet cell hyperplasia is highly indicative of the presence of a duodenal islet cell tumor in some cases, it may in fact represent the etiology of the ulcer disease in others. Information on this point may be forthcoming when gastrin determination of pancreatic tissue with islet cell hyperplasia can be made and compared with the content of gastrin in normal pancreatic tissue.

Diagnosis

The Zollinger-Ellison syndrome should be considered in patients who develop clinical symptoms of peptic ulcer or unexplained diarrhea after 40 years of age and who have a high gastric secretory rate under basal conditions. The study of such patients should include a gastric analysis under basal conditions and after maximal stimulation of the parietal cells with histamine or Histalog. A ratio of basal acid secretion to the maximal acid output greater than 0.6 is suggestive but not conclusive evidence that an islet cell tumor exists. A lower ratio does not necessarily exclude the diagnosis. The most conclusive preoperative evidence that the Zollinger-

Ellison syndrome exists is the presence of an elevated serum gastrin level. Such a finding was responsible for the preoperative diagnosis of the Zollinger-Ellison syndrome in cases 3 and 4 and the subsequent demonstration of gastrin-producing carcinoid islet cell tumors of the duodenum.

Studies in normal man have demonstrated that secretin competitively inhibits pentagastrin-stimulated gastric secretion. In our fourth patient, secretin infusion caused an elevation of the serum gastrin level and an increase in acid output equivalent to that seen after maximal stimulation with Histalog. A similar response in gastric secretion was also seen after calcium infusion. Isenberg, Walsh, Passaro, and Grossman (in press) have reported similar findings in patients with Zollinger-Ellison tumors. However, secretin did not cause an increase in gastric secretion in three additional patients with Zollinger-Ellison tumors. The mechanism for the stimulation rather than the inhibition of gastric secretion by secretin is unknown. This requires further investigation for it may provide a mechanism for the early detection of patients with Zollinger-Ellison tumors. These observations help to explain why Oberhelman (Oberhelman, Nelsen, Johnson, and Dragstedt, 1961; Oberhelman and Nelsen, 1964) failed to inhibit gastric secretion in his patients with duodenal islet cell tumors by the administration of secretin.

In all patients with marginal ulcers, the first consideration should be the possibility that the patient is harboring a Zollinger-Ellison tumor unless there is an obvious cause for recurrent ulcer such as: (1) a history of ingestion of drugs or alcohol, (2) a stressful situation due to severe illness, (3) an inadequate vagotomy demonstrated at reoperation, (4) an inadequate gastric resection, (5) an obstruction at the stoma, or (6) a retained antrum demonstrated by biopsy. Gastric analysis is less helpful in the diagnosis after gastric resection because of the increased difficulty encountered in making quantitative collections. However, any patient who produces significant gastric acid in the basal state after an apparently adequate gastric operation should be considered to have a Zollinger-Ellison tumor. The presence of an elevated serum gastrin level is almost conclusive evidence of the existence of such a lesion except under the unusual circumstance of pernicious anemia where, in the absence of acid gastric juice to inhibit gastrin released from the antrum, gastrin levels will be elevated to the same range as is seen in patients with Zollinger-Ellison tumors.

Before operation, the patient should be studied as thoroughly as possible because the preoperative diagnosis of a Zollinger-Ellison tumor entails a major commitment which may require a great deal of time in order to determine that the patient does or does not have this diagnosis. Exploration requires careful bimanual palpation of the entire pancreas. If a tumor is not located in the pancreas, a meticulous search should be made for a tumor in the duodenum. Multiple biopsies should be taken from the head, body, and tail of the pancreas for the identification of pancreatic islet cell hyperplasia which appears to suggest the presence of a duodenal carcinoid islet cell lesion. The duodenum should be thoroughly mobilized by the Kocher maneuver and palpated externally and internally. If there has been a previous gastric resection, the duodenal stump should be excised and examined for retained antrum as well as the possibility of a small carcinoid islet cell tumor. Lymph nodes from the area surrounding the pancreas and the celiac axis should be liberally removed in search of metastatic tumor. The number of islet cell tumors of the duodenum which has been reported by those who have made a special study of this lesion raises the question whether many lesions of this type are not being overlooked because of the difficulty encountered in their recognition.

TREATMENT

If a carcinoid islet cell tumor of the duodenum is found without evidence of lymph node or distant metastasis, Oberhelman (Oberhelman, Nelsen, Johnson, and Dragstedt, 1961) is of the opinion that treatment by local excision is justified. In our opinion, the difficulty has been the uncertainty that there is not an undetected metastatic lesion or that there is not a multiplicity of tumors which is unrecognized. We have not had experience that permits an evaluation of Oberhelman's (Oberhelman and Nelsen, 1964) observation that gastric secretion falls precipitously during anesthesia when all the tumor has been removed. This finding deserves further study.

Currently, if the patient has not been operated on previously, it is our practice to combine vagotomy and gastric resection with removal of the tumor. The radioimmunoassay of gastrin permits us to determine in the early postoperative period whether all tumor was removed. If the serum gastrin level and gastric acid secretion remain elevated, further operation can be undertaken before complications occur. For us, this is a more rational approach than the initial performance of total gastrectomy when all tumor appears to have been removed. Conversely, if extensive metastatic disease has occurred, total gastrectomy should be performed at the first operation. If the metastatic disease is limited, as in two of our patients (CASES 1 and 4), it may be adequate to remove the primary tumor and its metastases and perform limited gastric surgery. Again, if the serum gastrin level and acid secretory levels remain high or subsequently become elevated, the patient should be reexplored and total gastric resection probably performed at that time, unless there is limited recurrent disease that can be resected. These two cases demonstrate that the more conservative approach can now be undertaken safely if the patients are closely followed up for recurrence of excessive gastrin production.

If an adenoma cannot be found in the pancreas or duodenum of a patient suspected of having a Zollinger-Ellison tumor, the treatment of choice has been uncertain. In two patients (CASES 6 and 7) with virulent ulcer diathesis, pancreatic islet cell hyperplasia was present. It is unknown whether this was the source of gastrin production or indicative of an undiscovered adenoma, as was found at autopsy in a third patient (CASE 5). If these three patients had had total gastrectomy at an earlier time in their ulcerogenic history, very likely they would have each lived. Availability of a serum gastrin assay will in the future provide us with the information required to make the decision to perform total gastrectomy. Such a decision will be possible except in patients operated on for perforated marginal ulcer or emergency bleeding where there is insufficient time to acquire this information. In those instances, the decision to perform total gastric resection in the absence of tumor will rest on the clinical history, the virulence of the ulcer diathesis, and the presence of pancreatic islet cell hyperplasia. It is our opinion that if pancreatic islet cell hyperplasia can be documented by frozen section, this is sufficient indication of hypergastrin production by the pancreas or an unidentified islet cell tumor to warrant total gastrectomy.

Summary

A series of seven patients with a virulent peptic ulcer diathesis is reported. Five of these patients had carcinoid islet cell tumors in the duodenum. This diagnosis was made preoperatively in our most recent two patients on the basis of elevated acid secretion and elevated serum gastrin levels. Four patients had their tumor recognized and removed at operation. In two of these, a metastatic lymph node was also present. All four patients were treated by subtotal gastrectomy. They are under close surveillance to detect a rise in the serum gastrin level or an increase in acid secretion which would be indication for further operation. One patient with a tumor and an isolated metastatic lymph node died of recurrent ulcer disease because the lesions were not evident at operation and total gastrectomy was not performed. Two patients with pancreatic islet cell hyperplasia, in whom there was no known tumor, underwent multiple operations for recurrent ulcer and eventually died from complications of ulcer disease. It was not known whether the ulcer diathesis in these patients resulted from hypergastrinemia secondary to pancreatic islet cell hyperplasia. The availability of a gastrin assay should make it possible to answer this question.

REFERENCES

Forty, F., and Barrett, G. M.: Peptic ulceration of the third part of the duodenum associated with islet-cell tumours of the pancreas. *The British Journal of Surgery*, 40:60-63, July 1952.

Gregory, R. A., Tracy, H. J., French, J. M., and Sircus, W.: Extraction of a gastrin-like substance from a pancreatic tumour in a case of Zollinger-Ellison syndrome. *The Lancet*, 1:1045-1048, May 1960.

Isenberg, J. I., Walsh, J. H., Passaro, E., Jr., and Grossman, M. I.: The effects of secretin on serum gastrin, serum calcium and gastric acid secretion in a patient with Zollinger-Ellison syndrome. *The New England Journal of Medicine*. (In press.)

McGuigan, J. E.: Immunochemical studies with synthetic human gastrin. *Gastroenterology*, 54:1005-1011, June 1968.

Oberhelman, H. A., Jr., and Nelsen, T. S.: Surgical consideration in the management of ulcerogenic tumors of the pancreas and duodenum. *The American Journal of Surgery*, 108:132-141, August 1964.

Oberhelman, H. A., Jr., Nelsen, T. S., Johnson, A. N., Jr., and Dragstedt, L. R., II: Ulcerogenic tumors of the duodenum. *Annals of Surgery*, 153:214-227, February 1961.

Peterson, H., Myren, J., and Liavåg, I.: Secretory response to secretin in a patient with diarrhoea and the Zollinger-Ellison pattern of gastric secretion. *Gut*, 10:796-799, October 1969.

Porter, M. R., and Frantz, V. K.: Tumors associated with hypoglycemia—pancreatic and extrapancreatic. *The American Journal of Medicine*, 21:944-961, December 1956.

Stewart, M. J., and Hartfall, S. J.: Adenomata of pancreatic islet tissue in the pylorus and duodenum. *The Journal of Pathology and Bacteriology*, 31:137-139, January 1928.

Weichert, R., Reed, R., and Creech, O., Jr.: Carcinoid-islet cell tumors of the duodenum. *Annals of Surgery*, 165:660-669, May 1967.

Weichert, R. F., III: The neural ectodermal origin of the peptide-secreting endocrine glands. A unifying concept for the etiology of multiple endocrine adenomatosis and the inappropriate secretion of peptide hormones by nonendocrine tumors. *The American Journal of Medicine*, 49:232-241, August 1970.

Weichert, R. F., III, Roth, L. M., Krementz, E. T., Hewitt, R. L., and Drapanas, T.: Carcinoid-islet cell tumors of the duodenum. Report of twenty-one cases. *The American Journal of Surgery*, 121:195-205, February 1971.

Zollinger, R. M.: Discussion of: Weichert, R. F., III, Roth, L. M., Krementz, E. T., Hewitt, R. L., and Drapanas, T.: Carcinoma-islet cell tumors of the duodenum. Report of twenty-one cases. *The American Journal of Surgery*, 121:205, February 1971.

Zollinger, R. M., Elliot, D. W., Endahl, G. L., Grant, G. N., Goswitz, J. T., and Taft, D. A.: Origin of the ulcerogenic hormone in endocrine induced ulcer. *Annals of Surgery*, 156:570-578, October 1962.

Zollinger, R. M., and Ellison, E. H.: Primary peptic ulcerations of the jejunum associated with islet cell tumors of the pancreas. *Annals of Surgery*, 142:709-728, October 1955.

Radiologic Manifestations of the Zollinger-Ellison Syndrome

GERALD D. DODD, M.D.

*Department of Diagnostic Radiology, The University of Texas
at Houston M. D. Anderson Hospital and Tumor Institute,
Houston, Texas*

In 1969, a Congress was held in Erlangen, Germany, to discuss the most recent information available on the Zollinger-Ellison syndrome and related problems. The proferred papers have been published in monograph form (International Symposium at Erlangen, 1969). In the course of the introduction, it is stated that the volume contains information which should be of great interest to the internist, surgeon, pathological anatomist, biochemist, or physiologist concerned with the problems of gastroenterology. It is interesting that the radiologist is not included in this litany of specialists. In point of fact, patients suffering from the Zollinger-Ellison syndrome are frequently seen by a radiologist early in the course of their disease, usually with a provisional diagnosis of peptic ulceration. In the opinion of Zboralske and Amberg (1968), the responsibility of recognizing this syndrome devolves upon the radiologist in most instances. If he is familiar with the fluoroscopic and radiographic findings commonly associated with nonbeta islet tumors of the pancreas, the correct diagnosis may be suggested in the majority of patients.

The syndrome, as originally described, consisted of the classic triad of gastric hypersecretion, a fulminating ulcer diathesis, and the presence of a noninsulin-producing islet cell tumor (Zollinger and Ellison, 1955). The radiologic manifestations of this triad have been reported by Missakian, Carlson, and Huizenga (1965) and by Christoforidis and Nelson (1966).

As the result of hypersecretion, large amounts of nonopaque fluid are usually present in the stomach. When barium is given by mouth, it tends to gravitate into the dependent portions of the stomach with the less viscid, nonopaque secretions layering above the contrast material. The gastric mucous membrane pattern is also prominent and the folds tend to be large and to coat poorly with barium (Fig. 1). The fold thickening results from edema and an increase in the size and number of parietal cells in the gastric wall. These findings are, of course, not characteristic of the Zollinger-Ellison syndrome and may be observed with nonspecific gastroduodenal ulceration and/or gastritis. However, the sheer volume of the gastric secretions will frequently serve to alert the radiologist to the proper diagnosis. If the inflammatory changes are sufficiently intense, bizarre contraction patterns may be observed which may be described as irregular, segmental distortions of the gastric contour unrelated to orderly peristaltic contractions (Fig. 2A). Occasionally, the submucosal edema may be so intense as to virtually obliterate most of the mucous membrane folds, but double-

Fig. 1.—Zollinger-Ellison syndrome. Malignant nonbeta-cell tumor in a 43-year-old female. This erect film shows layering of the heavier barium in the dependent portions of the stomach and duodenum. The proximal stomach and duodenum are filled with nonopaque secretions.

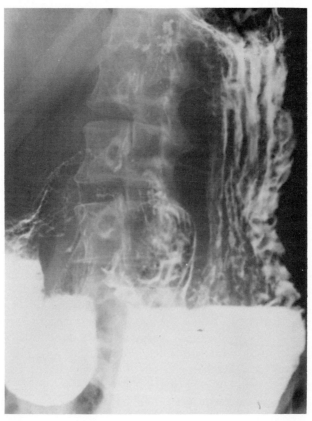

contrast techniques may reveal a granular pattern indicative of severe gastritis (Fig. 2B). Superficial or frank gastric ulceration may also be present (Figs. 2C and D).

Most ulcers which occur in the Zollinger-Ellison syndrome are found in the duodenal bulb; only a small number (4 to 5 per cent) are found in the stomach proper. The characteristic duodenal ulcer tends to be large and superficial; a zone of edema may be present (Fig. 3A). Since the craters are of relatively recent origin, it is commonplace to find little or no deformity.

Ulceration may also occur in the distal duodenum and proximal jejunum. The demonstration of an ulcer in these atypical areas should immediately suggest the possibility of the Zollinger-Ellison syndrome.

In the absence of atypical ulceration, the appearance of the duodenum distal to the superior genu is most significant. It is not uncommon for the folds of the mucous membrane to be grossly edematous and the duodenal wall atonic and dilated. The reasons for these changes are conjectural. Presumably, they are caused by the tremendous outpouring of acidic gastric secretions into the duodenum where the climate is normally alkaline; *i.e.*, a chemical duodenitis is produced with secondary neuromuscular phenomena resulting in dilatation of the lumen (Fig. 3B). Whether this hypothesis is correct is of no importance from the diagnostic standpoint. Of greater significance is the fact that the described changes are readily demonstrable radiographically. While not pathognomonic, their frequency in the Zollinger-Ellison syndrome is so great that the diagnosis must be considered when they are observed. Occasionally, a penetrating duodenal ulcer, unassociated with a pancreatic neoplasm, may produce similar findings in the descending limb of the duodenum. In such instances, differentiation is usually possible by means of gastric analysis. By and large, with the Zollinger-Ellison syndrome, the overnight secretions will be more voluminous. If the histamine stimulation test is employed, only a minimal response will be observed in the Zollinger-Ellison syndrome whereas a characteristic increase is usually obtained with nonspecific peptic ulceration.

Although the gastroduodenal findings are not entirely specific, concomitant changes in the small bowel are likely to occur with the Zollinger-Ellison syndrome. These can make the radiologic diagnosis fairly secure in many instances. In the usual peptic ulcer, there is no specific abnormality of the small intestine. In the full-blown Zollinger-Ellison syndrome, apparently because of the continuous outpouring of the highly acid gastric juice into the small intestine, the changes described in the duodenum may be observed to a greater or lesser degree in the jejunum and ileum. Instances

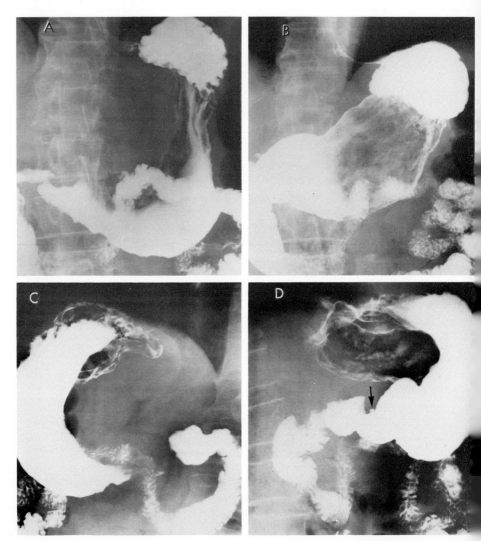

Fig. 2.—Zollinger-Ellison syndrome. Malignant nonbeta-cell tumor in a 72-year-old male. *A*, anteroposterior film of the stomach showing mucosal edema and hypersecretion. Note the shallow, irregular contractions along the greater curvature aspect of the antrum and distal body of the stomach. *B*, double-contrast study of the stomach showing mucosal edema and granularity. The mucosal folds are largely obliterated by underlying fluid. The mucosal surface has a granular appearance suggestive of gastritis. *C*, prone oblique film of the stomach showing retrogastric mass and superficial gastric ulceration. The large mass anteriorly displaces the stomach and ligament of Treitz anteriorly. Multiple shallow ulcerations are apparent on the lesser curvature aspect of the

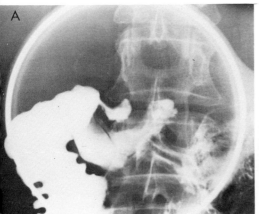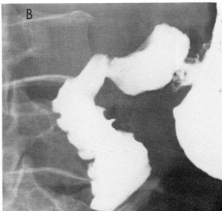

Fig. 3.—Zollinger-Ellison syndrome. Malignant nonbeta-cell tumor in a 38-year-old female. *A*, compression film of the duodenal bulb. A large ulcer is visualized with a pronounced surrounding zone of edema. There is little deformity. *B*, edema and dilatation of the descending duodenum. Note that the acute ulcer (*A*) is not seen without compression.

of involvement of the right side of the colon have also been reported (Zboralske and Amberg, 1968). The radiologic changes in the small bowel may vary from minor degrees of edema and dilution of the opaque material to virtual obliteration of the mucosal pattern (Figs. 4A and B). Clumping and flocculation of the barium may also occur in association with random areas of spasticity. Following passage of barium, one may see a feathery or lace-like pattern representing the opaque material trapped between individually thickened mucosal folds (Fig. 4C).

There is often no apparent relationship between the severity of the patient's symptoms and the size of the tumor. Marble-sized adenomas may be associated with notable hypersecretion and ulceration, whereas very large tumors may produce only minimal functional changes in the gastrointestinal tract. When large enough, nonbeta cell tumors may invade or displace adjacent organs. The radiographic findings in these cases are similar to those produced by other pancreatic neoplasms and are nonspecific (Fig. 5). However, the nonbeta cell tumors are commonly so small that no signs of mass can be elicited in the upper gastrointestinal examination. While the secondary findings of hypersecretion, ulceration, and en-

distal half of the stomach. *D*, lateral film of the stomach showing retrogastric mass and prepyloric ulcer. The ulcer is small, but has all the characteristics of a typical benign peptic ulcer.

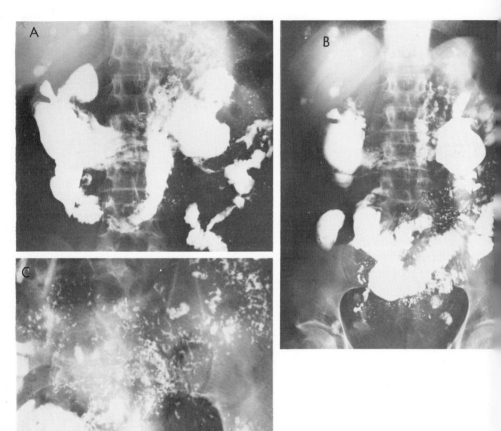

Fɪɢ. 4.—Zollinger-Ellison syndrome. Malignant nonbeta-cell tumor in a 52-year-old male. *A*, there is dilution of the gastric and duodenal contents by gastric secretions. Note the distinct mucosal edema of the proximal small bowel. The duodenal bulb is deformed and there is partial obstruction of the descending limb. *B*, the dilution, edema, and dilatation persist well into the jejunum and proximal ileum. *C*, residual barium trapped between mucosal folds in the distal small bowel produces a feathery pattern in the roentgenogram. This is the result of mucosal edema.

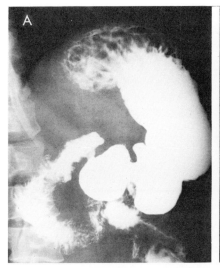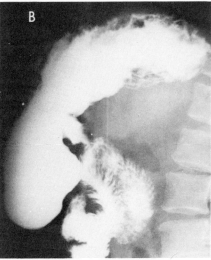

Fig. 5.—Zollinger-Ellison syndrome. Malignant nonbeta-cell tumor in a 60-year-old male. *A*, prone oblique film of the stomach showing distortion of the duodenal loop with invasion and fixation of the mucous membrane. *B*, lateral film showing anterior displacement of the stomach and duodenum. The findings are indistinguishable from those of other types of pancreatic neoplasms.

teritis are highly suggestive of the proper diagnosis, demonstration of the primary tumor is desirable. Approximately 10 per cent of ulcerogenic tumors are ectopic in location, *i.e.*, they may be found in the stomach, duodenum, splenic hilum, *etc.* (Nelson and Christoforidis, 1968). Additionally, the smaller masses in the body and tail may be extremely difficult for the surgeon to palpate (Fig. 6). Since it is estimated that about 63 per cent of the islet cell tumors larger than 1 cm. in diameter can be demonstrated arteriographically because of their hypervascularity (McKinnon, Malcolm, and Rosch, in press), selective arteriography may be considered the procedure of choice for both the diagnosis and localization of these masses. The celiac and superior mesenteric vessels may be individually or simultaneously catheterized, and supraselective injections of the pancreaticoduodenal and gastroduodenal arteries may be performed when necessary. Angiographic findings include not only displacement and encasement of vessels by mass in the case of the larger tumors, but also a "tumor stain" which is reasonably specific, particularly when taken in conjunction with the gastrointestinal findings noted above. Typically, the tumors appear as well-defined areas of radiopacity during the late arterial phase of the angiogram. Tumor vessels may or may not be present. Staining may occur

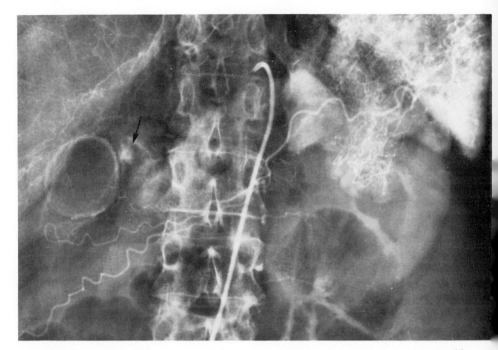

FIG. 6.–Zollinger-Ellison syndrome. Benign, nonbeta-cell adenoma in a 56-year-old female. A small tumor stain is seen in the arterial phase of the celiac angiogram (arrow). At operation, a 1 cm. mass was found in the anterior wall of the descending duodenum. Histologic examination revealed a benign, nonbeta-cell adenoma. (Courtesy of Dr. Josef Rosch, University of Oregon Medical School.)

with both benign and malignant tumors and is nonspecific for differential diagnosis (Figs. 6 and 7). The metastatic deposits are also highly vascular and most commonly are found in the liver and peripancreatic lymph nodes (Fig. 7). Occasionally the hepatic metastases will calcify and can be diagnosed preoperatively (Fig. 8). Calcifying metastases have been demonstrated in three of our 11 patients, a finding which has not previously been reported in the literature. In none of these patients could the hepatic calcification be ascribed to prior therapy.

Occasionally, a diffuse hyperplasia of the pancreas (microadenomatosis) may be encountered. Ellison and Wilson (1964) state that 10 per cent of cases are in this category. In such instances, an abnormal density of the pancreas is noted during the late arterial phase of the visceral angiogram. The finding is nonspecific and must be closely correlated with other clinical and laboratory findings.

As has been noted, there may be a disparity between the size of the tumor and the symptoms produced. According to Zollinger, about 6 per cent of patients with notable gastric hypersecretion have only diarrhea and do not develop an ulcer diathesis (Zollinger, 1970). Priest and Alexander (1957) and Verner and Morrison (1958) have also described patients with proven islet cell tumors and severe diarrhea but no peptic ulceration. Thus, it would seem that islet cell tumors may be associated with a syndrome quite distinct from that under discussion. Presumably, the basic difference lies in the production of gastrin by those tumors associated with the ulcerogenic syndrome as opposed to secretin production in those producing the primary diarrheogenic form of the disease. The latter may be associated with severe hypokalemia and low or absent acid values. Diabetes may also occur, and occasionally islet cell tumors may be associated with familial multiple endocrine adenomatosis. Although a discussion of the interrelationships of the various forms of islet cell tumor is not within the province of this article, it should be noted that the tumors have the potential to produce a variety of hormones. These include insulin, serotonin, gastrin, secretin, adrenocorticotropin, and glucogen. While the radiographic features of the various syndromes do not differ greatly except for the presence or absence of peptic ulceration, in those instances where multiple familial

FIG. 7.—Zollinger-Ellison syndrome. Malignant nonbeta-cell tumor in a 60-year-old male. *A*, celiac angiogram in the early arterial phase. Multiple hepatic masses are revealed by displacement of the hepatic artery subdivisions and the presence of abnormal tumor vessels. *B*, late arterial phase showing the dense staining characteristics of the hepatic metastases plus tumor stain in the region of the body of the pancreas and peripancreatic lymph nodes.

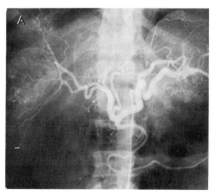
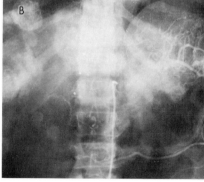

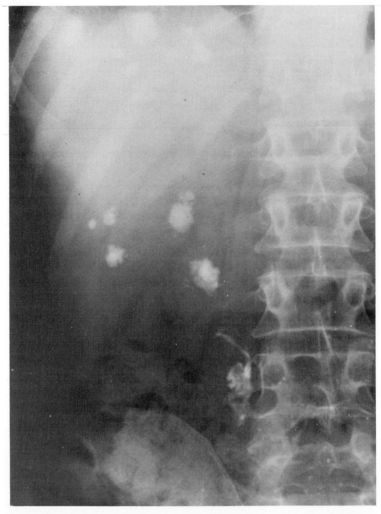

Fig. 8.—Zollinger-Ellison syndrome. Malignant nonbeta-cell tumor in a 60-year-old male. There are multiple calcifying metastases within the liver; these occurred independently of any form of treatment.

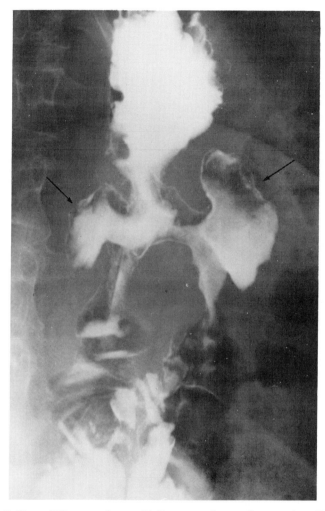

Fig. 9.—Zollinger-Ellison syndrome. Malignant nonbeta-cell tumor in a 63-year-old female. A prior subtotal gastrectomy had been performed. The spot film of the gastric remnant shows a hiatal hernia with an anastomosis between the gastric pouch and a loop of jejunum. Two very large ulcers appear on either side of the anastomotic loop below the stoma (arrows). Note that the small intestine below the level of the ulcers is dilated and edematous. (Courtesy of Drs. Joseph Medoff and Murray Dalinka, Thomas Jefferson University Hospital, Philadelphia, Pa.)

adenomatosis is suspected, roentgen evidence of sellar enlargement, parathyroid hyperplasia, adrenal pheochromocytoma, *etc.* should be searched for when indicated.

Total gastrectomy is considered the surgical procedure of choice in patients with ulcerogenic tumors. Even the smallest gastric remnant may be associated with massive recurrent ulceration (Fig. 9). As pointed out by Christoforidis and Nelson (1966), the ulcers tend to occur in the efferent loops rather than at the gastrojejunal stoma, particularly along the mesenteric border of the bowel. The ulcerations may be quite large and often very deep. Presumably, they result from the great quantities of highly acid gastric juice which gain direct access to the small intestine via the surgical stoma. The ulcerations may occur anywhere in the small intestine and have been identified well down in the jejunum. Their incidence is higher at operation or autopsy than one would anticipate from the radiologic literature. This is probably a result of the tendency on the part of radiologists not to explore carefully the small intestine distal to the stoma.

Recently, there has been some question as to the need for total gastrectomy in every instance. Cases are cited wherein subtotal gastric resection has not been followed by stomal ulceration. It is probable that these cases represent instances of nongastrin-producing islet cell tumors. Such cases, rather than vitiating the need for total gastrectomy in those patients with ulcerogenic tumors, merely underscore the need for thorough hormonal assays before selection of the proper surgical procedure.

Although 60 per cent of islet cell tumors are of the malignant variety and have in most instances metastasized by the time the diagnosis is established, many are remarkably indolent in their course. If the possibility of hemorrhage and/or perforation is controlled by adequate surgical procedures, the patients may pursue useful lives for years following diagnosis.

Summary

The radiologist plays a vital role in the diagnosis and management of islet cell tumors of the pancreas. Often, the primary responsibility for the diagnosis is his, both with those patients seen for the first time as well as with those who have had some prior form of therapy for intractable peptic ulceration. Frequently the findings on the conventional upper gastrointestinal series will indicate the probable diagnosis. Certainly, in those patients in whom the clinical and radiological findings are sufficiently suspicious to warrant visceral angiography, correct diagnosis should be achieved in the majority of patients.

Since these tumors may follow a relatively benign course after a suitable surgical procedure, the assistance of the radiologist in identifying those patients with ulcerogenic forms is indispensible. Because many of the ulcers are atypical in location, a thorough examination of the postbulbar and poststomal small bowel is essential in every case.

REFERENCES

Christoforidis, A. J., and Nelson, S. W.: Radiologic manifestations of ulcerogenic tumors of the pancreas. *The Journal of the American Medical Association,* 198:97-102, October 31, 1966.

Demling, L., and Ottenjann, R., Eds.: *Non-Insular Producing Tumors of the Pancreas: Modern Aspects on Zollinger-Ellison Syndrome and Gastrin.* Stuttgart, Germany, Georg Thieme Verlag, 1969, 213 pp.

Ellison, E. H., and Wilson, S. D.: The Zollinger-Ellison Syndrome: Re-appraisal and evaluation of 260 registered cases. *Annals of Surgery,* 160:512-530, September, 1964.

McKinnon, C. M., and Rosch, J.: Angiography in the diagnosis and management of extrapancreatic islet cell tumor. Case report. (In press.)

Missakian, M. M., Carlson, H. C., and Huizenga, K. A.: Roentgenographic findings in Zollinger-Ellison syndrome. *The American Journal of Roentgenology, Radium Therapy and Nuclear Medicine,* 94:429-437, June, 1965.

Nelson, S. W., and Christoforidis, A. J.: Roentgenologic features of the Zollinger-Ellison syndrome—Ulcerogenic tumor of the pancreas. *Seminars in Roentgenology,* 3:254-266, July, 1968.

Priest, W. M., and Alexander, M.: Islet-cell tumour of pancreas with peptic ulceration, diarrhea, and hypokalemia. *The Lancet,* 2:1145-1147, 1957.

Verner, J. V., and Morrison, A. B.: Islet cell tumor and a syndrome of refractory watery diarrhea and hypokalemia. *The American Journal of Medicine,* 25:374-380, 1958.

Zboralske, F. F., and Amberg, J. R.: Detection of the Zollinger-Ellison Syndrome: The radiologist's responsibility. *The American Journal of Roentgenology, Radium Therapy and Nuclear Medicine,* 104:529-543, November, 1968.

Zollinger, R. M.: The GI effects of Pancreatic Tumors. 39th Dacosta Oration. *Philadelphia Medicine,* 219-231, March 5, 1970.

Zollinger, R. M., and Ellison, E. H.: Primary peptic ulcerations of the jejunum associated with islet cell tumors of the pancreas. *Annals of Surgery,* 142:709-728, 1955.

Parathyroid Hormones and Parathyroid Neoplasms

L. J. DEFTOS, H. T. KEUTMANN, H. D. NIALL,
G. TREGEAR, J. F. HABENER, T. MURRAY,
D. POWELL, AND J. T. POTTS, JR.

*Department of Medicine, Massachusetts General Hospital and
Harvard Medical School, Boston, Massachusetts and
Veterans Administration Hospital and University of California,
San Diego School of Medicine, La Jolla, California*

RECENT PROGRESS in the biochemistry and immunochemistry of parathyroid hormones has resulted in significant advances of our understanding of the importance of the peptide in disorders of bone and calcium metabolism. By performing ion-exchange chromatography in the presence of 8M urea as the final step in the isolation of bovine parathyroid hormone (PTH), Keutmann *et al.* (1971) have demonstrated three variants or isohormonal forms of the hormone, termed PTH-1, PTH-2, and PTH-3 (Fig. 1). The amino acid sequence has been determined for the predominant form of the hormone, PTH-1 (Niall *et al.*, 1970; Brewer and Ronan, 1970; Keutmann *et al.*, 1971). Figure 2 shows the complete amino acid sequence of bovine PTH. The structure of porcine parathyroid hormone (Woodhead *et al.*, 1971) has also been determined (Potts *et al.*, 1972) (Fig. 2), and studies are currently underway to determine the structure and significance of bovine PTH-2 and bovine PTH-3.

The biological activity of bovine parathyroid hormone (PTH-1) has been shown to reside in the amino-terminal region of the molecule (Potts *et al.*, 1971; Potts *et al.*, 1972; Keutmann, Dawson, Aurbach, and Potts, in press). Studies with synthetic fragments indicate that the amino-terminal residue may also be necessary for biological activity, since deletion of the amino-terminal alanine abolishes all biological activity (Potts *et al.*, 1972). Figure 3 shows some of the other structure-function relations in PTH (Potts *et al.*, 1971; Potts *et al.*, 1972). Current information about

298 / *Deftos et al.*

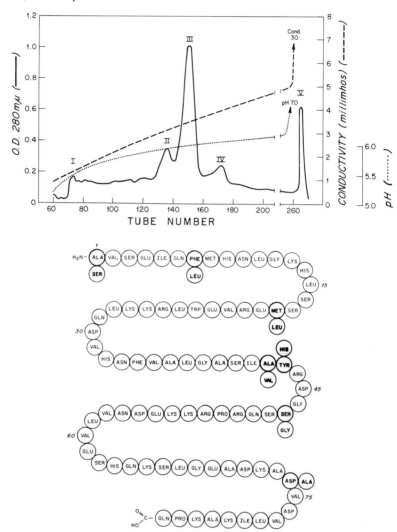

Fig. 1 (*top*).—Final step in purification of bovine PTH by ion-exchange chromatography on carboxymethyl cellulose using a linear ammonium acetate gradient in the presence of 8 M urea. The predominant form of the hormone (PTH-1) eluted in pure form as peak III. The minor variants of the hormone, PTH-2 and PTH-3, eluted in peaks II and IV, respectively.

Fig. 2 (*bottom*).—The complete amino acid sequence of bovine and porcine PTH. The backbone sequence is that of the bovine hormone; bold amino acids represent the positions in which the porcine and bovine sequences differ.

BIOLOGICAL ACTIVITY OF PTH FRAGMENTS

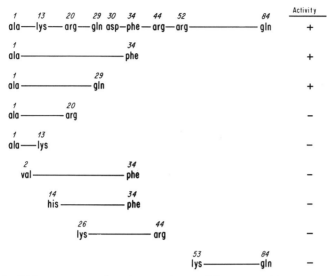

FIG. 3.—Biologic activity of synthetic and natural fragments of bovine PTH.

structure-activity relations suggests that all of the structural information necessary for expression of the biological activity of PTH on receptors in kidney and bone is found in a continuous peptide sequence beginning with residue number one and extending at least as far as residue number 20, but not necessarily as far as residue number 29.

Although the structure of human parathyroid hormone has not been determined, initial studies have shown a strong similarity in size and amino acid composition between human and bovine hormone (Potts *et al.*, 1972). Consequently, there is a significant degree of immunochemical similarity between the human and bovine molecules such that the two peptides cross-react very closely against antibodies prepared to the bovine peptide (O'Riordan, Potts, and Aurbach, 1971). Because of this, it has been possible to develop immunoassays for human PTH based on the bovine molecule (Potts *et al.*, 1971). These assays have been used to examine the control of secretion of PTH in both man and experimental animals (Potts and Deftos, 1969). However, the chemical nature and metabolic fate of circulating endogenous PTH are quite complex. This complexity arises in part from the persistence in the circulation of degradation products or peptide fragments of the originally biosynthesized 84 amino acid polypeptide (Habener *et al.*, 1971). These findings may explain the difference in absolute quantities of circulating immunoreactive hormone detected by various antiparathyroid hormone antisera, the lack of parallelism in dose dilution curves between standard hormone and plasma hormone (nonlinearity), and the paradoxical results sometimes encountered when stimulation or suppression tests are applied to test autonomy of gland secretion (Potts and Deftos, 1969; Deftos and Potts, 1969; Potts *et al.*, 1971; Deftos *et al.*, 1972; Berson and Yalow, 1971). However, when appropriate caution is observed, the immunoassay for PTH even in its present form, is quite useful in interpretation and diagnostic evaluation of patients with disorders of calcium homeostasis.

Differential Diagnosis of Hypercalcemic States

Most laboratories (Potts *et al.*, 1971; Berson and Yalow, 1971; Arnaud, Tsao and Littledike, 1971), but not all (Reiss and Canterbury, 1969) report an overlap between the levels of PTH in normal subjects and in patients with primary hyperparathyroidism. Figure 4 compares the basal concentrations of PTH, as determined by our immunoassay, in a group of

FIG. 4.—Plasma PTH concentrations in normal subjects, patients with hyperparathyroidism, and patients with nonparathyroid hypercalcemia. The overlap of hormone concentration between normal subjects and patients with hypercalcemia (*left*) can be minimized by plotting the PTH in relation to the blood calcium concentration (*right*). Although there is overlap in hormone concentration between normal subjects and patients with hyperparathyroidism, patients with hyperparathyroidism and patients with hypercalcemia not caused by hyperparathyroidism are readily distinguished; hormone is undetectable in patients with nonparathyroid hypercalcemia (*left*). Dashed line represents the detection limits of assay.

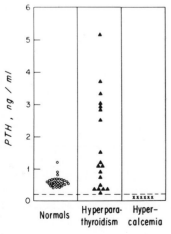
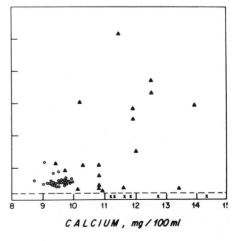

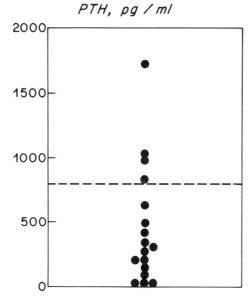

FIG. 5.—PTH concentrations in 17 patients with medullary thyroid carcinoma. Dashed line represents upper limits of normal hormone concentration. The majority of patients had normal basal levels of PTH and were normocalcemic. Only four patients had elevated PTH concentrations, and each of these four also had associated hyperparathyroidism and hypercalcemia.

normal subjects and a group of patients with primary hyperparathyroidism. The mean concentration of hormone in the normal group is 0.56 ng./ml., with a standard deviation of 0.15 ng./ml. The overlap between normal subjects and patients with hyperparathyroidism is apparent (Fig. 4, left). However, many of the patients with hyperparathyroidism have concentrations of hormone clearly elevated above the normal range; in these patients the assay can confirm the diagnosis. The discrimination between normal and hyperparathyroid subjects can be improved by plotting the concentration of PTH in relation to the blood calcium concentration (Fig. 4, right). When PTH concentration is plotted against serum calcium, the overlap between normal subjects and patients with primary hyperparathyroidism is minimized, and the two groups appear more distinct.

Despite the overlap in hormone concentration between normal subjects and patients with primary hyperparathyroidism, the immunoassay is uniquely valuable for making the distinction between hypercalcemia of parathyroid and nonparathyroid origin. It can be seen in Figure 4 (left) that in a group of patients with hypercalcemia not caused by parathyroid disease, the levels of PTH are undetectable. This presumably occurs since

the secretion of the normal parathyroid glands is suppressed by the hypercalcemia. Therefore, the patients with hyperparathyroidism, who have
easily detectable concentrations of hormone, can be readily distinguished
from the patients with hypercalcemia not resulting from hyperparathyroidism but from other causes, such as cancer metastatic to bone.

We have also applied our PTH assay to the measurement of hormone in
the plasma of patients with medullary carcinoma of the thyroid. Despite
the fact that this tumor secretes excessive amounts of the potent hypocalcemic peptide, calcitonin, most patients with this tumor are eucalcemic
(Deftos, Goodman, Engelman, and Potts, 1971). In agreement with the
findings of Berson and Yalow (1971), but in contrast to the findings of
Melvin, Miller, and Tashjian (1971), we have found that the majority of
patients with this tumor exhibit normal basal levels of PTH (Fig. 5).

Fɪɢ. 6.—Increase in PTH concentration following EDTA-induced hypocalcemia in
patients with primary hyperparathyroidism caused by an adenoma of the parathyroids,
chief-cell hyperplasia of the parathyroids, and subjects with idiopathic hypercalciuria.

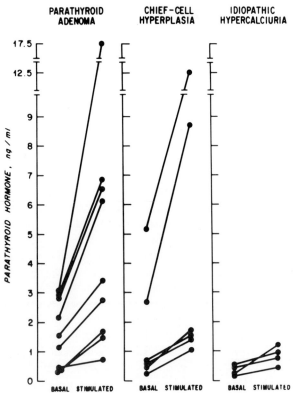

Secretion of PTH in Primary Hyperparathyroidism

Since there is overlap between basal parathyroid hormone concentrations in normal subjects and patients with primary parathyroidism, we attempted to distinguish between these two groups by measuring hormone concentration during functional tests of secretion. We compared the pattern of hormone secretion in a group of patients with primary hyperparathyroidism to a control group of subjects with idiopathic hypercalciuria (Potts *et al.*, 1971). Our findings revealed that hormone secretion was not autonomous in patients with primary hyperparathyroidism. Figure 6 shows that patients with hyperparathyroidism caused by both parathyroid adenomata and chief-cell hyperplasia exhibited a significant increase in PTH concentration during ethylenediaminetetraacetate (EDTA)-induced hypocalcemia. Figure 7 demonstrates, furthermore, that PTH secretion in patients with hyperparathyroidism can be suppressed by calcium infusion. These results do not support the view (Reiss and Canterbury, 1969) that PTH concentration is secreted in autonomous fashion in patients with primary hyperparathyroidism. The apparent discrepancy in reports (Potts *et al.*, 1971; Reiss and Canterbury, 1969) concerning autonomy probably results from the complex nature of circulating PTH (see below).

Fig. 7.—Decrease in PTH concentration following calcium infusion in eight patients with primary hyperparathyroidism.

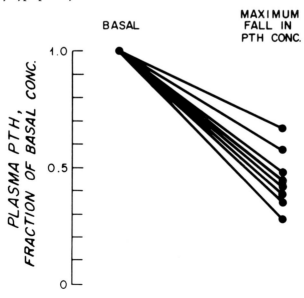

Localization of Abnormal Parathyroid Tissue

In addition to its usefulness for establishing the correct diagnosis in hypercalcemic states, the immunoassay for PTH is also useful for the preoperative localization of abnormal parathyroid tissue; we previously introduced a technique for the localization of such tissue (Reitz *et al.*, 1969). In this procedure, samples were collected for assay from jugular, innominate, and subclavian veins and at various levels below the heart. The site of abnormal parathyroid tissue could be correlated with a localized increase, in the order of several fold, of PTH in 50 to 60 per cent of such patients studied (Deftos *et al.*, in press). We have subsequently found that the diagnostic accuracy of this procedure can be improved by sampling the smaller blood vessels draining the parathyroid glands, notably the superior, middle, and inferior thyroid veins. The sampling of venous blood closer to the parathyroid glands accentuates the localized gradient in hormone production over basal levels and considerably improves the diagnostic accuracy of this procedure. The gradient of hormone between samples taken from the thyroid veins and other sites in the circulation can be 15 to 50-fold, in contrast to the two- to three-fold gradient found with our original technique. Figure 8 demonstrates a typical result in two patients with primary hyperparathyroidism whose samples collected in this manner

Fig. 8.—Plasma PTH concentrations in samples obtained at different points in venous circulation in two patients. Veins are jugular (*J*), innominate (*I*), superior vena cava (*SVC*), superior thyroid (*STV*), and inferior thyroid veins (*ITV, IT*). In patient J., samples also were obtained from medial and lateral branches of right inferior thyroid vein (*ITV-M* and *ITV-L*). Sites of sampling are indicated by •; adjacent numbers indicate PTH concentration in mμGm./ml.

PATIENT J.

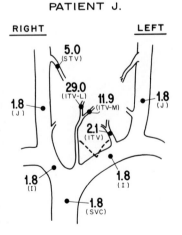

PATIENT R.

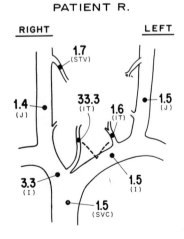

were assayed for PTH. In addition to demonstrating the marked step-up in hormone concentration found in the thyroid veins corresponding to the site of the abnormal parathyroid tissue, this figure also demonstrates that in patient J., localization by the original technique would not have been possible, since there was no step-up in hormone concentration in the larger vessels. Localization was quite easily accomplished in this patient by the small-vein catheterization technique. Application of this newer method has established the correct site of abnormal parathyroid tissue in each of 22 patients in whom proper sampling was possible. In addition to its usefulness as an aid in planning surgical approaches, early experience with the technique suggests it is useful as a diagnostic procedure *per se*. It has become possible to differentiate parathyroid hyperplasia from adenoma; multiple sites rather than a unilateral gradient are detected in chief-cell hyperplasia. In those patients in whom ectopic hyperparathyroidism is being considered in the differential diagnosis (symptoms or signs that suggest the possibility of an occult neoplasm), the application of the catheterization technique and the demonstration of a gradient of increased hormone concentration in the thyroid venous plexus greatly strengthens the diagnosis of primary hyperparathyroidism.

Molecular Size and Immunochemical Characteristics of Stored and Secreted PTH

The applications of the immunoassays for PTH to clinical studies in man and in animals have suggested that the biosynthesis and secretion, as well as the metabolism, of endogenous PTH is quite complex and that, in fact, the exact chemical nature of the active, circulating form of the hormone is not yet known (Habener *et al.*, 1971; Berson and Yalow, 1971; Potts *et al.*, 1972). Arnaud (Arnaud *et al.*, 1971) and Sherwood (Sherwood *et al.*, 1971) have recently reported that PTH secreted from parathyroid tissue during incubation *in vitro* consists of a fragment of the stored 84 amino acid peptide. They have further suggested that these fragments may represent the secreted form of PTH and that the 84 amino acid peptide represents stored or glandular hormone. However, recent *in vivo* studies in our laboratory indicate that PTH which is released from the parathyroid glands into the circulation is comparable in molecular size to PTH which is extracted from glands (Habener *et al.*, 1971). Once released into the circulation, PTH is probably metabolized into smaller fragments (Potts *et al.*, 1971; Habener *et al.*, 1971). Figure 9 shows the gel-filtration pattern of radioimmunoassayable PTH obtained simultaneously by venous catheterization from an inferior thyroid vein and the superior vena cava in a

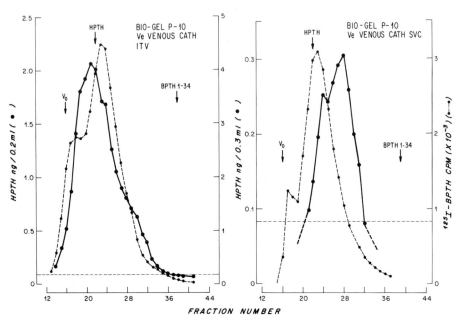

FIG. 9.—Gel-filtration (Bio-gel P-10) pattern of radioimmunoassayable PTH in plasma samples obtained simultaneously by venous catheterization of the inferior thyroid vein (*ITV*, *left*) and the superior vena cava (*SVC*, *right*) in a patient with a parathyroid adenoma (●—●). ^{125}I-labeled bovine PTH was cochromatographed in each filtration as a marker (●----●). Arrows mark elution position of first fraction containing plasma proteins (V_o), human parathyroid hormone (*HPTH*) standard, and synthetic bovine 1–34 amino-terminal peptide (*BPTH* 1–34). Dashed horizontal line indicates immunoassay detection limits.

patient with a parathyroid adenoma (Habener *et al.*, 1971). The hormone in plasma which was obtained directly from the parathyroid effluent blood eluted in a position closely coincident to the radioiodinated 1-84 bovine PTH marker. Therefore, the immunoreactive hormone secreted directly from the parathyroid glands is at least equal in molecular size to the 84 amino acid hormone marker. The hormone in the circulation superior vena cava is in the form of one or more smaller immunologically reactive fragments (Habener *et al.*, 1971). These results are consistent with the hypothesis that PTH secreted from the parathyroid glands is comparable in size to the molecule extracted from parathyroid glands. However, once secreted into the circulation PTH is metabolized into smaller fragments (Habener *et al.*, 1971).

Summary

Recent advances in the biochemistry and immunochemistry of parathyroid hormone (PTH) have had clinical implications important to the study of the secretion of hormone in patients with disorders of calcium homeostasis. The development of sensitive and specific radioimmunoassays for human PTH have provided an important diagnostic tool in the evaluation of patients with hypercalcemia. The application of the radioimmunoassay to preoperative localization techniques for abnormal parathyroid tissue has led to improvement in the surgical management of patients with primary hyperparathyroidism. Investigations of the structural features of PTH which influence its biological activity, in combination with immunochemical studies of glandular and circulating PTH, have led to an appreciation of the complex nature of PTH biosynthesis, storage, and secretion.

Acknowledgments

Supported in part by grants AM 15888, AM 11794, and AM 04501 of the United States Public Health Service and grants from the John A. Hartford Foundation, the Gebbie Foundation, and NASA. Dr. Deftos is a Research Scholar of the American Cancer Society (Massachusetts).

REFERENCES

Arnaud, C. D., Sizemore, G. W., Oldham, S. B., Fisher, J. A., Tsao, H. B., and Littledike, E. T.: Human parathyroid hormone: Glandular and secreted molecular species, *The American Journal of Medicine,* 50:630-638, 1971.

Arnaud, C. D., Tsao, H. S., and Littledike, E. T.: Radioimmunoassay of human parathyroid hormone in serum, *The Journal of Clinical Investigation,* 50:21-34, 1971.

Berson, S. A., and Yalow, R. S.: Clinical applications of radioimmunoassay of plasma parathyroid hormone. *The American Journal of Medicine,* 50:623-629, 1971.

Brewer, H. B., Jr., and Ronan, R.: Bovine parathyroid hormone: Amino acid sequence, *Proceedings of the National Academy of Sciences of the U.S.A.,* 67: 1862-1869, 1970.

Deftos, L. J., Goodman, A. D., Engelman, K., and Potts, J. T., Jr.: Suppression and stimulation of calcitonin secretion in medullary thyroid carcinoma, *Metabolism,* 20:428-431, 1971.

Deftos, L. J., Murray, T. M., Powell, D., Habener, J. F., Singer, F. R., Mayer, G. P., and Potts, J. T., Jr.: Radioimmunoassay for parathyroid hormones and calcitonins, *Proceedings of the Fourth International Parathyroid Conference,* Excerpta Medica, pp. 140-151, 1972.

Deftos, L. J., and Potts, J. T., Jr.: Radioimmunoassay for parathyroid hormone and calcitonin, *British Journal of Hospital Medicine*, 11:1813-1827, 1969.

Habener, J. F., Powell, D., Murray, T. M., Mayer, G. P., and Potts, J. T., Jr.: Parathyroid hormone: Secretion and metabolism *in vivo. Proceedings of the National Academy of Sciences of the U.S.A.*, 68:2986-2991, 1971.

Keutmann, H. T., Aurbach, G. D., Dawson, B. F., Niall, H. D., Deftos L. J., and Potts, J. T., Jr.: Isolation and characterization of the bovine parathyroid isohormones. *Biochemistry*, 10:2779-2787, 1971.

Keutmann, H. T., Dawson, B. F., Aurbach, G. D., and Potts, J. T., Jr.: A biologically active amino-terminal fragment of bovine parathyroid hormone prepared by dilate acid hydrolysis. *Biochemistry*. (In press.)

Melvin, K. E. W., Miller, H., and Tashjian, A. H., Jr.: Early diagnosis of medullary carcinoma, *The New England Journal of Medicine*, 285:1115-1119, 1971.

Niall, H. D., Keutmann, H., Sauer, R., Hogan, M., Dawson, B., Aurbach, G. D., and Potts, J., Jr.: The amino acid sequence of bovine parathyroid hormone I. *Hoppe-Seyler's Zeitschrift für physiologische chemie*, 351:1586-1588, 1970.

O'Riordan, J. L. H., Potts, J. T., Jr., and Aurbach, G. D.: Isolation of human parathyroid hormone. *Endocrinology*, 89:1, 234-239, 1971.

Potts, J. T., Jr., and Deftos, L. J.: Parathyroid hormone, thyrocalcitonin, Vitamin D and bone and bone mineral metabolism. In Bondy, P. K., Ed., Duncan's Diseases of Metabolism, 6th ed., Philadelphia, W. B. Saunders Co., 1969, pp. 904-1082.

Potts, J. T., Jr., Keutmann, H. T., Niall, H. D., Habener, J. F., Tragear, G. W., Deftos, L. J., O'Riordan, J. L. H., and Aurbach, G. D., The chemistry of the parathyroid hormones: Physiological and clinical implications. *Proceedings of the Fourth Parathyroid Conference*, Excerpta Medica, pp. 159-172, 1972.

Potts, J. T., Jr., Murray, T. M., Peacock, M., Niall, H. D., Tregear, G. W., Keutmann, H. T., Powell, D., and Deftos, L. J.: Parathyroid hormone: Sequence, synthesis, immunoassay studies. *The American Journal of Medicine*, 50:639-649, 1971.

Potts, J. T., Jr., Tregear, G. W., Keutmann, H. T., Niall, H. D., Sauer, R., Deftos, L. J., Dawson, B. F., Hogan, M. L., and Aurbach, G. D.: Synthesis of a biologically active n-terminal tetratriacontapeptide of parathyroid hormone. *Proceedings of the National Academy of Sciences of the U.S.A.*, 68:63-67, 1971.

Reiss, E., and Canterbury, J. M.: Primary hyperparathyroidism. *The New England Journal of Medicine*, 280:1381-1385, 1969.

Reitz, R. E., Pollard, J. J., Wang, C. A., Fleischli, D. L., Cope, O., Murray, T. M., Deftos, L. J., and Potts, J. T., Jr.: Localization of parathyroid adenomas by selective venous catheterization and radioimmunoassay. *The New England Journal of Medicine*, 281:348-351; 1969.

Sherwood, L. M., Lundberg, W. B., Jr., Targovnik, J. H., Rodman, J. S., and Seyfer, A.: Synthesis and secretion of parathyroid hormone *in vitro. The American Journal of Medicine*, 50:658-669, 1971.

Woodhead, J. S., O'Riordan, J. C. H., Keutmann, H. T., Stoltz, M. L., Dawson, B. F., Niall, H. D., Robinson, C. J., and Potts, J. T., Jr.: Isolation and chemical properties of porcine parathyroid hormone. *Biochemistry*, 10:2787-2792, 1971.

Surgical Management of Parathyroid Tumors

ROBERT C. HICKEY, M.D., AND
WILLIAM A. SCHEFTNER, M.D.

Department of Surgery, The University of Texas at Houston
M. D. Anderson Hospital and Tumor Institute,
Houston, Texas

THIS PAPER will deal with one facet of hypercalcemia, functioning adenoma, which is managed by surgeons. In the gamut of hypercalcemic difficulties, hyperparathyroidism is but one entity, but it has significant surgical connotations. Hyperparathyroidism can, through progressive organ system damage, bring about disability and death, and yet if surgical intervention is done in time, it may be synonymous with a return to health.

In all cases, other causes of hypercalcemia must be excluded. In fact, in a categorical cancer institution, the opportunity to observe a functioning adenoma is relatively infrequent. Indeed, surgical ablation is much more likely to inadvertently present parathyroprivia. There are several causes of the hypercalcemic disturbance which must be excluded. Among these are: other malignant tumors producing peptide hormones or causing bone destruction, vitamin D intoxication, sarcoidosis, acute atrophy of bone, idiopathic hypercalcemia of infancy, renal insufficiency, milk-alkali disease, myeloma, and lymphoma.

Historical Review

Attention was called to hyperparathyroidism for one of us (RCH) upon hearing, as a medical student, from Dr. Eugene F. DuBois, Professor of Medicine at Cornell Medical College, about one of his more interesting patients—Captain Charles E. Martell, whose medical history provides a foundation for physiologic understanding of hyperparathyroidism (Bauer and Federman, 1962).

Captain Martell, a 6-foot, 1-inch tall, 22-year-old man, was on active duty with the United States Merchant Marine in the North Atlantic in 1918. He had a fall and developed a sharp pain in his right loin, probably a fracture sequella. In 1919, he had become shorter and pigeon breasted, had kyphosis, and the jarring movement of walking caused pain. Within three years he had sustained a half dozen fractures. He passed fine gravel after urinating. Numerous therapies were prescribed without avail.

On January 15, 1926, he entered Bellevue Hospital under the care of Dr. DuBois. The patient's serum calcium level was 14.8 mg. per cent, the phosphorus level was 3.3 mg. per cent, and the radiographs showed a coarse trabeculation and decreased bone density. Urinary calcium excretion was high and fecal calcium excretion was low. With these data, Dr. DuBois referred the patient to Dr. Joseph C. Aub in Boston (Aub, Fairhall, Minot and Reznikoff, 1925), who had performed follow-up experiments on the parathyroid extract work done by Dr. J. B. Collip (1925) at the University of Alberta. Dr. Aub had shown that when the parathyroid extract was given in 100-unit lots to normal subjects, it caused a metabolic derangement similar to that identified in Captain Martell. (Aub and his colleagues had been testing the use of parathyroid hormone to hasten the elimination of lead from the skeleton. Patients who had been poisoned by lead could have the lead driven into the bones by large amounts of calcium, thus relieving the colic. Lead metabolism was shown to be similar to that of calcium. If the patient were put on a low calcium diet, then the lead was excreted with calcium in both the feces and urine; however, if the process of deleading were done too rapidly, colic was precipitated.) When Martell entered Massachusetts General Hospital, the first American diagnosis of primary overfunction of the parathyroid gland was postulated and made.

By April 1926, the patient had shrunk a total of 7 inches, had had eight fractures, had extreme muscle hypotonia, marked kyphosis, elevated serum calcium (15.1 to 16.3 mg. per cent) and depressed serum phosphorus. The radiographs showed decalcification. The patient was prepared for an operation to determine if there was abnormal parathyroid tissue in the neck.

Three cervical explorations were unsuccessful. He was discharged on a high calcium diet. This may have brought his metabolism into better balance, but could have been ruinous to his kidneys. Within five years, he was on crutches and was unable to lift his legs.

He returned to Massachusetts General Hospital and underwent three additional cervical explorations, all of which were negative. Upon the patient's insistence and after the studied concurrence of his physicians, the mediastinum was explored in 1932—14 years after his illness started. Dr.

Edward D. Churchill, assisted by Dr. Oliver Cope, performed the sternal-splitting procedure. A brown tumor, 3× 3 cm. was removed. The patient's serum calcium level fell rapidly, but he developed signs of tetany. Although he improved, the tetany was poorly controlled. A renal calculus which became lodged in a ureter required surgical intervention. He died of the combination of the hypocalcemic tetany and the urinary tract difficulties.

A clear understanding of Martell's case history will aid any surgeon to gain understanding of the disease. The metabolic studies in this case were many and a few are reviewed:

1. Serum calcium was persistently high.

2. Serum phosphorus was low until renal disease developed.

3. Urinary excretion of calcium was high—70 per cent of the intake.

4. Fecal excretion of calcium was low (the opposite of normal excretory patterns).

5. Parathormone (380 units administered over a period of two weeks) increased serum calcium slightly, but caused pain while the disease was active.

6. Normal parathyroid tissue removed during the early explorations had no effect of the disease.

7. High calcium diet (3.2 Gm./day) maintained the patient in calcium balance.

8. High phosphorus diet lowered the serum calcium level.

9. The threshold of phosphorus for renal excretion purposes was lowered. (This later became a diagnostic procedure for diagnosing the disease.)

10. Radiographs showed characteristic decreased density and coarse trabeculations.

In America, the understanding of parathyroid function came through physiological studies, while in Europe the understanding of hyperparathyroid disease was channeled through studies of anatomical and surgical pathology. As reviewed by Bauer and Federman (1962), the classic bone disease was described by Frederick D. von Recklinghausen, a pathologist at Strasbourg. In 1903, Askanazy, a pathologist at Tübingen, found a parathyroid tumor in a patient dying of von Recklinghausen's disease. Erdheim associated parathyroid enlargement with an osseous disease, but it was inferred that the parathyroid enlargement was sequential or secondary. In July, 1926, Mandl, a surgeon of Vienna, tried parathyroid pills and then a parathyroid graft on a patient with classic bone disease. Next he explored the neck and removed a large parathyroid tumor, after which the patient's osteitis fibrosa cystica improved. This communication had not reached the

United States, however, at the time that Martell's neck exploration was contemplated.

Through the years an appreciation has arisen for the theory that the "stone and bone" disease has ramifications. After 1926, the so-called osseous von Recklinghausen's disease, or osteitis fibrosa generalista, attracted attention; in the 1930's, aided by Albright's data, renal calcareous disease was studied. With Rogers' observations with Keating at the Mayo Clinic (1947), the digestive tract became a focal interest. Keating (1961 and 1970) noted "an objective evidence of peptic ulcer in 59 of 380 parathyroid patients, 15.5%" and stressed the diagnostic significance of hyperparathyroid in relation to recalcitrant acid peptic disease, especially in young women; in one series of patients credited to Cope as reviewed by Keating (1961), acid peptic disease accounted for the initial diagnostic clue of hyperparathyroidism in eight per cent of the patients. The same was true of pancreatitis (Cope *et al.*, 1957)! Wermer (1954) better defined the association of the parathyroid adenoma with other altered endocrine states, and the syndrome of multiple endocrine adenomatosis was more clearly identified.

In 1962, Copp *et al.* challenged the classic concept that parathyroid hormone alone maintained the constancy of serum calcium by a negative feedback mechanism; Hirsch, Gauthier, and Munson (1963) suggested that the thyroid gland contained a hypocalcemic hormone, thyrocalcitonin. Thyrocalcitonin is a polypeptide hormone which lowers serum calcium levels in animals and man. It may conceivably be of value in human studies, but results are inconstant.

A concomitant major addition to an understanding of hyperparathyroidism was by mass screening tests. Patients seemingly healthy but with hypercalcemia were discovered; obviously, not all required operation, but some might. Which ones? Next came the assessment of parathormone level by radioimmunoassay; this technique promises to be another milestone in study of the disease. Still another addition is the recognition that neoplastic tissue unrelated to parathyroid can produce a peptide substance physiologically identical to the parathyroid hormone. It is an excess of this peptide substance which causes alterations most frequently of significance in a categorical cancer hospital.

Clinical Review

We reviewed a group of 29 patients with hyperparathyroid adenomas at the University of Wisconsin (seen between 1933 and 1967). These ranged in age from 12 to 67 years; the average age was 49 years (Table 1).

TABLE 1.—HYPERPARATHYROIDISM
29 Patients

SEX	AGE	AVERAGE
Male—8	20–61 yrs.	49 yrs., of 6
Female—21	12–67 yrs.	49 yrs., of 21

TABLE 2.—SPECIFIC IDENTIFIABLE
CLINICAL ENTITIES

ENTITY		NUMBER
Proved renal calculi	7 ⎱	19
Proved bilateral calculi	12 ⎰	
Proved bladder calculi		2
Fracture°		4
Bone cysts (brown tumor)		4
Osteoporosis		13
Proved duodenal ulcer		6
Late duodenal ulcer		2
Neurologic disease		1

°One patient had 2 fractures.

TABLE 3.—TYPE AND DURATION OF PRIMARY SYMPTOMS

PRIMARY	PATIENTS	DURATION	AVERAGE
Renal	14	¾–24 yr.	6½ yr.
G.I.	11	½–27 yr.	5¼ yr.
Osseous	8	1 wk.–6 yr.	16½ mo.
Fatigue	4	½–2 yr.	1 yr.
Neurologic	2	2 yr.	2 yr.
Psychologic	2	3 mo.	3 mo.

TABLE 4.—HYPERPARATHYROIDISM
Adenoma Sites

Cervical:	R.U.	1	Mediastinal:	Digital	1
	R.L.	9		Split (4)	2
	L.U.	3			
	L.L.	3	Not stated:		3
	Paraesophageal	1 (R)	Multiple:		3
			Cancer:		0

The sex ratio was 21 women to 8 men. The single child attests to the rarity of the disease in childhood.

The more pertinent clinical findings in the 29 patients are summarized in Tables 2–5.

We have reviewed the charts of 13 patients with parathyroid abnormalities, two of which were neoplastic, seen at The University of Texas at Houston M. D. Anderson Hospital and Tumor Institute. The typical parathyroid tumor is shown in Figure 1. The patient illustrated in Figure 2 has physical changes which simulate those of Captain Martell.

Some brief case presentations will highlight pertinent features which identify the illness and its management:

CASE 1.—Aberrant location and bone "hunger" postoperatively: This 34-year-old woman entered the hospital having had a biopsy performed on the ulna. When a giant cell bone lesion was correctly diagnosed as a "brown" tumor, biochemical and discriminatory studies were undertaken; she had a high serum calcium and low serum phosphorus level, and also from the pyelograms, a unilateral renal calculus was discovered. The neck was explored, and an adenoma was found behind the esophagus.

Comment.—The parathyroid adenoma can localize nearly any place in the anterior neck and/or mediastinum, and diligent surgical search is essential. This patient suffered severe postoperative muscle irritability as a consequence of protracted hypocalcemia. She was maintained on supportive vitamin D and calcium therapy for nearly 15 months.

CASE 2.—Failure to find adenoma surgically and patient's failure to return. A treatment failure: This 20-year-old boy was admitted to the Urology Service having had a left ureteral calculus removed eight months previously and a calculus removed from the right kidney two months be-

TABLE 5.—THERAPY FAILURES

TYPE OF THERAPY	NUMBER	TOTAL
No operation		2
Refusal	1	
Crisis upon hospitalization	1	
Exploratory failure		3
Double adenoma	1	
Adenoma not found		
(all glands not identified)	1	
Tissue misidentified		
(no frozen-section histology)	1	
Death		2
Crisis	1	
Re-exploration	1	

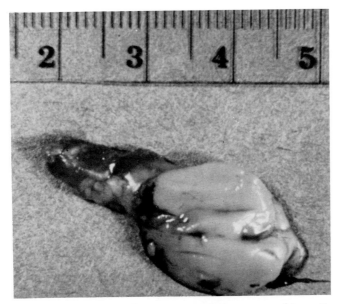

Fig. 1.—Typical parathyroid adenoma on cut section, measured in centimeters.

fore admittance. He had bilateral renal calculi on admission and the serum calcium level was 14 mg. per cent; phosphorus, 2.2 mg. per cent; and, excessive amounts of calcium were excreted in the urine. Cervical exploration was done, and a right upper, right lower, and left upper normal parathyroid were identified. Postoperatively, a bladder calculus was removed, and shortly thereafter, three other calculi were removed from the right kidney. The patient was readmitted five months after the first exploration; the mediastinum was explored and no tumor was found. The patient was rescheduled for another cervical anatomical search and a left lower thyroid lobectomy. He failed to return.

Comment.—The parathyroid was probably in the left thyroid lobe, but the patient could not be persuaded to return.

Case 3.—Hypercalcemic Crisis and Death: This 67-year-old woman complained for nine months of fatigue, insomnia, nausea, vomiting, and frequent dizziness. She had some signs during this time of early congestive failure. She was thought to have developed some dark cutaneous pigmentation and was given adrenocorticotropic hormone (ACTH) gel and corticoids. On admission the patient was acutely ill and vomiting; she suddenly became febrile and confused. Within 72 hours, she became hypotensive and anuric, regurgitated food and bile, suffered a cardiac arrest, and ex-

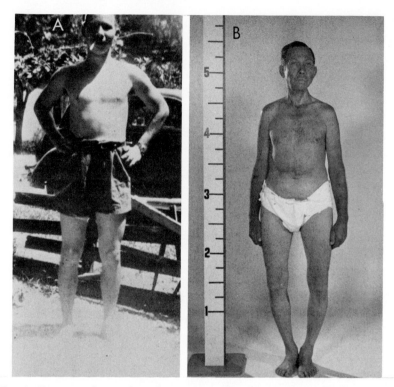

Fig. 2.—Patient with parathyroid carcinoma. The photograph on the left (*A*) was taken 24 years earlier when the disease started. He is shown on the right (*B*) at age 52 years. He has had multiple operations and treatment by oral phosphate and calcitonin (Hill, Ouais, and Leiser, 1972).

pired. The serum chemistry values returned after death showed 19.2 mg. per cent of calcium and 5.3 mg. per cent of phosphorus. The autopsy showed notable nephrosclerosis, renal calcific deposits, minimal fibrosis of the pancreas, an antemortum thrombosis of the renal vein, and a tan, elongated structure, 4 × 2 × 1.5 cm. below the right lower pole of the thyroid gland and attached to its capsule. Microscopically, this consisted of dark chief cells and hyperchromic nuclei, consistent with a parathyroid adenoma.

Comment.—This patient died in hyperparathyroid crisis. Patients with hypercalcemia from malignant disease also suffer hypotension, anuria, central nervous system change, and cardiac arrest.

CASE 4.—Multiple Adenomas: This 60-year-old woman was admitted after a fall drew attention to a lesion in the left shoulder. A diagnosis of hyperparathyroidism was made on the basis of the notable osseous changes, elevated serum calcium, depressed serum phosphorus, and elevated alkaline phosphatase, among other studies. Cervical exploration uncovered a proved parathyroid adenoma, and postoperatively (at one week) the serum calcium was 15.2 mg. per cent; it remained elevated over a protracted period of time. The likelihood of a second adenoma was recognized, but the patient was lost to follow-up at that time. She was admitted two years later with a fractured left hip, following a minor fall. She was operated on, and a second parathyroid adenoma was removed following which the blood serum calcium level fell and the phosphorus level rose. However, the patient died after a long and complicated hospital course punctuated by delayed hypocalcemia, inanition, and exhaustion.

Comment.—This case shows that more than one adenoma can be present in a patient.

CASE 5.—Associated Acute Acid-Peptic Disease and Parathyroid Adenoma: This 37-year-old woman entered the hospital with a typical acid-peptic ulcer history of nine months' duration. She had signs and symptoms of an acute duodenal perforation which had sealed. The upper gastrointestinal series showed two duodenal ulcers; a subhepatic abscess was drained and the pleural effusion resolved. The blood chemistry determinations showed a high calcium (12.3 mg. per cent) level and a low serum phosphorus level (2.9 mg. per cent); the radiograph showed no lamina dura about the teeth. The neck was explored, and three adenomas were removed.

Comment.—The gastrointestinal tract was not operated on. Notable gastric acidity levels existed preoperatively and decreased postoperatively with lessened calcium levels. The patient has been described in detail by Barreras and Donaldson (1967) who relate elevated serum calcium levels to increased acid secretion and potentially acid-peptic disease as shown here.

Discussion

Successful extirpation of an offending parathyroid adenoma with amelioration of the chemical and clinical abnormalities confirms the diagnosis. An array of diagnostic tests has been suggested, and each of these has some clinical significance; fundamentally, however, excessive secretion by the parathyroid tissue causes hypercalcemia, hypophosphatemia, hypercaluria, and hyperphosphaturia. Persistent hypercalcemia and hypophosphatemia as a recurrent finding is the mainstay of the clinical diagnosis.

Radioimmunoassay methods of assessing parathormone are also available in some laboratories but are not routine procedures generally.

In the presence of established renal change with structural tubular damage from calcium deposition, blood nitrogen increases and there is an insidious loss of renal function; there is a reduction in phosphate excretion with an elevation of serum phosphorus, and this lowers the previously elevated levels of calcium. At this stage, judicious clinical judgment is needed to determine if there is a hyperfunctioning adenoma and to remove it to stay the progression of kidney damage. It is difficult to differentiate this hyperfunctioning adenoma from renal failure with secondary hyperparathyroidism. Other diseases have been mentioned in differential diagnosis.

PREOPERATIVE IDENTIFICATION

Despite numerous maneuvers, there is no effective method to assuredly identify location of an adenoma. Only infrequently can an adenoma be clinically palpated, and the correlation of esophageal deviation by a parathyroid adenoma with barium swallow is also infrequent, but does occur (Wyman and Robbins, 1954).

Arteriography is helpful if the adenoma is large. Seldinger (1954) identified four of seven adenomas by this technique, and several patients have had such studies, using both aortic arch and thyrocervical arteriography, at M. D. Anderson Hospital. The method would be most applicable in a second search and before mediastinal exploration. Krementz, Yeager, Hawley, and Weichert (1971) report one death from stroke upon using arteriography. Selenomethionine is the only gamma ray-emitting amino acid analog that can be incorporated into the parathyroid synthesis of protein. To enhance ^{75}Se uptake by the parathyroid, thyroid uptake is suppressed with liothyronine sodium (Cytomel). At the Peter Bent Brigham Hospital, 40 patients had ^{75}Se scans and 20 of 24 operated on had a positive correlation (Potchen, Watts, and Awwad, 1967). It has been our experience, however, that false-negative scans plague the use of this technique.

Selective venous catheterization with massage of the thyroid area and timely sampling for parathyroid hormone could offer a clue with respect to tumor location. Reitz *et al.* (1969) used this technique on six patients (see also Deftos *et al.*, pages 297 to 308, this volume), and they were able to locate cervical adenomas in five. At open operation, we have measured blood parathormone levels in one patient with bilateral adenomas: from the right middle thyroid vein > 50 ng./ml., left lower thyroid vein > 38 ng./ml., right carotid artery < .8 ng./ml., all at approximately the same time. (Belatedly a second left lower adenoma was discovered so that the left side was not the control for the visualized right-sided adenoma as intended.) We plan to study the use of catheterization technique further, especially before reexploratory surgical procedures.

INTRAOPERATIVE MANAGEMENT

The adenoma can be extremely small and the lessons enumerated by Cope (1966) should be followed. The search should be orderly and careful and done in a dry field with a knowledge of where the parathyroid normally rests and with a familiarity of its appearance. The parathyroids are bilateral, usually four in number, and rest in or on the posterior part of the thyroid capsule. The superior parathyroids are posterior to the recurrent nerve; the inferior parathyroids are anterior. On the involved side the inferior parathyroid artery may be larger, but any anatomical predescription is inconstant.

Embryologically, the superior parathyroid descends with the thymus; if these are present, a mediastinal parathyroid is perhaps less likely. A mediastinal search (2–5 per cent) by sternal split is not usually scheduled as part of the first procedure. A mediastinal digital search is part of the first procedure. When one adenoma is found, a diligent search for others in the field should be done.

The surgeon must never perform an operation to look for parathyroid adenomas without quick-section surgical histologic help. Orderly confirmation of every piece of tissue removed or examined is essential. The parathyroid is normally tan, and it bruises easily, assuming a darker brown color; no other tissue behaves in an identical manner.

Preoperative staining or operative localization by toluidine blue has been helpful to others, but our experience with staining is limited. If the dye is given intravenously, as 7 mg./kg. of toluidine blue in 500 mg. of physiological saline with the induction of the anesthetic, it may selectively identify the parathyroid tissue. It is not to be used in patients with cardiac disease or renal disease, or in those with an irritable myocardium. During a second exploration (mediastinotomy and radical resection for cancer) the dye has its place. The technique is described by Skjoldborg and Nielsen (1971).

Summary

Data on parathyroid adenoma have been gathered from two types of institutions. We have chosen to excerpt the studies in more detail from one institution, because they are more applicable to clinical practice and this conference.

The physiological lesson from the case history of Captain Martell is very real: An adenoma not removed may lead to disability and death. In contrast, with mass screening or chemical biopsy, as now commonly done, the physician may be warned of an elevated serum calcium level and a depressed phosphorus level in his patient. However, this is not synonymous with a call for immediate exploration.

The diagnosis is by exclusion. In a cancer institution, a hyperfunctioning adenoma is rarely a proved cause of hypercalcemia. The functioning adenoma should be removed with the following surgical aids and points in mind:

1. Bloodless, clean field.
2. Orderly search with anatomical and embryological knowledge.
3. Frozen-section histological confirmation; this is essential, and there may be more than one adenoma present.
4. Unpredictability of adenoma sites, whether neck or mediastinum, is the rule.
5. Aids such as preoperative, radioisotopically tagged amino acids, arteriography, radiography, and intraoperative vital dye staining may be useful.

The association of multiple endocrine adenomatoses should not be overlooked.

REFERENCES

Aub, J. C., Fairhall, L. T., Minot, A. S., and Reznikoff, P.: Lead poisoning. *Medicine*, 4:1-250, 1925.

Barreras, R. F., and Donaldson, R. M.: Role of calcium in gastric hypersecretion, parathyroid adenoma and peptic ulcer. *The New England Journal of Medicine*, 276:1122-1124, May 1967.

Bauer, W., and Federman, D. D.: Hyperparathyroidism epitomized: The case of Captain Charles E. Martell. *Metabolism*, XI:21-29, January 1962.

Collip, J. B.: The extraction of parathyroid hormone which will prevent or control parathyroid tetany and which regulates the level of blood calcium. *The Journal of Biological Chemistry*, 63:395-438, 1925.

Cope, O.: The story of hyperparathyroidism at the Massachusetts General Hospital. *The New England Journal of Medicine*, 274:1174-1182, May 1966.

Cope, O., Culver, P. J., Mixter, C. G., Jr., and Nardi, G. L.: Pancreatitis, a diagnostic clue to hyperparathyroidism. *Annals of Surgery*, 145:857-863, June 1957.

Copp, D. H., Cameron, E. C., Cheney, B. A., Davidson, A. G. F., and Henze, K. G.: Evidence for calcitonin—a new hormone from parathyroid that lowers blood calcium. *Endocrinology*, 70:638-649, May 1962.

Hill, C. S., Jr., Ouais, S. G., and Leiser, A. E.: Long-term administration of calcitonin for hypercalcemia secondary to recurrent parathyroid carcinoma. *Cancer*, 29:1016-1020, 1972.

Hirsch, P. F., Gauthier, G. F., and Munson, P. L.: Thyroid hypocalcemic principle and recurrent laryngeal nerve injury as factors affecting response to parathyroidectomy in rats. *Endocrinology*, 73:244-252, August 1963.

Keating, F. R., Jr.: The clinical problem of primary hyperparathyroidism. *Medical Clinics of North America*, 54:511-529, March 1970.

————: Diagnosis of primary hyperparathyroidism. Clinical and laboratory aspects. *The Journal of the American Medical Association*, 178:547-555, November 1961.

Krementz, E. T., Yeager, R., Hawley, W., and Weichert, R.: The first 100 cases of parathyroid tumor from Charity Hospital of Louisiana. *Annals of Surgery*, 173:872-883, June 1971.

Potchen, E. J., Watts, H. G., and Awwad, H. K.: Parathyroid scintiscanning. *Radiologic Clinics of North America*, V:267-275, August 1967.

Reitz, R. E., Pollock, J. J., Wang, C. A., Fleischli, D. L., Cope, O., Murray, T. M., Deftos, L. J., and Potts, J. T., Jr.: Localization of parathyroid adenomas by selective venous catheterization and radioimmunoassay. *The New England Journal of Medicine*, 281:348-351, August 1969.

Rogers, H. M., Keating, F. R., Jr., Morlock, C. G., and Barker, N. W.: Primary hypertrophy and hyperplasia of the parathyroid glands associated with duodenal ulcer. Report of an additional case, with special reference to metabolic, gastrointestinal and vascular manifestations. *Archives of Internal Medicine*, 79:307-321, 1947.

Seldinger, S. I.: Localization of parathyroid adenomata by arteriography. *Acta radiologica*, 42:353-366, April 1954.

Skjoldborg, H., and Nielsen, H. M.: Preoperative staining of parathyroid adenomas by intravenous infusion of toluidine blue. *Acta chirurgica scandinavica*, 137:213-219, 1971.

Wermer, P.: Genetic aspects of adenomatosis of endocrine glands. *The American Journal of Medicine*, 16:363-371, March 1954.

Wyman, S. M., and Robbins, L. L.: Roentgen recognition of parathyroid adenoma. *The American Journal of Roentgenology, Radium Therapy and Nuclear Medicine*, 71:777-784, May 1954.

Malignant Thyroid Tumors: Their Manifestations

C. STRATTON HILL, JR., M.D.

Department of Medicine, The University of Texas at Houston
M. D. Anderson Hospital and Tumor Institute,
Houston, Texas

CLINICALLY, thyroid cancer can no longer be considered a single disease. It can be categorized into three distinct clinical groups. Fortunately, these groups also fall into distinctive histological categories.

The tumors of clinical Group I are histologically classified as pure papillary, pure follicular, mixed papillary, and follicular and Hürthle cell carcinomas. These four morphological types of thyroid cancer are composed of cells, and in some cases have structural characteristics, which resemble those of the normal thyroid gland. Because of this, it is reasonable to categorize them under the term "differentiated carcinomas;" 85 per cent of the thyroid cancers seen at M. D. Anderson Hospital fall into this category. The majority of these tumors are biologically indolent. Some, however, are aggressive in their behavior with early recurrence or metastasis after initial treatment. Factors which account for this difference in biological activity are unclear.

The clinical Group II tumor is characterized by an extremely rapid growth rate and early demise of the patient after the diagnosis is made. In our series, the median survival of these patients from diagnosis to death is three months. This tumor accounts for approximately 5 per cent of all the patients with thyroid cancer seen at M. D. Anderson Hospital and is histologically classified as anaplastic (spindle and giant cell) carcinoma. It occurs most frequently in patients in the seventh and eighth decades of life. Our studies indicate it is related to the differentiated types, as will be discussed subsequently.

The clinical Group III tumor is characterized by an intermediate grade of biological behavior; that is, intermediate in severity, both from the standpoint of aggressiveness in local invasion of tissue and of survival, between the two previous groups. It accounts for 9 per cent of all the patients with thyroid cancer seen at M. D. Anderson Hospital and is histologically classified as medullary or solid carcinoma (MCT) of the thyroid gland.

Detailed clinical features which justify the separation of thyroid tumors into these groups will be outlined subsequently, but there are general features that apply to all malignant thyroid tumors. The vast majority produce no systemic symptoms. If a tumor has obtained sufficient size to destroy the gland, there will be symptoms of hypothyroidism, and if it produces excess thyroid hormone, there are manifestations of hyperthyroidism. Altered thyroid function in these patients, however, rarely occurs. There may be symptoms related to the presence of the mass in the neck. Usually this does not occur in the differentiated carcinomas but it may in medullary and anaplastic tumors. When present, the symptom is usually a sense of discomfort with deglutition. The degree of discomfort is directly related to the size of the mass, except in those instances in which there has been direct invasion of the esophagus by the tumor. Esophageal invasion by the differentiated variety is rare.

Occasionally, hoarseness may be a symptom of thyroid cancer. It may be temporary or permanent. Temporary hoarseness occurs when the tumor produces pressure on the recurrent laryngeal nerve without causing permanent damage. Permanent hoarseness occurs when the pressure actually causes the nerve to deteriorate or when the tumor invades the nerve. Permanent hoarseness in patients with differentiated tumors occurs most frequently when there is extensive disease in the neck at the time of diagnosis. It usually occurs in patients who have neglected their disease or who have had poor medical advice. It is more likely to occur in patients having medullary or anaplastic carcinoma because of their more rapid growth rate and greater invasiveness.

Painless neck enlargement, when it occurs suddenly, is frequently a symptom of anaplastic carcinoma. This symptom rarely occurs in the other clinical groups. Sudden painful neck enlargement may occur when there is bleeding into either a benign or malignant goiter. Skin ulceration has been observed in rapidly growing anaplastic tumors but is seldom seen in the other groups.

Diarrhea may be a prominent symptom of medullary carcinoma. In some instances, this has preceded discovery of the neck mass. Severe, unexplained diarrhea should alert the physician to carefully examine the thyroid gland.

In general, one may state that symptoms from thyroid cancer are observed far more frequently in the anaplastic and medullary carcinomas than in the tumors of the differentiated category. These symptoms are usually confined to the neck area and related to the bulk of the tumor mass itself. Constitutional symptoms such as anorexia, weight loss, and fatigue are surprisingly minor, and when they occur, it is as a terminal event. The differentiated carcinoma is most frequently accidentally discovered by the patient while rubbing the neck, applying makeup, or shaving, or the tumefaction is pointed out by a neighbor or friend.

There are no reliable findings on physical examination of the thyroid gland which distinguish one group of thyroid cancer from the others. In general, the anaplastic tumors are larger and severely distort the normal contour of the thyroid gland. Similar findings hold for examination of the neck outside of the thyroid gland; that is, the anaplastic variety tends to invade the soft tissues of the neck more frequently than the other varieties.

Until recently, there was no laboratory test which could directly assess whether a thyroid nodule was malignant or benign, and certainly none that could distinguish the various clinical groups. With the development of a sensitive radioimmunoassay for measurement of calcitonin in human serum, it is now possible to diagnose MCT with certainty preoperatively (Hill *et al.*, 1971; Melvin, Miller, and Tashjian, 1971).

All thyroid tests which measure thyroid hormone production or iodine metabolism by the gland are not definitive in distinguishing either a malignant from a benign nodule or the various clinical types of thyroid cancer. Since most patients with thyroid cancer are euthyroid, these tests are normal. The physician should keep in mind that these tests assess the function of the gland only and do not help in any way to differentiate benign from malignant lesions or one variety of malignant tumor from another. The thyroid scan is helpful in assessing whether a thyroid nodule is malignant, but it cannot distinguish between the types of malignant tumors.

Clinical Manifestations of the Three Groups of Thyroid Cancer

DIFFERENTIATED CARCINOMAS

Of the four morphological types of thyroid cancer in this category, the pure follicular and Hürthle cell carcinomas have more specific clinical features characteristic for them than do the other types. The most frequently occurring characteristic of these tumors is bone involvement. A significant number of these patients will present with pathological fractures as the first manifestation of their disease. In addition, those who do not present this way are more likely to develop bone metastasis than patients with pure papillary or mixed papillary and follicular carcinomas.

The follicular carcinoma is more likely to concentrate radioactive iodine than the other types (Pochin, 1970). In spite of this concentration, however, the therapeutic effect is not always of significant benefit to the patient (Pochin, 1971). The following case report illustrates the above mentioned features:

F. O., a 62-year-old black woman, was referred because of a large tumor mass involving the right upper arm. Three years earlier, she had sustained a fracture of the right humerus after minor stress on the extremity. An X-ray film revealed a pathological fracture, and an intermedullary nail was placed in the humerus. A biopsy of the lesion was taken at that time and revealed highly differentiated metastatic thyroid carcinoma. Either no advice for further treatment of thyroid cancer was given at that time or the patient failed to understand it, because no treatment to the thyroid was done at that time. Shortly after the acute episode, the patient's arm began to enlarge and continued to do so progressively over the next three years.

The physical examination at the time of admission revealed a notably enlarged right upper arm with obvious evidence of venous obstruction (Fig. 1A) and single nodules in the left upper lobe and the right lobe of the thyroid. A radiograph of the right humerus revealed bone destruction (Fig. 1B).

A total thyroidectomy was performed, and follicular carcinoma was found in the nodule in the left lobe only. It was completely encapsulated, and no spread within the gland was detected by subserial sectioning.

The lesion in the arm had demonstrated a significant uptake of radioactive iodine before the thyroidectomy. After the thyroidectomy, the amount of uptake in the arm had increased. The patient was treated with radioactive iodine, and there was evidence of healing of the lesion in the humerus as indicated by thickening of the bone trabeculae. The size of the arm, however, did not diminish.

The patient did well for a period of approximately nine months, at which time she developed weakness of her right leg and loss of bladder control. A myelogram showed complete obstruction at the level of T_5. A laminectomy was done, but the patient progressed to complete paralysis of her lower extremities and died approximately four months after laminectomy. The total dose of radioactive iodine the patient received before the development of her paraplegia was 390 mc.

Although the factors which account for the characteristically favorable course in most of these patients are not clear, one possible significant observation may be the age factor. In general, the patients with an aggressive course are in the age group past 40 at the time of initial diagnosis. The

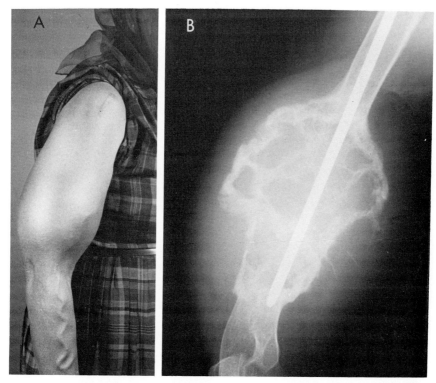

Fig. 1.—*A*, metastatic follicular carcinoma of the thyroid gland involving the distal humerus and soft tissue of upper arm. Note dilated vein of forearm secondary to venous obstruction by the tumor. (See also Figure 3, Russell and Ibanez, this volume.) *B*, roentgenograph of lesion illustrated in A. Intramedullary nail was applied at the time of initial fracture three years before this roentgenograph was made.

aggressive course in our patients did not seem to be related to any one of the specific types more frequently than to the others. We cannot definitely relate survival to the type of initial treatment, except that the highest percentage of survivors have had surgical removal of their disease as initial treatment; those having total thyroidectomy as the initial surgical procedure had less recurrence than those with lesser surgical procedures.

ANAPLASTIC (SPINDLE AND GIANT CELL) CARCINOMA

A typical clinical course of anaplastic carcinoma is illustrated by the following patient:

B. D., a 72-year-old white woman, presented with a history of having a thyroid nodule, "for as long as I can remember." At least 20 years previously she was advised to have the tumor removed; however, she failed to heed this advice.. In January 1971, the tumor mass began to grow rapidly and the patient became alarmed. She consulted her physician who advised removal of the gland. A total thyroidectomy was attempted, but apparently all of the gland could not be removed. After operation, she was treated with external irradiation. The exact amount was not known.

In July, 1971, the tumor mass reappeared, and ulceration through the skin occurred. There was notable progression of disease during the ensuing six weeks (Fig. 2).

We have observed 61 patients with anaplastic carcinoma at M. D. Anderson Hospital during the past 26 years. More than twice as many were observed during the second half of this period than the first, although the number of all types of thyroid cancer has increased only moderately. In 50 of these patients, we have observed a combination of differentiated and anaplastic pathology in the same specimen on histological examination. In six of the 11 patients who did not exhibit this phenomenon, we had limited material for histological study; therefore, we could not rule out the possibility that they too had combined pathology. This high percentage of patients exhibiting differentiated carcinoma and anaplastic carcinoma in the same tumor leads us to believe the two are related. Evidence for this belief is derived from the following: 11 of the 61 patients had been treated for the differentiated variety of thyroid cancer for a median of 96 months and an average of 104 months before the development of the anaplastic tumor. An additional 22 patients had a history of an undiagnosed thyroid nodule for a median of 240 months and an average of 228 months before diagnosis of anaplastic carcinoma. In this latter group, 15 (68 per cent) had combined pathology in their tumor. In four of the six in which no combined pathology could be demonstrated, the diagnosis of anaplastic carcinoma was made from the limited histological material for study. Failure to demonstrate combined pathology in all of our patients could easily be explained by the growth characteristics of this tumor which is highly invasive and could destroy all evidence of the differentiated component.

Additional evidence for this transition is found in the morphological features seen both in the primary tumor and the metastatic deposits. A more detailed discussion of this aspect of this characteristic of the tumor appears elsewhere (see pages 363 to 397, this volume).

It has been suggested by others that development of anaplastic carcinoma in a patient with the differentiated variety occurs as a result of exposure to irradiation from radioiodine for the treatment of the differentiated carcinoma (Crile and Wilson, 1959). Of the 22 patients with long-stand-

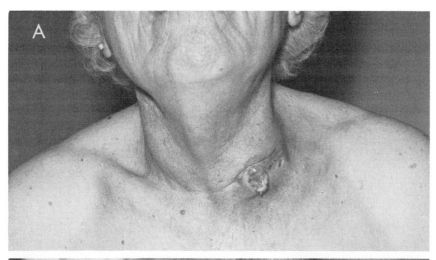

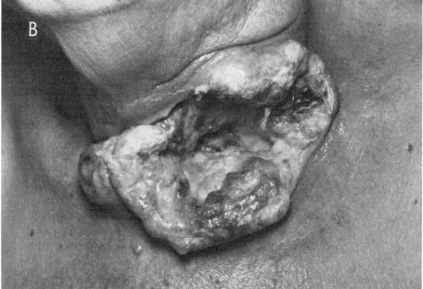

FIG. 2.—A, small ulcerating lesion at the left border of the thyroidectomy scar present when patient was initially referred for treatment. B, tumor has progressed into large, fungating, necrotic lesion in period of six weeks.

ing, undiagnosed thyroid disease, only one gave a history of radiation exposure before diagnosis of anaplastic carcinoma. Of 11 patients who were treated for the differentiated carcinoma before diagnosis of anaplastic carcinoma, five had either external X-ray therapy or radioactive iodine as the treatment for the differentiated carcinoma. These data suggest that the development of anaplastic carcinoma may be a natural result of the chronicity of untreated or perhaps inadequately treated differentiated carcinoma rather than being directly related to an additional insult such as irradiation.

Medullary (Solid) Carcinoma

Hazard and his colleagues, in 1959, were first to point out that medullary carcinoma (MCT) deserved recognition as a separate clinicopathological entity (Hazard, Hawk, and Crile, 1959). Features which they felt were sufficient to justify this recognition were the characteristic histological picture, an intermediate grade of malignancy, and its propensity for early cervical and mediastinal lymph node involvement.

On gross examination, MCT may be sharply demarcated from the surrounding normal thyroid tissue or may infiltrate it, forming no definite border. The tumor is grey-white in color and firm in consistency. The histological features, however, are the most distinctive. There are sheets of polyhedral cells separated by fibrous stroma containing amyloid. This is the only thyroid tumor which contains this substance. Tissue culture studies have shown that the tumor cells produce the amyloid, and it is found both intra- and extracellularly (Albores-Saavedra *et al.*, 1964). There may also be a component of spindle cells present in the tumor, and some have related the prognosis to the degree to which these cells are present; *i.e.*, the greater the number of spindle cells present, the worse the prognosis is (Williams, 1967). The pathologist, unfamiliar with this specific tumor, may categorize it as an "undifferentiated" thyroid carcinoma. This diagnosis should be accepted by the clinician only if it is certain that MCT has been considered in the differential diagnosis by the pathologist and has been rejected. A delay in diagnosis to obtain special stains of the tissue to assure accuracy in the final diagnosis is acceptable.

Figure 3 illustrates that MCT is intermediate in its grade of malignancy between the differentiated and anaplastic types.

Our MCT patients did not have a higher percentage of early cervical lymph node involvement at the time of diagnosis, as reported by Hazard, Hawk, and Crile (1959); however, there was a significantly higher percentage of patients with mediastinal lymph node involvement at the time of diagnosis than of the other types. Figure 4 shows a chest X-ray film of

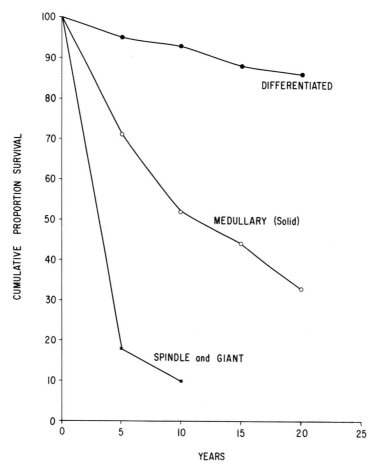

SURVIVAL BY HISTOLOGY ONLY
(BERKSON-GAGE)

FIG. 3.—Survival curves of the three clinical groups of thyroid cancer based on histologic evidence only.

a patient with minimal disease in the neck and extensive mediastinal involvement at the time of diagnosis.

Since Hazard's report, many new features about this tumor have been observed. They fall into three major categories: (1) familial occurrence, (2) association with other tumors, and (3) hormone and enzyme production. In addition to these, we have observed several other features, some of

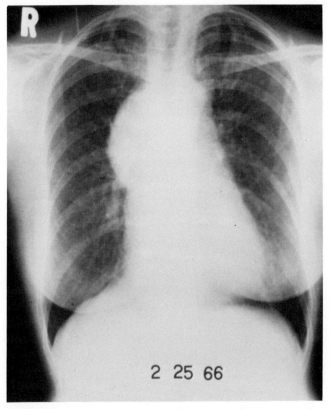

Fɪɢ. 4.—Large hilar mass representing early lymph node metastasis from minimal lesion in right lobe of thyroid. Note slight deviation of trachea to left.

which have been alluded to by others, which we feel are worthy of reporting. They are as follows: (1) desmoplastic reaction, (2) peptic ulceration, (3) visceral diverticulum, and (4) Marfanoid habitus.

Many reports have appeared in which this tumor occurs on a familial basis. The mode of inheritance is autosomal dominant (Steiner, Goodman, and Powers, 1968). Of 67 families with this disease seen at M. D. Anderson Hospital, three have exhibited the familial occurrence. Our data suggest that the sporadic variety of this tumor occurs more frequently than the familial type. The familial occurrence of the tumor may confer special features to it. In all of our patients with the familial type, the tumor has occurred bilaterally. This has also been reported in the literature (Keynes and Till, 1971). We have observed the pheochromocytoma and parathyroid adenomas only in patients with the familial variety.

Sipple (1961) pointed out the unusually high association of thyroid cancer with pheochromocytomas. Many reports of this association have appeared since Sipple's initial report, and significantly all of the thyroid cancers have been of the medullary variety (Huang and McLeish, 1968; Ljungberg, Cederquist, and von Studnitz, 1967; Mowar, 1966; Slavotinek, de la Lande, and Head, 1968). The incidence of pheochromocytoma in patients with MCT followed up at our institution and specifically examined for this association was 18 per cent (8/44). It is difficult to draw conclusions concerning this incidence from our data because not all MCT patients have yet developed pheochromocytoma, and deceased patients may have died before it could develop. Either the thyroid cancer or the pheochromocytoma may occur first, and the interval between the tumors may be variable from patient to patient. Generally, however, and in all but one of our patients, the thyroid cancer appeared first. In this one patient, the first pheochromocytoma preceded the thyroid tumor by 12 years. Two pheochromocytomas were discovered simultaneously in the opposite adrenal gland 18 months after the thyroid tumor was removed. A sister of another patient has had removal of a unilateral pheochromocytoma but has not as yet developed MCT. Pheochromocytoma associated with MCT is bilateral in a high percentage of cases (Urbanski, 1967). The incidence of bilaterality in our series was 50 per cent. This compares closely with the incidence of 46 per cent bilaterality in familial pheochromocytoma not associated with MCT and is much higher than the 5 per cent bilaterality observed in spontaneous pheochromocytoma (Huang and McLeish, 1968). A diagnosis of pheochromocytoma can be made with certainty in almost all cases by the measurement of urinary catecholamines and/or their metabolites. Once the diagnosis is established, some method of localization is necessary because of the high incidence of bilaterality. Knowledge about bilaterality allows for proper surgical planning. We are not aware of pheochromocytoma developing in sites other than the adrenal gland when it occurs in association with MCT. However, pheochromocytoma occurring in an accessory gland has been reported in association with this tumor (Ljungberg, Cederquist, and von Studnitz, 1967). Several methods are available for localizing pheochromocytomas; namely, arteriography, selective adrenal arteriography, selective adrenal venography, and analysis of plasma samples obtained by caval catheterization for epinephrine and norepinephrine. We prefer selective adrenal venography since it is technically relatively simple and the results are immediate. Venography has the disadvantage of failing to detect any extra-adrenal lesions. However, as stated previously, no extra-adrenal pheochromocytoma has been reported in association with MCT.

It has been speculated that parathyroid adenoma and hyperplasia develop as a compensatory reaction to the excessive calcitonin production by MCT (*cf.* calcitonin following) (Finegold and Haddad, 1963; Manning *et al.*, 1963; Melvin, Miller, and Tashjian, 1971). The possibility of a genetic basis, however, cannot be ignored. Two of our patients had histologically proven parathyroid adenomas. Both were discovered in patients with the familial variety of MCT. Neither of the parathyroid adenomas was clinically active. However, no measurements of serum parathyroid hormone were done.

Mucosal neuromata were not observed in any of our living patients, and review of the records of those who died before this association was appreciated make no mention of neuromata. One patient, who is dead, had megacolon. It is possible this patient had ganglioneuromatosis, which may have accounted for his megacolon, involving the myenteric and submucosal plexuses by the same neuromatous process as that seen on the eyelids, buccal mucosa, tongue, and lips by other investigators. Unfortunately, he died outside of the hospital and no postmortem examination was done. That none of our patients exhibited neuromata can be explained genetically by the fact that instances of MCT in association with pheochromocytoma and neuromata are more probably the result of a different allele than are instances of the syndrome in which neuromata are not observed (Knudson and Strong, in press).

In 1968, several investigators reported almost simultaneously that MCT produced large quantities of calcitonin when compared to the normal thyroid gland of man (Meyer and Abdel-Bari, 1968; Tashjian and Melvin, 1968; Tubiana *et al.*, 1968). The development of the radioimmunoassay to measure calcitonin has made it possible to measure conveniently the concentration of this substance in the serum. This has proven to be diagnostic for MCT (Tashjian, Howland, Melvin, and Hill, 1970). The significantly elevated serum calcitonin concentration which occurs with extensive MCT seems to produce surprisingly little effect on the patient. Since the primary action of calcitonin is to inhibit calcium resorption from bone, one would expect increased bone density in these patients, but we have observed no radiographic evidence of increased bone density.

Calcitonin is also purported to lower the serum concentration of calcium, and excessive concentrations of calcitonin would be expected to produce hypocalcemia. We have not observed this nor has it been the general experience of others in patients with metastatic MCT and high levels of calcitonin, although it has been reported (Tashjian and Melvin, 1968).

The calcitonin assay is useful in (1) diagnosing MCT in patients with a thyroid nodule, (2) possible monitoring of patients with MCT who have been treated for the development of recurrent and metastatic disease, and (3) the detection of MCT in high-risk individuals (children and sibs of patients) whose thyroid glands are normal on physical and laboratory examination.

Baylin showed that patients with MCT have high levels of histaminase in the tumor compared to normal thyroid tissue (Baylin, Beaven, Engelman, and Sjoerdsma, 1970). In addition, these patients have elevated serum levels of this enzyme when the disease spreads outside the confines of the gland; this is useful in detecting metastatic disease. This laboratory test is a complement to the measurement of serum calcitonin concentration for full evaluation of any patient's tumor status.

Williams and Bernier *et al.*, were the first to focus attention on the symptom of diarrhea as a component of the MCT syndrome (Williams, 1966; Bernier, Bouvry, Cattan, and Prost, 1966). Thirty-three per cent of our patients had diarrhea. It is suspected that this symptom is the result of some type of humoral substance elaborated by the tumor; however, no consistent findings have been observed. Studies done at M. D. Anderson Hospital suggest that the diarrhea occurs when the patient has widespread metastatic disease. The type of diarrhea is compatible with that seen in disturbances of motility, and, like Bernier and colleagues (1966), we found that the diarrhea could be controlled with small doses of antispasmodics and opiates.

MCT has been associated with two endocrine syndromes which are caused by hormones not produced by the thyroid gland, *viz.*, Cushing's syndrome and the carcinoid syndrome (Melvin, Tashjian, Cassidy, and Givens, 1970; Moertel, Beahrs, Woolner, and Tyce, 1965). Additionally, one patient was reported to have pigmentation which disappeared when the thyroid tumor was removed (Cunliffe *et al.*, 1970). The symptom of "flushing" without any detectable cause has also been reported in patients with MCT.

We have observed severe desmoplastic reactions involving fibrotic reaction in the lungs. Peptic ulcers were observed in five of our patients, and in two of them, one with a duodenal and one with a gastric ulcer, the ulcers were multiple. We noted diverticula in several of our patients, and this has also been reported in some case reports in the literature. Finally, one of our patients had a Marfanoid habitus, and this too has been reported sporadically in the literature (Cunliffe *et al.*, 1970; Mielke, Becker, and Gross, 1965; Nankin, Hydovitz, and Sapira, 1970; Normann and Otnes, 1969). We cannot claim that the last four observations have occurred in our patients more frequently than one would expect by chance alone but merely suggest that these features be looked for in future patients with MCT.

There is increasing evidence that MCT is a tumor of the so-called "C cell," which is derived from the neural crest and travels with the ultimobranchial body into the thyroid gland in man (Le Douarin and Le Lievre, 1970; Pearse, 1970). This would best explain this tumor's ability to produce a polypeptide hormone and probably accounts for its distinct clinical behavior.

Summary

Evidence has been presented that thyroid cancer may be divided into three groups based upon clinical behavior. These clinical groups also fall into three distinctive histological categories. The most commonly occurring thyroid cancer, differentiated carcinoma, is characterized by prolonged survival for the majority of patients. The follicular and Hürthle cell varieties of differentiated carcinoma have a propensity for bone metastasis, and indeed this may be the presenting symptom for these tumors. The rarest thyroid cancer, anaplastic (spindle and giant cell) carcinoma, usually occurs in patients in the seventh and eighth decades of life and is characterized by an extremely short survival. The third thyroid cancer type, MCT, is characterized for most patients by a survival intermediate between the other two types. In certain instances, which are probably genetically determined, MCT is associated with special features. This is the only malignant thyroid tumor that can be diagnosed before histological examination. The basis of this diagnosis is the tumor's ability to produce a polypeptide hormone, calcitonin, and the development of a sensitive radioimmunoassay which makes it possible to detect elevated levels of this hormone in the serum of patients with MCT. The assay is useful in (1) diagnosing MCT in patients with thyroid nodules, (2) possibly monitoring patients with MCT who have been treated for the development of recurrence and/or metastasis, and (3) detection of MCT in high-risk individuals (children and sibs of patients with MCT) who have normal thyroid glands on clinical and laboratory examination.

Acknowledgments

Portions of this work were supported by U.S.P.H.S. Grants No. CA 05831-01, CA 12521-01 and RR 00254, and a grant from the Kelsey and Leary Foundation for the Advancement of Medicine.

REFERENCES

Albores-Saavedra, J., Rose, G. G., Ibanez, M. L., Russell, W. O., Grey, C. E., and Dmochowski, L.: The amyloid in solid carcinoma of the thyroid gland. Staining characteristics, tissue culture, and electron microscopic observations. *Laboratory Investigation*, 13:77-93, January 1964.

Baylin, S. B., Beaven, M. A., Engelman, K., and Sjoerdsma, A.: Elevated histaminase activity in medullary carcinoma of the thyroid gland. *The New England Journal of Medicine*, 283:1239-1244, December 1970.

Bernier, J. J., Bouvry, M., Cattan, D., and Prost, A.: Diarrhee motrice par cancer medullaire thyroidien. Nouvelle entite anatomo-clinique. *Bulletins et Memoires de la Societe Medicale des Hopitaux de Paris*, 117:1191-1197, 1966.

Crile, G., Jr., and Wilson, D. H.: Transformation of a low grade papillary carcinoma of the thyroid to an anaplastic carcinoma after treatment with radioiodine. *Surgery, Gynecology and Obstetrics*, 108:357-360, March 1959.

Cunliffe, W. J., Hudgson, P., Fulthorpe, J. J., Block, M. M., Hall, R., Johnston, I. D. A., and Shuster, S.: A calcitonin-secreting medullary thyroid carcinoma associated with mucosal neuromas, Marfanoid features, myopathy and pigmentation. *The American Journal of Medicine*, 48:120-126, January 1970.

Finegold, M. J., and Haddad, J. R.: Multiple endocrine tumors. Report of an unusual triad in a family. *Archives of Pathology*, 76:449-455, October 1963.

Hazard, J. B., Hawk, W. A., and Crile, G.: Medullary (solid) carcinoma of the thyroid—A clinicopathologic entity. *The Journal of Clinical Endocrinology and Metabolism*, 19:152-161, January 1959.

Hill, C. S., Jr., Tashjian, A. H., Ibanez, M. L., Samaan, N. A., and Clark, R. L.: Diagnostic value of plasma calcitonin in patients with medullary carcinoma of the thyroid. In Fellinger, K., and Hofer, R., Eds.: *Further Advances in Thyroid Research*. Vienna, Austria, Verlag der Weiner Medizinischen Akademie, 1971, pp. 1245-1252.

Huang, S., and McLeish, W. A.: Pheochromocytoma and medullary carcinoma of thyroid. *Cancer*, 21:302-311, February 1968.

Keynes, W. M., and Till, A. S.: Medullary carcinoma of the thyroid gland. *Quarterly Journal of Medicine*, New Series, Vol. XL, 159:443-456, July 1971.

Knudson, A. G., and Strong, L. C.: Mutation and Cancer: Neuroblastoma and pheochromocytoma. *The American Journal of Human Genetics*. (In press.)

Le Douarin, N., and Le Lievre, C.: Démonstration de l'origine neurale des cellules à calcitonine du corps ultimobranchial chez l'embryon de poulet. *Comptes Rendus Hebdomadairds des Seances de l'academie des Sciences* (D) Paris, 270:2857-2860, June 8, 1970.

Ljungberg, O., Cederquist, E., and von Studnitz, W.: Medullary thyroid carcinoma and phaeochromocytoma: A familial chromaffinomatosis. *British Medical Journal*, 1:279-281, February 1967.

Manning, P. C., Molnar, G. D., Black, B. M., Priestley, J. T., and Woolner, L. B.: Pheochromocytoma, hyperparathyroidism and thyroid carcinoma occurring coincidentally. Report of a case. *The New England Journal of Medicine*, 268:68-72, January 1963.

Melvin, K. E. W., Miller, H. H., and Tashjian, A. H., Jr.: Early diagnosis of medullary carcinoma of the thyroid gland by means of calcitonin assay. *The New England Journal of Medicine*, 285:1115-1120, November 1971.

Melvin, K. E. W., Tashjian, A. H., Jr., Cassidy, C. E., and Givens, J. R.: Cushing's syndrome caused by ACTH and calcitonin-secreting medullary carcinoma of the thyroid. *Metabolism*, 19:831-838, October 1970.

Meyer, J. S., and Abdel-Bari, W.: Granules and thyrocalcitonin-like activity in medullary carcinoma of the thyroid gland. *The New England Journal of Medicine*, 278:523-529, March 1968.

Mielke, J. E., Becker, K. L., and Gross, J. B.: Diverticulitis of the colon in a young man with Marfan's syndrome. *Gastroenterology*, 48:379-382, March 1965.

Moertel, C. G., Beahrs, O. H., Woolner, L. B., and Tyce, G. M.: "Malignant carcinoid syndrome" associated with noncarcinoid tumors. *The New England Journal of Medicine*, 273:244-248, July 1965.

Mowar, S. N.: Pheochromocytoma with thyroid cancer. *Indian Medical Journal*, 60:73-74, April 1966.

Nankin, H., Hydovitz, J., and Sapira, J.: Normal chromosomes in mucosal neuroma variant of medullary thyroid carcinoma syndrome. *Journal of Medical Genetics*, 7:374-378, December 1970.

Normann, T., and Otnes, B.: Intestinal ganglioneuromatosis, diarrhoea and medullary thyroid carcinoma. *Scandinavian Journal of Gastroenterology*, 4:553-559, 1969.

Pearse, A. G. E.: The characteristics of the C cell and their significance in relation to those of other endocrine polypeptide cells and to the synthesis, storage and secretion of calcitonin. In Taylor, S., and Foster, G., eds.: *Calcitonin 1969, Proceedings of the Second International Symposium.* London, England, Heinmann, 1970, pp. 125-140.

Pochin, E. E.: Criteria for selecting thyroid cancers as suitable for radioiodine treatment. *Indian Journal of Cancer*, 7:191-199, September 1970.

————: Radioiodine therapy of thyroid cancer. *Seminars in Nuclear Medicine*, 1:503-515, October 1971.

Sipple, J. H.: The association of pheochromocytoma with carcinoma of the thyroid gland. *The American Journal of Medicine*, 31:163-166, July 1961.

Slavotinek, A., de la Lande, I. S., and Head, R.: Medullary thyroid carcinomas with bilateral pheochromocytomas. *Australian Annals of Medicine*, 17:320-326, November 1968.

Steiner, A. L., Goodman, A. D., and Powers, S. R.: Study of a kindred with pheochromocytoma, medullary thyroid carcinoma, hyperparathyroidism and Cushing's disease: Multiple endocrine neoplasia, Type 2. *Medicine*, 47:371-409, 1968.

Tashjian, A. H., Jr., Howland, B. G., Melvin, K. E. W., and Hill, C. S., Jr.: Immunoassay of human calcitonin: Clinical measurement, relation to serum calcium and studies in patients with medullary carcinoma. *The New England Journal of Medicine*, 283:890-895, October 1970.

Tashjian, A. H., Jr., and Melvin, K. E. W.: Medullary carcinoma of the thyroid gland: Studies of thyrocalcitonin in plasma tumor extracts. *The New England Journal of Medicine*, 279:279-283, August 1968.

Tubiana, M., Milhaud, G., Coutris, G., Lacour, J., Parmentier, C., and Bok, B.: Medullary carcinoma and thyrocalcitonin. *British Medical Journal*, 4:87-89, October 1968.

Urbanski, F. X.: Medullary thyroid carcinoma, parathyroid adenoma, and bilateral pheochromocytoma. An unusual triad of endocrine tumors. *Journal of Chronic Diseases*, 20:627-636, 1967.

Williams, E. D.: Diarrhea and thyroid carcinoma. *Proceedings of the Royal Society of Medicine*, 59:602-603, July 1966.

————: Medullary carcinoma of the thyroid. *Journal of Clinical Pathology*, 20:395-398, 1967.

Calcitonin, The Significance of Its Measurement and Its Metabolic Effects

NAGUIB A. SAMAAN, M.D., M.R.C.P., Ph.D., F.A.C.P.

Department of Medicine, The University of Texas at Houston
M. D. Anderson Hospital and Tumor Institute,
Houston, Texas

About 12 years ago, Harold Copp of Vancouver (Copp and Davidson, 1961) postulated the presence of a serum calcium-lowering hormone in the parathyroid gland.

Two years later, Paul Munson and his group at Boston (Hirsch, Gauthier, and Munson, 1963) found that the crude extract from the thyroid gland injected into an intact young rat produced a significant fall in the serum calcium level. Similar findings were observed in the goat and reported by MacIntyre's group at London (Foster et al., 1964). Thus, it was established that the origin of the hypocalcemic factor is the thyroid gland rather than the parathyroid gland. This hypocalcemic substance was then called calcitonin.

The cells of origin of calcitonin were found to be the parafollicular or C cells which are present between the follicles of the thyroid gland (Young and Leblond, 1963; Pearse, 1968; Bussolati and Pearse, 1967; Pearse, 1969). These cells can be easily observed by the immunofluorescent technique (Bussolati and Pearse, 1967; Pearse, 1969).

Embryological Origin of the C Cells

It is of clinical interest to look into the embryological origin of the parafollicular C cells. The parathyroid glands come from the third and fourth pharyngeal pouches. There is a region below this, called the ultimobranchial region of the pharynx, which gives rise to cells which migrate and fuse with the thyroid in mammals and which in submammalian vertebrates remain a separate body. Many people thought that these ultimobranchial cells were the source of the C cells; that is, that they were pharyngeal derivatives, and that calcitonin could be looked upon as an ultimobranchial hormone. However, it has been found that the C cells are of neuroectodermal origin, although they are located in the ultimobranchial body. Pearse (1969) and Johnston (1966) showed the migration of the neural crest cells in the embryo to the thyroid gland.

There is an extension of this theory in which a similar origin is postulated for many other endocrine cells such as gastrin, secretin, glucagon, and also the cells of the adrenal medulla. This, in fact, provides an explanation for the clinical association of pheochromocytoma with medullary carcinoma of the thyroid (MCT) or carcinoma of the C cells (Sipple, 1961; Williams, 1967; Samaan, Hill, Beceiro, and Ouais, 1971).

In man, calcitonin was found in high concentrations in patients with MCT, both in the tumor extract and the peripheral blood.

The recognition of MCT in man as an endocrine syndrome with excess production of calcitonin (Neher *et al.*, 1968; Tubiana *et al.*, 1968; Meyer and Wagih, 1968; Riniker *et al.*, 1968) led to the isolation of calcitonin M (Neher *et al.*, 1968; Riniker *et al.*, 1968). The sequence of calcitonin M was rapidly deduced and confirmed by total synthesis (Neher, Riniker, Rittel, and Zuber, 1968; Sieber *et al.*, 1968). In addition to calcitonin M, which is a monomer, another molecule was also found in MCT which is a dimer form of calcitonin M (Neher, Riniker, Rittel, and Zuber, 1968; Sieber *et al.*, 1968).

Chemistry of Calcitonin

The chemical structure of calcitonin from different species such as pig and salmon has been established (Neher, Riniker, Rittel, and Zuber, 1968). It was found that calcitonin peptides prepared from different species have similar biological activities but different potencies. Because of the notable difference in the immunological behavior of calcitonin obtained from different species, the radioimmunoassay methods from nonhuman calcitonin have not been useful for clinical studies.

Radioimmunoassay of Human Calcitonin

We developed a highly specific and sensitive radioimmunoassay for human calcitonin. A potent antibody was prepared in our laboratory by injecting a purified extract of MCT into rabbits. Synthetic human calcito-

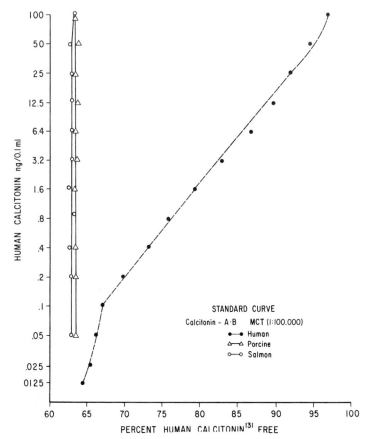

Fig. 1.—Standard dose-response curve for human calcitonin and lack of cross-reaction of porcine and salmon calcitonin in the assay is shown: 0.1 ml. of the standard calcitonin was present in each tube; 0.1 ml. of unknown serum is similarly measured; thus, the results are read as ng./ml.

nin (Ciba) was labeled with ^{131}I according to the method of Greenwood, Hunter, and Glover (1963). The measurement of the calcitonin in serum was achieved by the double antibody technique. The details of the procedure are essentially the same as those previously described (Samaan, Yen, Friesen, and Pearson, 1966; Samaan, Hill, Beceira and Schultz, in press). With this method, we could measure amounts as low as 0.0032 ng./ml. incubate (Fig. 1). Both porcine and salmon calcitonin (Armour) did not cross-react in the human calcitonin assay.

Calcitonin Levels in Normal Subjects and
Patients with Thyroid Disease

HEALTHY SUBJECTS.—Twelve healthy subjects and 16 patients with thyroid disease other than cancer had basal levels of calcitonin ranging from 0.05 to 0.5 ng./ml., and levels did not exceed 1 ng./ml. during the calcium stimulation. Calcium in a dose of 15 mg./kgm. of body weight, given intravenously over a period of four hours was used to provoke the release of calcitonin from the parafollicular C cells.

FIG. 2.—Serum calcitonin levels at fasting and during calcium infusion in eight patients with MCT. Some of the patients were studied more than once during the course of the disease. These values were compared to those found in control normal patients.

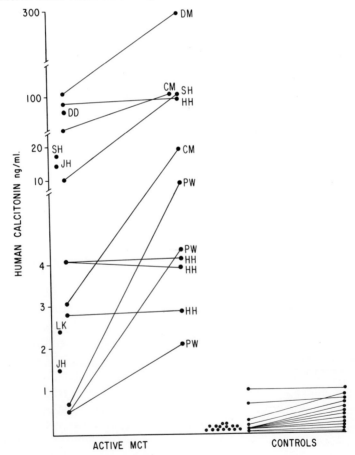

MEDULLARY CARCINOMA

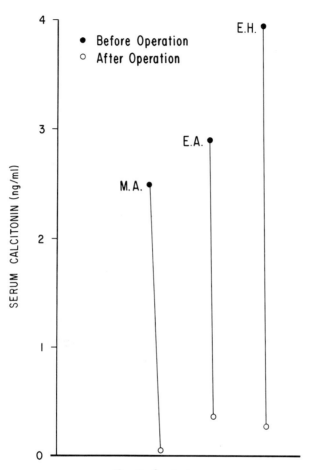

FIG. 3.—See text.

PATIENTS WITH MEDULLARY CARCINOMA OF THE THYROID.—Eight patients with clinically active MCT showed an increase in calcitonin levels in serum either basally or in response to calcium infusion (above 1 ng./ml.). All patients also showed a significant rise of calcitonin levels during calcium infusion, except for one patient who had a high basal level (patient H. H., Fig. 2). Three patients with active disease, who were investigated at various intervals, showed progressive rise of calcitonin levels with progression of the disease. One patient (P. W.), who had clinically active disease with metastases, showed a normal basal calcitonin level but a notable rise during calcium infusion. There was also a progressive incremental rise of calcitonin with progression of the disease, as assessed clinically and radiologically (Fig. 2). In contrast, calcitonin levels fell precipitously after the removal of the MCT (Fig. 3).

Of 11 patients with MCT (Fig. 4) who were previously treated surgically and showed no clinical signs of recurrence of the disease, five showed normal calcitonin levels either basally or during calcium stimulation. The

FIG. 4.—Serum calcitonin levels in 11 patients with MCT who were previously treated surgically and in whom there are no clinical signs of recurrence of the disease.

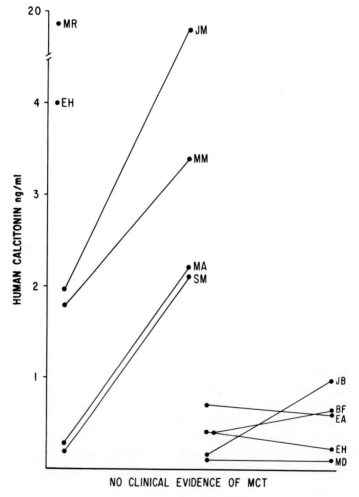

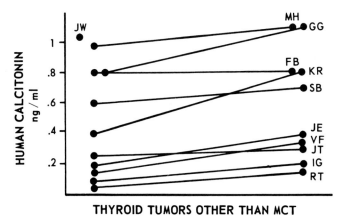

Fig. 5.—Serum calcitonin level basally and during calcium infusion in 11 patients with thyroid carcinoma other than MCT.

remaining six patients showed high levels of calcitonin either basally or during calcium stimulation; this may indicate active disease which cannot be detected clinically. Follow-up of these cases is warranted.

PATIENTS WITH NONMEDULLARY CARCINOMA.—In the patients with nonmedullary carcinoma, the serum level of calcitonin did not exceed 1 ng./ ml. either basally or during calcium infusion (Fig. 5).

Our data, as well as that of others (Melvin, Miller, and Tashjian, 1971), indicate that the serum calcitonin measurement is useful for: (1) diagnosis of MCT in patients with thyroid nodules, (2) monitoring patients after treatment for MCT to detect recurrence or metastasis, (3) diagnosis of MCT in high-risk individuals (family members) with normal thyroid glands upon physical and laboratory examination.

The Metabolic Effects of Calcitonin

Different effects of calcitonin have been described in both man and animals. The various known effects of calcitonin compared to those of parathyroid hormone are shown in Table 1. However, the main action of calcitonin is inhibition of calcium mobilization from the bone. The second organ that calcitonin affects is the kidney (Robinson, Martin, and Mac-Intyre, 1966; Robinson, Martin, Mathews, and MacIntyre, 1967). Calcitonin inhibits reabsorption of phosphorus by the renal tubules, resulting in phosphaturia.

However, we must consider that man differs from other mammals in

TABLE 1.—Comparison Between Parathyroid
and Calcitonin Effects

	Parathyroid Hormone	Calcitonin
Urinary phosphorus	↑ ↑ ↑	↑ ↑ ↑
Urinary calcium	↓ ↓	↑
Urinary sodium	↑ ↑	↑ ↑
Urinary potassium	—	↑
Urinary pH	—	↑
Urinary magnesium	↓	—
Serum calcium	↑ ↑	↓ ↓
Fecal calcium	↓	↓
Bone resorption	↑ ↑	↓ ↓

↑ Increase
— No change
↓ Decrease

several ways, with respect to calcitonin. Pearse (1967, 1969) has shown that the C cells are rather sparse in the normal adult thyroid but are present in a small number in the fetal thyroid.

While searching for parathyroid tumors in two patients, we obtained blood from the thyroid veins during thyroid operation in one and by catheterization in the second. We found that calcitonin levels in the thyroid veins were only slightly higher than those in the peripheral blood while there was a highly significant difference in the parathyroid hormone levels. This leads us to believe that calcitonin production by the thyroid gland of the adult must be very low.

The evidence that calcitonin's real action is homeostasis of the skeleton is provided by some excellent experiments by Robinson and associates (Lewis, Rafferty, Shelley, and Robinson, 1970) in which they used thyroidectomized rats which were maintained on normal amounts of thyroxin and allowed to become pregnant. When these investigators compared rats which had a thyroid and also C cells with rats which were thyroidectomized and therefore had a calcitonin deficiency, they found that the thyroidectomized rats lost 10 per cent of their skeletal weight. This suggests that under stress the absence of calcitonin leads to greater calcium loss. This experiment probably provides a clue to the most likely physiological role of calcitonin. It is possible that it is a hormone which protects the skeleton under calcium stress. It is also most likely that its role in plasma calcium homeostasis is a minor one especially under normal circumstances.

When calcitonin is injected into rats, a tremendous fall in plasma calcium occurs in young rats; in old rats, however, it has hardly any calcium-lowering effect. Thus the effect of calcitonin is more notable when there is rapid turnover of bone such as in young animals, young children, or in conditions such as Paget's disease of the bone (Woodhouse *et al.*, 1971).

We should always consider that calcitonin acts not by driving calcium out of the blood but by stopping the calcium from coming back from the bone to the blood. It is not the hormone to use to lower serum calcium in man since it has little effect in normal adult subjects.

When one takes a situation such as Paget's disease of the bone where there is a tremendous increase in the bone turnover, calcitonin has the same effect as it does in young experimental animals. Salmon calcitonin has been used in the Endocrinology Section at M. D. Anderson Hospital to treat patients who have Paget's disease. The dosage used was 100 MRC (British Medical Research Council) units intramuscularly daily for a period of four to 24 months. Bone pain was relieved and skin temperature over the affected limbs was reduced. Elevated total urinary hydroxyproline levels fell to within normal range and serum alkaline phosphatase to normal or near normal value (Fig. 6). This indicates inhibition of bone destruction.

The Joplin and MacIntyre group (Woodhouse *et al.*, 1971) used human synthetic calcitonin to treat Paget's disease. Their results showed complete healing of the bone. They demonstrated by histological studies that the

Fig. 6.—Effect of intramuscular salmon calcitonin on serum alkaline phosphatase and 24-hour urinary hydroxyproline in a patient with Paget's disease.

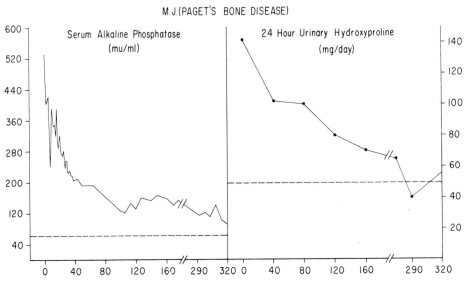

number of osteoclasts was significantly reduced and that new bone, having a normal lamellar structure, formed after calcitonin treatment.

The daily calcitonin dose used by the London group (Woodhouse *et al.*, 1971) and our Houston group (Hill, Saaman, and Ouais, in preparation) may be more than is required. It is possible that smaller doses of calcitonin or injections at less frequent intervals may prove to be equally effective. The human calcitonin may be more advantageous to use than salmon calcitonin since some of our patients treated with salmon calcitonin developed antibodies which may have interfered with the biological action of calcitonin. We must also consider that prolonged administration of calcitonin may induce hypertrophy of the parathyroid gland and raise the parathyroid hormone level in the circulation.

Relationship between Calcitonin and Parathyroid Hormone

In MCT with high circulating calcitonin level, the parathyroid glands are usually enlarged. To investigate this phenomenon further, we administered 4,000 MRC units of salmon calcitonin intravenously over a period of four hours to a patient with parathyroid carcinoma. This patient had his hypercalcemia maintained for several months at a level of 12 to 13 mg./ 100 ml. by using oral phosphate, 1.5 Gm./day plus 100 MRC units of

Fig. 7.—Effect of 4,000 MRC units of salmon calcitonin IV on serum calcium and parathyroid hormone levels in a patient with parathyroid carcinoma.

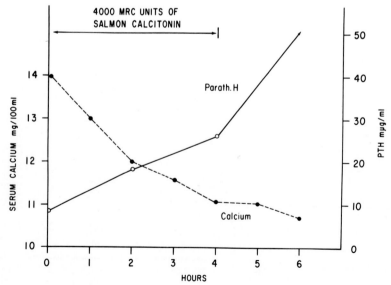

salmon calcitonin daily. We noticed a definite fall in his serum calcium level, while the parathyroid hormone level rose significantly (Fig. 7). The following few days, the patient felt ill, nauseated, and lethargic. Ten days after this procedure, when the patient returned to the hospital, his serum calcium level was found to be 18 mg./100 ml. although he was receiving the same therapy (1.5 Gm. phosphorus by mouth plus 100 MRC units of salmon calcitonin daily) which had maintained his serum calcium at 12 to 13 mg./100 ml. a few months previously. Therefore, it is quite apparent that there is a reciprocal relationship between calcitonin and parathyroid hormone action.

Summary

1. Calcitonin preserves the integrity of the skeleton while under calcium stress.
2. Human calcitonin does produce complete remission in Paget's disease.
3. Calcitonin is a neuroectodermal hormone.
4. Medullary carcinoma of the thyroid (MCT) can be detected by calcitonin measurement.

Acknowledgments

This study was supported by U.S.P.H.S., N.I.H. Grants No. CA 12521-01 and CA 05831-10 and the American Cancer Society Grant No. T-558.

REFERENCES

Bussolati, G., and Pearse, A. G. E.: Immunofluorescent localization of calcitonin in the "C" cells of pig and dog thyroid. *The Journal of Endocrinology*, 37:205-209, February 1967.

Copp, D. H.: Parathyroids, calcitonin, and control of plasma calcium. *Recent Progress of Hormone Research*, 20:59-88, 1964.

———: Simple and precise micromethod for EDTA titration of calcium. *The Journal of Laboratory and Clinical Medicine*, 61:1029-1037, June 1963.

Copp, D. H., and Davidson, A. G. F.: Direct humoral control of parathyroid function in the dog. *Proceedings of the Society for Experimental Biology and Medicine*, 107:342-344, June 1961.

Foster, G. V., Baghdiantz, A., Kumar, M. A., Slack, E., Soliman, H. A., and MacIntyre, I.: Thyroid origin of calcitonin. *Nature*, 202:1303-1305, June 1964.

Greenwood, F. C., Hunter, W. M., and Glover, J. S.: The preparation of ^{131}I-labelled human growth hormone of high specific radioactivity. *Biochemical Journal*, 89:114-123, October 1963.

Hill, C. S., Jr., Samaan, N. A., and Ouais, S. G.: Salmon calcitonin in the treatment of Paget's bone disease. (In preparation.)

Hirsch, P. F., Gauthier, G. F., and Munson, P. L.: Thyroid hypocalcemic principle and recurrent laryngeal nerve injury as factors affecting the response to parathyroidectomy in rats. *Endocrinology*, 73:244-252, August 1963.

Johnston, M. C.: A radioautographic study of the migration and fate of cranial neural crest cells in the chick embryo. *Anatomical Record*, 156:143-150, October 1966.

Lewis, P., Rafferty, B., Shelley, M., and Robinson, C. J.: A suggested physiological role of calcitonin: The protection of the skeleton during pregnancy and lactation. *The Journal of Endocrinology*, 49:ix-x, 1971 (reprinted from *The Proceedings of the Society for Endocrinology 19-20, November, 1970.*)

Melvin, K. E. W., Miller, H. H., and Tashjian, A. H., Jr.: Early diagnosis of medullary carcinoma of the thyroid gland by means of calcitonin assay. *The New England Journal of Medicine*, 285:1115-1120, November 1971.

Meyer, J. S., and Wagih, A.: Granules and thyrocalcitonin-like activity in medullary carcinoma of thyroid gland. *The New England Journal of Medicine*, 278:523-529, February 1968.

Neher, R., Riniker, B., Maier, R., Byfield, P. G. H., Gudmundsson, T. V., and MacIntyre, I.: Human calcitonin. *Nature*, 220:984-986, 1968.

Neher, R., Riniker, B., Rittel, W., and Zuber, H.: Menschliches Calcitonin III. Struktur von Calcitonin Mund D. *Helvetica chim Acta*, 51:1900, 1968.

Pearse, A. G. E.: Common cytochemical and ultrastructural characteristics of cells producing polypeptide hormones (the A P U D series) and their relevance to thyroid and ultimobranchial C cells and calcitonin. *Proceedings of the Royal Society of London B*, 170:71, 1968.

————: The characteristics of the C cells and their significance in relation to those of other endocrine polypeptide cells and to the synthesis, storage and secretion of calcitonin. In *International Symposium on Calcitonin*. London, England, July 21-24, 1969, pp. 125-140.

————: The thyroid parenchymatous cells of baber and the nature and function of their C cell successors in thyroid parathyroid and ultimobranchial bodies. In *Calcitonin 1967; Proceedings of Symposium on Thyrocalcitonin and the C cells*. London, England, July 17-20, 1967, pp. 98-109.

Riniker, B., Neher, R., Maier, R., Kahnt, F. W., Byfield, P. G. H., Gudmundsson, T. V., Galante, L., and MacIntyre, I.: Menschliches Calcitonin I. Isolierung and Charakterisierung. *Helvetica chim Acta*, 51:1738-1742, October 31, 1968.

Robinson, C. J., Martin, T., and MacIntyre, I.: Phosphaturic effect of thyrocalcitonin. *The Lancet*, 2:83-84, July 1966.

Robinson, C. J., Martin, T. J., Mathews, E. W., and MacIntyre, I.: Mode of action of thyrocalcitonin. *The Journal of Endocrinology*, 39:71-79, September 1967.

Samaan, N. A., Hill, C. S., Jr., Beceiro, J. R., and Ouais, S. G.: Medullary carcinoma of the thyroid and calcitonin. *The Cancer Bulletin*, 23:2-5, January-February 1971.

Samaan, N. A., Hill, C. S., Jr., Beceiro, J. R., and Schultz, P. N.: Serum immunoreactive calcitonin in medullary carcinoma of thyroid. Accepted for publication in *The Journal of Laboratory and Clinical Medicine*, August, 1972.

Samaan, N. A., Yen, S. C. C., Friesen, H., and Pearson, O. H.: serum placental lactogen levels during pregnancy and in trophoblastic disease. *The Journal of Clinical Endocrinology and Metabolism*, 26:1303-1308, December 1966.

Sieber, P., Brugger, M., Kamber, B., Riniker, B., and Rittel, W.: Menschliches Calcitonin IV. Die Synthese von Calcitonin M. *Helvetica chim Acta,* 51:2057, 1968.

Sipple, J. H.: Association of pheochromocytoma with carcinoma of thyroid gland. *The American Journal of Medicine,* 31:163-166, July 1961.

Tubiana, M., Milhaud, G., Coutris, G., Lacour, J., Parmentier, C., and Bok, B.: Medullary carcinoma and thyrocalcitonin. *British Medical Journal,* 4:87-89, October 1968.

Williams, E. D.: Medullary carcinoma of the thyroid. *Journal of Clinical Pathology,* 20:395-398, 1967.

Woodhouse, N. J. Y., Reiner, M., Bordier, P. H., Kalu, D. N., Fisher, M., Foster, G. V., Joplin, G. F., and MacIntyre, I.: Human calcitonin in the treatment of Paget's bone disease. *The Lancet,* 1:1139-1142, 1971.

Young, B. A., and Leblond, C. P.: The light cell as compared to the follicular cell in the thyroid gland of the rat. *Endocrinology,* 73:669-686, December 1963.

Thyroid Tumors:
Surgical Management

E. C. WHITE, M.D.

Department of Medicine, The University of Texas at Houston
M. D. Anderson Hospital and Tumor Institute,
Houston, Texas

ONE OF THE QUESTIONS commonly posed regarding the surgical management of thyroid tumors concerns the advisability of removing all thyroid tumors for histologic study. Because of the relatively low incidence of thyroid cancer in relation to that of thyroid nodules, physicians have been hesitant to make such a blanket recommendation, especially in patients from endemic goiter areas. Methods of preoperative clinical and laboratory differentiation between benign and malignant disease have been of little value with the exception of the specific diagnosis of medullary or solid carcinoma in the relatively few patients harboring this disease.

It is probable that no harm is done in attempting a trial suppression of the specific dominant nodule of relatively small size by administration of thyroid medication. Our experience has been that few of the nodules in question will resolve in this situation. We believe that the thyroid gland should be surgically explored in all patients with a nontoxic solitary nodule and in the majority of those with multinodular goiters. Should the nodule in question be demonstrable by scintigram and fail to take up ^{131}I, the so-called "cold nodule" will prove to be cancer in approximately 25 per cent of cases.

Upon exploration, small and superficial lesions may be biopsied by simple wedge excision, including a section of the surrounding normal tissue. Large nodules require that the entire lobe be removed. In the latter situation, total lobectomy possesses two advantages: (1) the danger of injury to the recurrent laryngeal nerve and parathyroid glands is reduced, and (2) the possibility that recurrent or subsequent tumors will develop is eliminated. This is important to both the patient and the surgeon since a secondary surgical procedure is usually both tedious and harassing and greatly increases the danger of injury to the recurrent nerve and parathyroid glands. In patients with multinodular goiter, if no cancer is found on frozen-section study, a total lobectomy should be performed on the side of the more extensive disease. The problem here is that the involvement may be so extensive as to require an almost total intracapsular dissection on the opposite side. Benign tumors of the thyroid are predominantly adenomas or lesions falling into the category of Hashimoto's disease (Table 1).

The pathologist, using the cryostat technique, can give an unequivocal diagnosis from frozen-section studies in almost all instances. At the time of diagnosis of thyroid cancer of one of the differentiated types, *i.e.*, follicular, papillary, mixtures of the two, or solid, it is generally agreed that the treatment of choice is surgical removal. There is further agreement that extensive surgical procedures are of little value in the management of spindle and giant cell variants of this tumor. The controversial issue concerns the extent of the operation to be performed. There are advocates of lobectomy, lobectomy with isthmusectomy, and total or near-total thyroidectomy. Each of these procedures may be accompanied by a neck dissection of varied extent.

Before 1950, the surgical staff of M. D. Anderson Hospital considered that thyroid lobectomy, with or without neck dissection on the homolateral side, was the surgical procedure of choice. Two events then occurred in rather rapid succession which radically altered our opinion. The first of these was the introduction of ^{131}I as a new modality for both the diagnosis and treatment of thyroid disease. It soon became apparent that in treating patients with thyroid cancer metastatic to the lung or other sites, maximum uptake of the radioactive drug by the metastasis could only be achieved by total removal of all thyroid tissue. Thus, the patient who previously had had a lobectomy or lobectomy and radical neck dissection, and who now had metastatic disease, required the removal of the remaining lobe and isthmus before administration of therapeutic doses of radioactive iodine. Our pathologists reported that routine examinations of the tissue removed at these secondary procedures revealed that one in three patients had residual cancer in the supposedly normal lobe.

TABLE 1.—BENIGN TUMORS OF THE THYROID

NUMBER OF PATIENTS		TYPE OF TUMOR
421	—	Adenoma
153	—	Adenomatous goiter
64 115	>	Hashimoto's disease and others

TABLE 2.—THYROID GLANDS STUDIED BY
WHOLE-ORGAN SUBSERIAL SECTION
130 Cases

HISTOLOGIC TYPE	BILATERAL		UNILATERAL		TOTAL
Follicular	11	64%	6	36%	17
Papillary	11	68%	5	32%	16
Mixed papillary and follicular	50	67%	25	33%	75
Hürthle	1				1
Solid	8	67%	4	33%	12
Spindle and giant	9				9
Totals	90	69%	40	31%	130

It logically followed that perhaps it would be better to remove the entire gland at the first operation. A series of patients with thyroid cancer were then treated by total thyroidectomy, a radical neck dissection being added only if there was clinical evidence of disease in the cervical nodes.

With the entire gland as a specimen, the pathologist was afforded an unusual opportunity to study dissemination of the disease within the thyroid tissue. The second event of importance was the utilization of whole-organ subserial sections to do an in-depth study of the disease within the gland. The specimens from 142 patients who had primary total thyroidectomy at M. D. Anderson Hospital were studied; one of three showed dissemination of a tumor beyond the primary site when studied by routine methods, while four of five showed dissemination when studied by subserial review of the whole gland. Similar results were obtained upon study of the remaining lobe or tissue from each of 76 patients who had previously undergone total lobectomy or subtotal thyroidectomy. Again, dissemination was shown in one-third by routine study and in three-fourths by subserial sections. (Clark, White, Russell, and Ibanez, 1965).

There are surgeons who believe that the extent of excision of the thyroid gland can, or should be, varied according to the histologic characteristics of the primary lesion in differentiated carcinoma; they advocate extensive resection or total thyroidectomy only in follicular lesions or in solid or medullary lesions. A study of 130 specimens by whole-organ section demonstrates that there is no significant difference in the occurrence of dissemination through the gland between the various cell types of differentiated thyroid cancer (Table 2). This led to the conclusion that one can not allow the histologic type of the lesion to be the determinant of the extent of resection. Nor is it generally possible to clinically determine the extent of the disease. This point is demonstrated in Figure 1.

The patients concerned are members of a family presently under study. Figure 1A shows solid carcinoma of the thyroid in a gland obtained at autopsy from a 53-year-old woman treated for malignant pheochromocytoma of the right adrenal gland in 1962. After considerable difficulty, her son was persuaded to undergo exploration of the thyroid gland after appropriate studies in February 1969. At operation, the inferior pole of the left lobe (shown on the left in Fig. 1B) contained gross tumor which proved to be a medullary carcinoma. The lesion in the opposite, or right

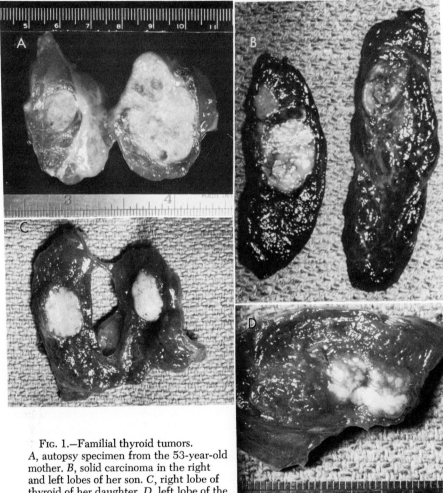

Fig. 1.—Familial thyroid tumors. A, autopsy specimen from the 53-year-old mother. B, solid carcinoma in the right and left lobes of her son. C, right lobe of thyroid of her daughter. D, left lobe of the daughter (C). See text for fuller discussion.

pole, was not palpable although in the photograph, it would appear to be easy to demonstrate. Figures 1C and 1D show the right and left lobes of the thyroid gland of her daughter who, in addition to a large pheochromo-cytoma which was asymptomatic, also had solid carcinoma in the left lobe of the thyroid. To the surgeons, the right lobe (Fig. 1C) appeared com-pletely innocuous. The tumor was not palpable, even to the internist who had the excised lobe in his hands and to the pathologist who performed the frozen-section study; but, again, the same pattern was repeated.

Further support of total thyroidectomy was evident in a review, con-ducted here in 1963 by Rose and associates, of 116 patients who were fol-lowed up after receiving a lobectomy for the management of thyroid carcinoma. Most of these patients had been operated on in other hospitals. Of the 116 patients, 20 developed clinical recurrence and required further surgical treatment; 34, at some point during the study, received prophy-lactic removal of the remaining portion of the gland. Of these, 21, or 60 per cent, contained residual cancer. Thus, of the 116 patients, 41 were proved to have carcinoma in the remaining lobe—again an incidence of one in three.

Total thyroidectomy would be universally accepted as the treatment of choice were it not for the complications that can ensue. Hypothyroidism, often listed as a complication, is not a complication at all, but rather one of the goals of the operation. Injury to the recurrent nerve can occur but is rare when the nerve is carefully exposed and traced to its entry into the cricothyroid membrane. Of the 218 patients, 142 primarily operated on and 76 secondarily operated on, there was evidence of preoperative nerve injury in 6 patients and in 10 patients the nerves were intentionally severed because of involvement with disease. Bilateral nerve injury did not occur (Clark, White, Russell, and Ibanez, 1965). The chief objection to total thyroidectomy is the possibility of producing permanent hypocalcemia or tetany. The incidence of this complication in thyroidectomy for hyper-thyroidism is fairly well established and appears to average approximately 3 per cent, with permanent tetany occurring in less than 1 per cent (Bar-tels, 1952).

When total thyroidectomy is performed for carcinoma, the occurrence of permanent hypoparathyroidism varies in several reports from 4.2 per cent of patients to almost 50 per cent (Block, Horn, and Brush, 1960; Thompson and Harness, 1970; Beahrs, Ryan, and White, 1956). In our own experience with 218 patients reported several years ago, 17 of 142 who were operated on primarily developed permanent tetany, a frequency of 12 per cent. When the operation was performed secondarily, permanent tetany occurred in 14.5 per cent, resulting in an over-all average of 12.8

per cent. Patients with tetany are usually easily managed by the use of vitamin D_2 and calcium lactate. These data are presently being updated. The total experience now includes 369 patients, 282 of whom had primary total thyroidectomy at M. D. Anderson Hospital and 87 of whom received secondary completion of previously incomplete procedures.

It may be redundant to point out that a patient, competent, and careful dissection is necessary to minimize complications. The recurrent nerve is variable in position and may pass behind the main trunk of the inferior thyroid artery, behind its terminal branches, or between its terminal branches. Unfortunately, in most anatomical and surgical texts, it is depicted in a cadaveric position well behind the location at which it appears at operation (Fig. 2A). When the gland is rotated medially after ligation of the middle thyroid vein, the recurrent nerve almost invariably splits the 90° angle formed between the planes of the trachea and the inferior thyroid artery (Fig. 2B). If the nerve is not palpable, this is the area in which to begin one's search. It must be traced to its entry through the cricoid thyroid membrane. Once the terminal branches of the inferior artery are severed, the recurrent nerve can be pushed posteriorly and traced quite easily to the "ligament of Berry." This is usually described as a definite ligamentous structure but appears to the surgeon as an area in which the posterior capsule is deficient and the thyroid tissue becomes quite adherent at the level of the first and second tracheal ring. In this area, the nerve must be posteriorly retracted quite cautiously and the thyroid tissue cut away if a tell-tale "smudge" on the postoperative scintigram indicating remaining thyroid tissue is to be prevented. Unfortunately, in this area of difficult dissection, one or two small branches of the inferior thyroid artery appear just behind the nerve with considerable constancy. When these small vessels are severed, surprising hemorrhage results. Attempts to control this hemorrhage are perhaps the most common cause of nerve injury during total thyroidectomy.

Also depicted in this diagram (Fig. 2B) is a small group of nodes occurring rather constantly almost level with the lower pole of the thyroid and closely associated with the recurrent nerve. These should be closely inspected, and should there be any doubt about the diagnosis of primary disease, a biopsy of one of these nodes will often confirm the presence of cancer of the thyroid. This group of nodes should always be biopsied in the case of solid or medullary carcinoma since the disease so frequently descends directly down the chain.

Once the diagnosis of carcinoma is established, the regional nodes, particularly those along the recurrent laryngeal nerve, should be carefully palpated in the area exposed through the wound. If only the nodes along

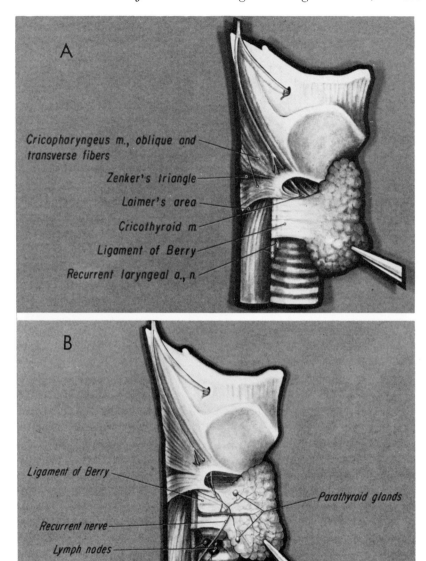

Fig. 2.—*A*, usual depiction of the position of the recurrent nerve. *B*, actual position of recurrent nerve as seen at operation.

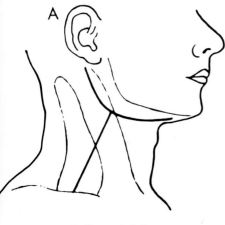

Crile, 1905

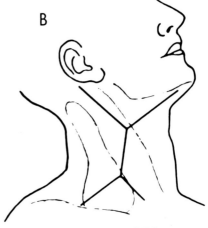

Martin, 1951

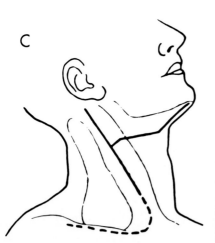

Semken, 1932

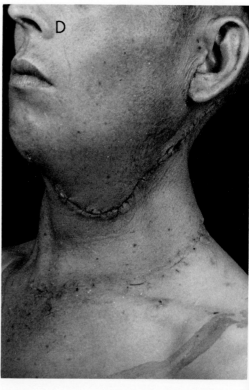

FIG. 3.—Radical neck dissection. *A*, the Crile technique of incision. *B*, the Semken incision. *C*, the Martin double Y incision. *D*, postoperative appearance of a patient with "double collar" incision.

the recurrent nerve appear to contain metastasis, a compartmental dissection between the two carotid sheaths from the suprasternal notch to the upper limits of the thyroid cartilage should be added to the thyroidectomy. A radical neck dissection is performed if the lateral nodes of the neck are involved. The presence of bilateral nodes requires a bilateral radical neck dissection.

In our experience, one third of our patients have had node dissection, less than a radical neck and usually a compartmental dissection. One-third have had a radical neck dissection, and 7 per cent have required laryngectomy as a result of the invasiveness of their disease.

Various incisions are used for the performance of a radical neck dissection. Illustrated are those of Crile, 1905 (Fig. 3A), and Semken, 1932 (Fig. 3B), as well as the double Y of Martin, 1951 (Fig. 3C). Gaining in favor today is the double collar incision which gives a good cosmetic result (Fig. 3D). One word of warning here: Should the patient have received previous irradiation in any significant dosage, a single incision extending from the mastoid process downward and forward to terminate in the usual collar incision for removing the thyroid should be used. The advantage is that the carotid artery is crossed low in the neck and in a transverse plane rather than being subjected to a compound angle as occurs in the double Y or other variants thereof. This has been found to significantly reduce the incidence of necrosis with subsequent rupture of the carotid artery.

Summary

1. With few exceptions, tumors of the thyroid gland of a size sufficient to be detectable by the physician should be explored surgically and biopsied.

2. Total lobectomy on the affected side is the biopsy procedure of choice in all but a few small lesions which are quite advantageously placed.

3. The various differentiated forms of thyroid cancer are equally prone to intraglandular dissemination.

4. The extent of the disease within the gland cannot be determined by inspection or palpation.

5. Total thyroidectomy best assures ablation of the primary lesion of the thyroid cancer together with its immediate area of spread within the gland. With the exception of solid or medullary carcinoma, a further advantage is gained in that the physician responsible for follow-up may render the patient myxedematous at any time and thereby improve both the

diagnostic and therapeutic efficiency of radioiodine. In theory at least, it may prevent further seeding of the regional lymph nodes, and finally, it should prevent the transformation of a differentiated type of thyroid cancer into the anaplastic and fatal forms. This transformation is being reported with increasing frequency by pathologists.

REFERENCES

Bartels, E. C.: Hyperthyroidism—Evaluation of treatment with antithyroid drugs followed by subtotal thyroidectomy. *Annals of Internal Medicine,* 37:1123-1134, 1952.

Beahrs, O. H., Ryan, R. F., and White, R. A.: Complications of thyroid surgery. *The Journal of Clinical Endocrinology and Metabolism,* 16:1456-1469, 1956.

Block, M. A., Horn, R. C., and Brush, B. E.: The place of total thyroidectomy in surgery for thyroid carcinoma. *Archives of Surgery,* 81:236-243, 1960.

Clark, R. L., White, E. C., Russell, W. O., and Ibanez, M. L.: Clinicopathologic studies in 218 total thyroidectomies for thyroid cancer. In *Proceedings of the Fifth International Thyroid Conference, Rome, Italy.* New York, New York, Academic Press, 1965, pp. 1045-1050.

Rose, R. G., Kelsey, M. P., Russell, W. O., Ibanez, M. L., White, E. C., and Clark, R. L.: Follow-up study of thyroid cancer treated by unilateral lobectomy. *The American Journal of Surgery,* 106:494-500, 1963.

Thompson, N. W., and Harness, J. K.: Complications of total thyroidectomy for carcinoma. *Surgery, Gynecology and Obstetrics,* 131:861-868, 1970.

Primary Thyroid Carcinoma: Histogenesis, Classification and Biologic Behavior Based on Studies of 777 Patients

WILLIAM O. RUSSELL, M.D., AND
MICHAEL L. IBANEZ, M.D.

*Department of Anatomic Pathology, The University of Texas
at Houston M. D. Anderson Hospital and Tumor Institute,
Houston, Texas*

PRIMARY MALIGNANT TUMORS of the thyroid gland represent only 1.4 per cent of all malignant lesions reported in Public Health Service cancer morbidity figures (United States Department of Health, Education, and Welfare, 1959) and only 1.1 per cent of all cancers seen at this institution in a 28-year period through August 1971. Despite their relative infrequency, thyroid tumors have been a subject of intense interest to pathologists and clinicians concerned with diagnosis and treatment of cancer patients. Although many differing opinions appear in the medical literature regarding classification, diagnosis, therapy, and prognosis, definite trends are now evolving toward more simplified concepts of nosology, greater emphasis on correlations of histologic type with biologic behavior and response to treatment, as well as agreement on histogenesis of the principal types of primary thyroid tumors. These developments all support a multidisciplinary team approach to more satisfactory management of this disease.

M. D. Anderson Hospital has been conducting comprehensive studies of patients with thyroid carcinoma since March 1944. The series now includes 777 patients (the series was updated to a total of 887 patients as of January 1972) with primary thyroid carcinoma whose records form the basis of this communication concerning histogenesis, classification, and biological behavior of these lesions.

Classification Related to Histogenesis of Primary Thyroid Carcinomas

The functional parenchymal tissues of the thyroid gland are divisible into two categories: (1) The thyroid follicles which produce colloid and thyroxin and (2) the interfollicular cells which produce thyrocalcitonin. Each of these two types of tissues has a different histogenesis and characteristic morphology and produces functionally distinct hormones. The differentiated carcinomas arise from the cells of follicular derivation while solid, or medullary carcinoma arises from the parafollicular cells of the thyroid gland. The histogenesis of each of these two tumor types is discussed separately.

DIFFERENTIATED THYROID CARCINOMAS

Differentiated thyroid carcinomas, comprising approximately 89 per cent of tumors in this series, typify the classical image of thyroid cancer. These are the malignant tumors which show varying degrees of differentiation of thyroid follicular cells. Tumors of this type have a clearly established histogenesis from cells derived from the thyroglossal duct, a primary foregut midline structure (Arey, 1965).

SOLID CARCINOMAS

Solid carcinomas represent approximately 9 per cent of the primary thyroid tumors in this series. In 1959, Hazard, Hawk, and Crile definitely established what they called "medullary (solid) carcinoma" of the thyroid as a distinct pathologic and clinical entity to be distinguished from the anaplastic form of differentiated carcinoma. Various terms such as medullary carcinoma, solid carcinoma with amyloid stroma, medullary (solid) carcinoma, solid carcinoma, C cell carcinoma and parafollicular cell carcinoma (reflecting hormonal function) have been applied to this tumor. The term solid carcinoma, although not ideal, seems most appropriate because it is brief and descriptive of the solid type of mass produced by the tumor. This term is used throughout this communication.

Morphologically, solid carcinoma of the thyroid gland is so distinct from the differentiated tumors of follicular derivation that entirely differing histogeneses would be expected. Solid carcinoma characteristically is poorly differentiated, shows great variation in cell morphology, and has amyloid deposition among the cells and supporting stroma (Ibanez, Cole, Russell, and Clark, 1967). Its origin from the parafollicular cell of the thyroid gland, after an early period of controversy, now has been clearly established (Williams, 1966; Gonzalez-Licea, Hartmann, and Yardley, 1968). The parafollicular cells are derived from the foregut entodermal ultimobranchial bodies which migrate into the neck. Cells from these structures then enter the thyroid lobes which develop from the thyroglossal duct anlage.

On the basis of observations in chick and quail embryos, it has been postulated that neural crest cells migrate into the primitive stomodeum and are incorporated into the ultimobranchial body (Johnston, 1966; Le Douarin and Le Lievre, 1970). Although this remains to be confirmed in the human fětus, the hypothesis does offer a plausible explanation for the fact that while the ultimobranchial bodies are entodermal in origin, the tumors (solid carcinomas) derived from the parafollicular cells are morphologically and functionally similar to other tumors derived from neural crest structures. This mechanism of transport of neural crest cells is identical to the early embryonic migrations of neural crest cells into the gastrointestinal tract, the pituitary, pancreas, lung, and soft tissues (Arey, 1965; Eisenberg and Wallerstein, 1932).

Moreover, solid carcinoma of the thyroid gland is associated with numerous genetically determined benign and malignant lesions of neuroectodermal tissues such as von Recklinghausen's disease, Sipple's syndrome, and multiple carcinoid tumors (Sipple, 1961; Williams, Brown, and Doniach, 1965; Williams and Pollock, 1966; Block *et al.*, 1967; Schimke, Hartmann, Prout, and Rimoin, 1968; Ljungberg, Cederquist, and von Studnitz, 1967).

The parafollicular cells are known to be functional and are analogous to the argyrophilic cells in the pituitary corticotrophs producing adrenocorticotropic hormone, melanotrophs producing melanocyte-stimulating hormone, and alpha cells in the pancreas producing gastrin. Demonstration of the production of thyrocalcitonin in the interfollicular cells and by the cells of solid carcinoma, with characteristic secretory granules containing calcitonin in both types of cells, was the convincing morphophysiologic evidence supporting neuroectodermal histogenesis of the tumor (Braunstein, Stephens, and Gibson, 1968; Meyer and Abdel-Bari, 1968).

Therefore, although the differentiated and the solid thyroid tumors are primary lesions of one organ, they must be considered histogenetically as two entirely different neoplasms, each with distinctly characteristic diagnostic and therapeutic aspects, biological behaviors, and histologic patterns.

HISTOLOGIC TYPES EXCLUDED FROM THIS STUDY

Neoplasms such as malignant lymphoma, angiosarcoma, soft tissue sarcomas, and squamous carcinoma have been reported as primary in the thyroid gland (Prakash, Kukreti and Sharma, 1968; Fries, Chamberlin, and Vandivier, 1961). At this institution, these tumors are viewed as rare fortuitous occurrences of lesions totally unrelated to the two functional parenchymal components of the thyroid gland. The so-called small cell carcinoma (Warren and Meissner, 1953) also has been described as a poorly differentiated anaplastic tumor of thyroid follicular cell origin. However, in the nearly 30 years' experience of this institution, the only small cell carcinomas of the thyroid gland observed were believed to be morphologically and biologically related to lymphomatous disease rather than to represent primary tumors arising from the parenchymal elements of the gland. Therefore, these various unusual tumors are not included in this discussion of primary thyroid carcinoma as herein defined.

Anaplastic (spindle and giant cell) thyroid carcinoma is excluded from this section on histogenesis because studies have demonstrated that this form does not arise *de novo* in the gland but, rather, represents highly malignant transformation of a precursor differentiated tumor (Russell, Ibanez, Clark, and White, 1963). This concept is discussed and illustrated in subsequent sections of this paper.

CLASSIFICATION OF THYROID CARCINOMA AND ANALYSIS OF STUDY SAMPLE

The previously expressed concept of two histologic groups of primary malignant neoplasms of the thyroid gland has made possible a simplified and more meaningful classification of these tumors. The two basic categories are (1) differentiated carcinoma and (2) solid carcinoma. The differentiated carcinomas include four subtypes, each of which is capable of developing anaplastic change (Table 1). In solid carcinoma, the variations observed in morphologic patterns of growth are not sufficiently meaningful to justify designation of subtypes. Accumulated experience has shown this classification to be sufficiently descriptive to serve as the basis for lucid communications between the pathologist and the clinician for deci-

TABLE 1.—Primary Thyroid Cancer by Histologic Type

	No. of Patients	% of Series	Differentiated Tumors with Anaplastic Change	
			Number	% of Histologic Type
Differentiated Carcinoma				
Follicular	106	13.6	10	10.4
Papillary	120	15.4	5	04.3
Mixed papillary and follicular	432	55.6	16	03.8
Hürthle cell	18	2.3	2	12.5
Materials inadequate for precise identification of differentiated subtype	14	1.8	14	
Totals	690	88.8	47	06.8
Solid Carcinoma	70	09.0		
(Cases receiving histologic review)	17	2.2		
Total Series	777	100.0	47	06.8

sions regarding selection of therapy for the morphologic variations recognized within the two histologic groups of primary thyroid tumors.

Distribution by Histologic Type

Among the 690 patients with differentiated thyroid carcinoma, 55.6 per cent had mixed papillary and follicular lesions, 15.4 per cent had pure papillary tumors, 13.6 per cent had the pure follicular form, and 2.3 per cent had Hürthle cell carcinoma. As shown in Table 1, these figures include 47 patients with differentiated tumors which developed anaplastic change. Materials available for histologic study were inadequate to permit precise identification of the precursor differentiated tumor in 14 of these patients.

The 70 patients (9.0 per cent of the series) with solid carcinoma include two who also had discrete, entirely separate, differentiated primary thyroid lesions. The occurrence of these two types of primary lesions within the same gland is believed to be fortuitous since the intermingling of differentiated and solid carcinoma has not been observed in this series. Furthermore, the phenomenon of anaplastic change has not been observed in solid thyroid carcinoma at this institution; this attests further to the entirely different biologic behavior and embryologically distinct histogenesis of the solid tumors.

AGE AT DIAGNOSIS BY HISTOLOGIC TYPE

Table 2 shows that 84 per cent of the thyroid tumors in this series were initially detected in patients between ages 20 to 69. The 30 to 39 decade predominates with 157 patients (20.2 per cent); the 20 to 29 group is next with 132 patients (17.0 per cent). However, no age group is spared, including children under 10 and adults over 80.

When age at diagnosis was tabulated by histologic type (Table 3), mixed papillary and follicular thyroid tumors showed a distinct 44.2 per cent peak in patients aged 20 to 39, and 12 per cent of these lesions were detected in patients under 20 years of age. In other words, 56 per cent of the mixed tumors were initially diagnosed in patients less than 40 years old and 87.5 per cent were diagnosed in patients under age 60. These percentages are considerably higher than those shown in the younger age groups for the other subtypes of differentiated carcinoma.

Papillary thyroid carcinoma also showed a peak in the 20 to 39 age group, but only 43 per cent were diagnosed in patients under 40; the remaining percentages were more evenly distributed between the older age groups than for the mixed lesions. Only 36 per cent of follicular carcinomas were diagnosed in patients under 40 years old and the peak was in the 40 to 59 age group (34.4 per cent).

Hürthle cell carcinoma is the only differentiated subtype in which no tumors were initially diagnosed in patients under 20 years of age. With only a total of 16 patients involved, the numbers become too small to have real significance, but the peak of 37.4 per cent observed in the 20 to 39 age group is almost equalled by the percentages for the older patients.

The highest peak in the entire table is seen in the column representing

TABLE 2.—777 PATIENTS WITH PRIMARY THYROID CANCER

Age at Diagnosis

AGE IN YEARS	NUMBER OF PATIENTS	PER CENT OF TOTAL SERIES	
0–9	6	0.8	
10–19	62	8.0	
20–29	132	17.0	
30–39	157	20.2	
40–49	130	16.7	84%
50–59	126	16.2	
60–69	108	13.9	
70–79	47	6.0	
80–89	9	1.2	
Total	777	100%	

TABLE 3.–777 PATIENTS WITH PRIMARY THYROID CANCER

AGE AT DIAGNOSIS BY HISTOLOGIC TYPE

AGE IN YRS.	Papillary		Follicular		Mixed Papillary and Follicular		Hürthle Cell		Anaplastic Change in Differentiated Tumors		Solid (Medullary)	
	Pts.	%	Pts.	%	Pts.	%	Pts.	%	Pts.	%	Pts.	%
Over 80	2	1.7	1	1.0	2	0.5	—	—	3	6.0	1	1.5
60–79	22	19.1	27	28.1	50	12.0	5	31.2	28	59.0	15	22.0
40–59	42	35.7	33	34.4	129	31.0	5	31.2	14	29.0	28	38.8
20–39	45	39.1	28	29.1	184	44.2	6	37.4	2	4.0	23	32.5
0–19	5	4.3	7	7.2	51	12.3	—	—	—	—	3	4.4
Totals	116		96		416		16		47		70	

differentiated tumors with anaplastic change where 59 per cent were diagnosed in patients over 60. Also, comparison of the percentages in the 20 to 39 age group shows only 4 per cent with anaplastic change while all other histologic types, including solid carcinoma, are in the 30 to 40 per cent range. This supports the observation that anaplastic carcinoma represents further malignant change in a slow-growing precursor differentiated type.

Solid carcinoma again is distinguished from the differentiated lesions when viewed from the standpoint of age at diagnosis. Over 70 per cent of the solid tumors were first detected in patients between 20 and 59 years of age. This is comparable to the distribution for the mixed thyroid lesions, which have the most favorable prognosis among the differentiated types. However, solid carcinoma has a significantly less favorable prognosis, as will be seen in the survival data which follow.

SURVIVAL BY HISTOLOGY

The current status of the study sample is summarized in Table 4. In Table 5 deaths from thyroid cancer and from all other causes are analyzed by histology in the 221 deceased patients in the series. The 119 patients who succumbed to their disease represent 53.8 per cent of total deaths. With percentages calculated on the basis of total deaths within each differentiated category, follicular carcinoma again appears to have the least favorable prognosis with 43 per cent of patients dead of their disease, compared to 29 per cent of those with papillary tumors and 27 per cent of those with mixed carcinomas. Of the eight deaths among patients with Hürthle cell carcinoma, five, or 62.5 per cent, were due to the disease. Among the differentiated tumors with anaplastic change, 95 per cent of deaths were from the disease. In patients with solid carcinoma, 28 of 36 deaths (80 per cent) were caused by the tumors. While more than 50 per cent of the deaths in this series were attributed to primary thyroid disease,

TABLE 4.—DEATHS IN SERIES OF 777 PATIENTS

	NUMBER OF PATIENTS	PER CENT
Total Series	777	100.0
Living	556	71.6
Deceased	221	28.3
Deceased of thyroid cancer	119	15.3 (of series)
		53.8 (of deceased)
Deceased of thyroid cancer within five years of diagnosis	77	09.9 (of series)
		34.8 (of deceased)

TABLE 5.—CAUSES OF DEATH IN 221 DECEASED PATIENTS OF 777 PATIENTS
WITH PRIMARY THYROID CARCINOMA

HISTOLOGY (TOTAL PATIENTS)		TOTAL DEATHS	% BY HISTOLOGY	THYROID CANCER[*]		ALL OTHER CAUSES
				Patients	% of Deceased by Histology	
Differentiated Carcinoma						
Follicular	(96)	30	31.2	13	43.3	17
Papillary	(115)	27	23.6	8	29.6	19
Mixed	(416)	69	16.2	19	27.5	50
Hürthle cell	(16)	8	50.0	5	62.5	3
Anaplastic change in differentiated tumors	(47)	42	89.2	40	95.1	2
Solid Carcinoma	(70)	36	51.3	28	80.0	8
(Cases being reviewed)	(17)	9	52.2	6	66.7	3
Total	777	221	28.3	119	53.8	102

[*]Includes 12 patients probably dead of thyroid cancer.

the 119 deceased represent only approximately 15 per cent of the 777 patients.

Pathologic Anatomy of Primary Thyroid Carcinoma

DIFFERENTIATED THYROID CARCINOMA

The tumors in this category replicate the various phases and degrees of differentiation seen in the follicular anlage cells carried to the neck by the thyroglossal duct. Solid masses and sheets of cells may be interspersed between differentiating cells forming papillations or follicles or both. These varying patterns give rise to the four subtypes used to classify differentiated thyroid carcinoma at this institution (Table 1). This classification, with the distinct separation of differentiated carcinomas from solid carcinoma, was developed on the basis of whole-organ studies of excised glands from patients with primary thyroid carcinoma (Russell, Ibanez, Clark, and White, 1963) and from individual studies of selected tumor types (Albores-Saavedra *et al.*, 1964; Ibanez *et al.*, 1966; Ibanez, Cole, Russell, and Clark, 1967; Russell *et al.*, 1969a; and Russell *et al.*, 1969b).

The histologic characteristics of the four subtypes of differentiated carcinoma will be discussed individually, with consideration of anaplastic transformation observed in each type.

FOLLICULAR CARCINOMA.—This type has a propensity for metastasizing to bone, frequently from an occult primary tumor in the gland. The primary site may be encapsulated and difficult to distinguish histologically from an adenoma (Figs. 1 and 2). These tumors are composed of replicating differentiated thyroid follicles which may vary in size from microfollicles to large, colloid-filled macrofollicles. These tumors show the highest degree of differentiation of all the differentiated types. In fact, it may be impossible to distinguish neoplastic from normal follicles if the specimen is observed out of context without knowledge of stromal invasion or without information that the tissue actually represents an extraglandular metastasis (Figs. 3 and 4).

Both follicular and papillary thyroid carcinoma may contain scattered solid masses and sheets of cells. These areas represent the solid phase of each type which will eventually show follicular or papillary differentiation. These areas are not to be confused with solid thyroid carcinoma which has a distinct histologic pattern and histogenesis (Russell *et al.*, 1969b).

Transformation of follicular thyroid carcinoma to the anaplastic phase

FIG. 1.—Large section of the left lobe of a thyroid gland showing primary follicular carcinoma replacing a portion of the lobe. A broad fibrous capsule surrounds the lesion (hematoxylin and eosin, × 2). (Courtesy of Russell *et al.*, 1969.)

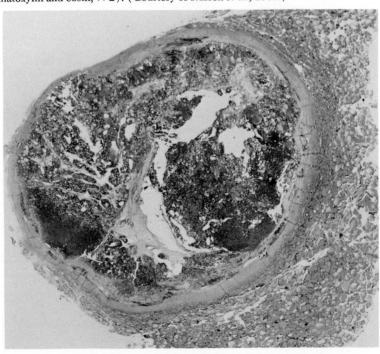

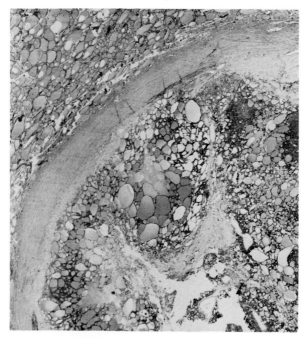

Fig. 2.—Higher magnification of Figure 1 showing the fibrous capsule composed of lamellar connective tissue surrounding masses of normal-appearing differentiated thyroid follicles, resembling those seen outside the capsule. This tumor had metastasized to the right humerus and produced the mass illustrated in Figures 3 and 4 (hematoxylin and eosin, × 9). (Courtesy of Russell *et al.*, 1969.)

has been well demonstrated by the whole-organ serial sectioning technique (Russell, Ibanez, Clark, and White, 1963) and further discussed in a review of this subtype (Russell *et al.*, 1969a). The sequence of transformation begins with the appearance of atypical follicular cells with altered nuclear chromatin and greatly increased numbers of mitotic figures. In approximately 50 per cent of tumors, these atypical cells will next show squamoid differentiation and finally, a totally disorganized, highly anaplastic neoplasm will emerge which bears no morphologic resemblance to the former follicular lesion.

Slightly more than 10 per cent of patients with follicular thyroid carcinoma developed anaplastic change. This percentage is more than double the rate of change seen for the other two major subtypes of differentiated tumors and is consistent with the less favorable prognosis for follicular carcinoma demonstrated by data on survival (Russell *et al.*, 1969b).

PAPILLARY CARCINOMA.—This type of tumor is composed of replicating

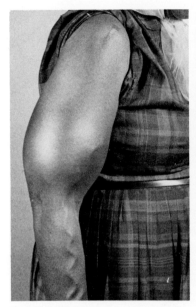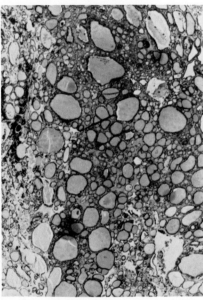

FIG. 3 (*left*).—Patient with metastatic thyroid carcinoma in right arm. The flail limb has a pathologic fracture in the midportion of the humerus and prominent distended veins resulting from obstruction by the metastatic tumor. (See also Figure 1B, Hill, this volume.)

FIG. 4 (*right*).—Photomicrograph of the biopsy specimen taken from the pathologic fracture. The well-differentiated follicles resemble normal thyroid tissue with histologic patterns similar to those seen in the primary lesion shown in Figure 2 (hematoxylin and eosin, × 80). (Courtesy of Russell *et al.*, 1969.)

follicular-type cells growing in fronds and cords which rarely form colloid. These cells closely resemble the papillary parenchymal cells seen in developing thyroid tissue. They are columnar, and the majority have round to oval nuclei with slightly granular cytoplasm. A rare follicle may be formed but usually these tumors are composed entirely of papillary growth. A loose, inconspicuous, fibrous supporting stroma accompanies these tumors which, in the fronds, may show edematous change (Fig. 5). Compared to follicular carcinoma, primary papillary tumors generally are larger and may replace a considerable portion of the gland (Fig. 6). These tumors frequently metastasize to regional lymph nodes, lungs, and liver.

In contrast to follicular thyroid carcinoma, the papillary lesions are always readily identifiable as neoplastic, but they may be confused with primary papillary tumors of other organs such as ovary, kidney, or lung.

In papillary carcinoma, anaplastic transformation follows the same sequence as described for follicular carcinoma—atypical cells with altered nuclear chromatin, numerous mitotic figures, optional squamoid phase, and ultimately, total, highly anaplastic dedifferentiation. In the M. D. Anderson Hospital series, 4 per cent of the papillary thyroid tumors showed anaplastic change.

MIXED FOLLICULAR AND PAPILLARY CARCINOMA.—This type generally shows diffuse involvement of the gland with early and massive extension to the deep cervical lymph nodes (Fig. 7). Microscopically these tumors are composed of follicles and papillations growing in a continuous intermingled pattern (Fig. 8). Degrees of differentiation may vary from typical papillations to fully mature follicles with colloid and vacuoles in juxtaposition between cells and colloid. This mixed growth of two morphologic types of differentiating cells corresponds to the known sequence of development of thyroid parenchyma from papillations and follicles. Whereas exhaustive sampling and studies of other areas are required to establish an

FIG. 5.—High power photomicrograph of primary papillary carcinoma of the thyroid gland with branching fronds of loose connective tissue covered by low cuboidal cells. A small follicle is formed with a trace of colloid indicated by the arrow (hematoxylin and eosin, $\times$ 100).

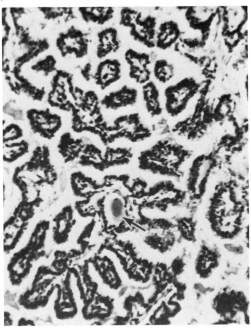

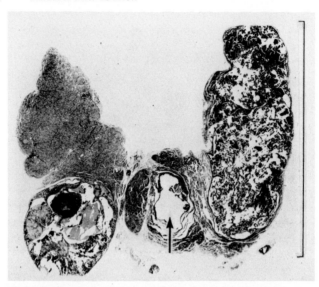

Fig. 6.—Whole-organ section of thyroid gland with the right lobe entirely replaced by papillary carcinoma. The mass in the isthmus (arrow) is metastatic tumor with cystic change. The lower part of the left lobe is displaced by a large macro- and micro-follicular adenoma. Despite massive replacement of the right lobe, no papillary carcinoma was found in subserial sections of the left lobe (hematoxylin and eosin, × 2.5).

unequivocal diagnosis of the pure papillary or pure follicular thyroid carcinomas, one specimen showing intermingled growth of both types is all that is necessary to establish the diagnosis of a mixed thyroid tumor.

Development of anaplastic change in mixed tumors is in all respects identical to that observed in the pure follicular and pure papillary types. The incidence of anaplastic transformation was only 3.8 per cent in patients with mixed thyroid tumors, which is slightly lower than for the other differentiated lesions. The mixed forms also are associated with the most favorable prognosis, as previously noted in discussion of survival.

HÜRTHLE-CELL CARCINOMA.—This carcinoma is composed of round, oval, or polygonal cells with eosinophilic cytoplasm (Fig. 9). The cells may grow in cordlike trabecular patterns or form alveolar arrangements. The vascular stroma has a conspicuous endocrine-like pattern with close relationships between the individual cells and the vascular endothelium. The tumor cells may show foci of differentiation to small follicles lined with cuboidal cells; they may store small amounts of atypical-appearing colloid substances.

Hürthle cells have a characteristic ultrastructural pattern showing large mitochondria filling the cytoplasm (Fig. 10). This feature is seen in both

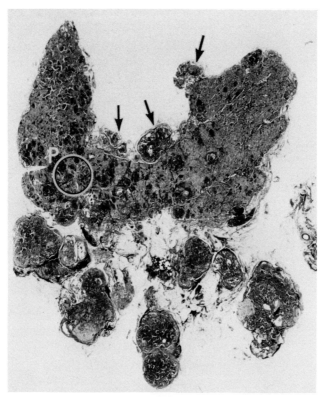

Fig. 7.—Whole-organ section of thyroid gland with deep cervical lymph nodes attached. Mixed follicular and papillary carcinoma is seen as the darker stained areas throughout both lobes and the isthmus. The heaviest concentration of tumor with stromal reaction is in the lower pole of the left lobe (white circle). This area is interpreted as the most likely primary site (P). Metastases in pericapsular lymph nodes are marked by arrows. The eight deep cervical lymph nodes (lower portion of specimen) are diffusely involved with tumor. Lymphoid tissue is replaced by the metastases which are forming follicles and papillations. This is an exceptionally clear demonstration of extensive dissemination of mixed carcinoma to all parts of the gland, the pericapsular and the deep cervical lymph nodes on both sides (hematoxylin and eosin, ×2.7).

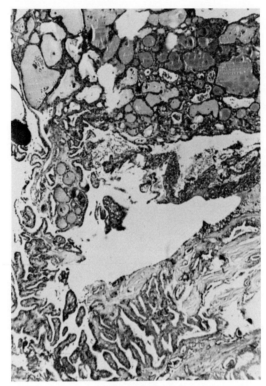

FIG. 8.—Pure follicular and pure papillary patterns as well as intermingled growth are shown in this high power photomicrograph of a section from the right lobe of a thyroid gland. The upper right half of the field is composed of closely packed follicles filled with colloid of varying staining qualities. Characteristic papillary patterns are seen in the lower portion. Transition from follicles to papillations is evident in the central area (hematoxylin and eosin, × 90).

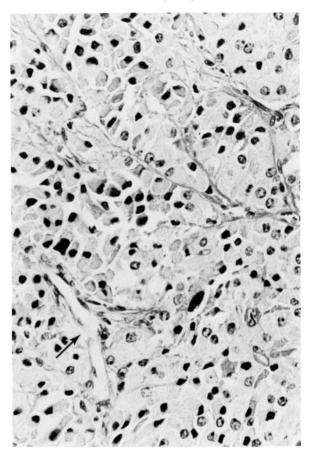

FIG. 9.—High power photomicrograph of Hürthle-cell carcinoma showing cuboidal or polygonal cells arranged in cords separated by thin strands of connective tissue. These strands are connected with thin-walled blood spaces typical of most endocrine tissues (*arrow*). Hyperchromatic irregular giant nuclei are seen in the central and midleft areas, exhibiting cytologic evidence of a malignant state (hematoxylin and eosin, × 150).

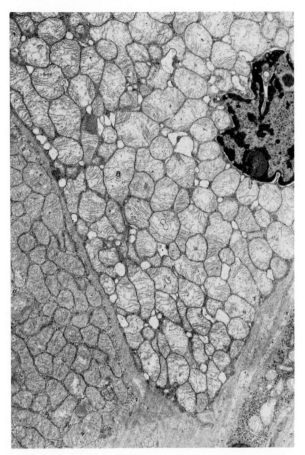

FIG. 10.—Electron micrograph showing mitochondria characterizing Hürthle cells. The nucleus in the upper right field is surrounded by large, closely packed mitochondria filling the cytoplasm to the nuclear membrane. Similarly arranged mitochondria appear in cells adjacent to the nuclear membrane (× 26,000).

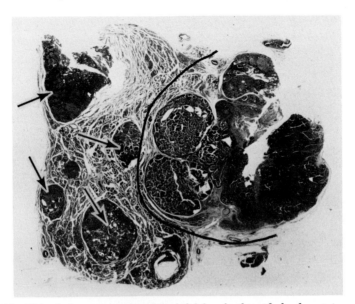

Fig. 11.—This whole-organ section of the left lobe of a thyroid gland contains multiple cellular masses including adenomas (arrows). The largest mass outlined on the right is Hürthle-cell carcinoma with anaplastic change. The homogeneous, deeply stained portion of the mass (right) represents anaplastic carcinoma. Differentiated Hürthle-cell carcinoma is seen as the two lobulated granular areas to the left (hematoxylin and eosin, × 2.5). (Courtesy of Russell, Ibanez, Clark, and White, 1963.)

the benign Hürthle cell adenomas and in the Hürthle-cell carcinomas, so it cannot be used as a basis for establishing the benign or malignant nature of a lesion. Nevertheless, electron microscopy can aid in identifying the cell type in small biopsy specimens.

Thus, differentiation between Hürthle-cell adenoma and carcinoma may be difficult on the basis of morphology alone because no completely distinguishing histologic criteria have been established. Observations such as absence of capsule, intraglandular dissemination, extension beyond the capsule, and metastases to lymph nodes or parenchymatous organs may be required for definitive diagnosis of the malignant lesion. Figure 11 illustrates the lobe of a gland with multiple adenomas, Hürthle-cell carcinoma, and anaplastic transformation.

Hürthle-cell carcinoma develops the same sequential changes to the anaplastic form as have been described for the other subtypes of differentiated thyroid lesions. Two of the 18 patients with Hürthle-cell carcinoma developed anaplastic changes. This yields an incidence of approximately

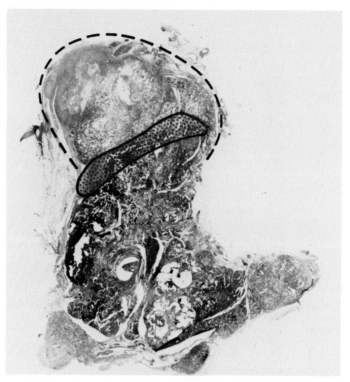

Fɪɢ. 12.—This large section shows the left lobe of the thyroid gland and part of the isthmus largely replaced by tumor. The area in the superior pole of the lobe indicated by the broken line shows a homogeneously cellular mass expanding the lobe beyond the normal configuration. The stippled area marks a broad zone of transition between mixed carcinoma and anaplastic tumor with squamoid growth (hematoxylin and eosin, × 2.5).

12 per cent, but these figures are too small for meaningful comparison with incidence of anaplasia in the other subtypes of differentiated thyroid carcinoma.

Aɴᴀᴘʟᴀsᴛɪᴄ ᴛʀᴀɴsғᴏʀᴍᴀᴛɪᴏɴ.—Anaplastic transformation in primary differentiated thyroid carcinomas has been conclusively demonstrated by whole-organ subserial sectioning techniques. Sequential development of anaplastic transformation in a mixed carcinoma is shown in a large section of a lobe in Figure 12. Direct transformation to anaplastic disease was observed in approximately half of these tumors. A final phase of this type of direct transformation of follicles to anaplastic carcinoma is seen in Figure 13. In the tumors showing an intermediate phase of squamoid metaplasia,

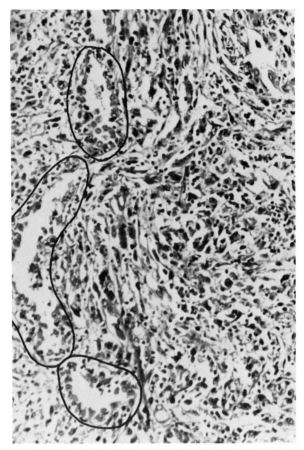

FIG. 13.—High power photomicrograph illustrating transformation of follicles to anaplastic carcinoma with conspicuous loss of most formed structures. The remaining poorly formed follicles are outlined in three areas to the left. Most of the section shows total disorganization of malignant cells with hyperchromatic nuclei and manifest pleomorphism (hematoxylin and eosin, × 100).

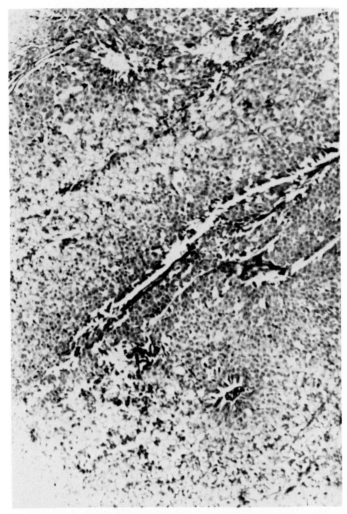

FIG. 14.—Squamoid phase of transformation to anaplastic carcinoma. Squamoid cells are differentiating from the more deeply stained basal zone in the central area of the photomicrograph. Immediately adjacent to the area from which this section was taken, follicles and papillations undergoing atypical change could be found, as well as the typically disorganized, bizarre patterns characterizing complete anaplasia (hematoxylin and eosin, × 150).

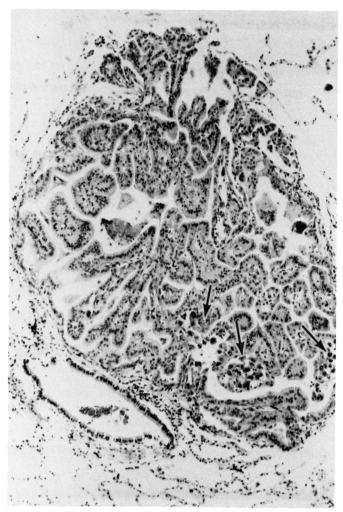

Fig. 15.—Photomicrograph of metastatic papillary thyroid carcinoma in the lung, showing marked atypical cellular changes. The tall, irregular epithelium has many pleomorphic hyperchromatic nuclei. Three foci of anaplastic change with giant cells and bizarre nuclei are indicated by arrows. This section demonstrates direct transformation of papillations to anaplastic carcinoma in a metastatic site without the intermediate phase of squamoid metaplasia (hematoxylin and eosin, × 175).

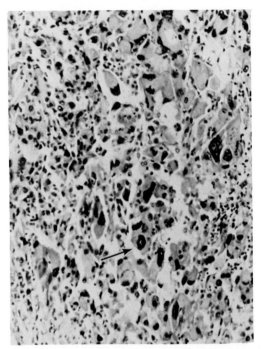

F<small>IG</small>. 16.—The typical morphologic patterns of anaplastic thyroid carcinoma demonstrate giant cells with enlarged nuclei mixed with smaller pleomorphic cells. Lethal forms are represented by the giant cells with huge, bizarre, hyperchromatic nuclear masses. An atypical mitotic figure is marked by the arrow (hematoxylin and eosin, × 175).

the atypical follicles and papillations dedifferentiate to anaplastic carcinoma. The squamoid phase is illustrated in Figure 14.

Anaplastic change has been observed in metastatic foci of differentiated thyroid carcinoma 20 years after removal of the gland. The metastatic papillary lesion in the lung illustrated in Figure 15 progressed directly to anaplasia without an intermediate squamoid phase. The highly malignant pattern of anaplastic thyroid carcinoma characterized by extreme cellular pleomorphism, giant cells with bizarre hyperchromatic nuclear masses, and atypical mitotic figures is shown in Figure 16.

S<small>OLID</small> T<small>HYROID</small> C<small>ARCINOMA</small>

These tumors are composed of cells which vary remarkably in form and arrangement. Subtyping these various patterns has been attempted on a

purely morphologic basis, but no meaningful relationship to biological behavior has been established. These tumors infiltrate all parts of the gland
and, similarly to the differentiated tumors, metastasize to the pericapsular
and deep cervical lymph nodes (Fig. 17).

The cells may be oval and spindled and have giant nuclei. An organoid
pattern is consistently observed, suggesting paraganglioma, islet cell tumor
of pancreas, carcinoid tumor, or a pleomorphic neurogenic sarcoma (Fig.
18). True follicular or papillary structures are never seen. Pseudopapilla-
tions may be found, but they represent arrangements of cells on tufts of
stroma rather than primary papillary growth. In keeping with their previously discussed histogenesis from the parafollicular cells of neural crest
derivation, ganglion-like cells with dendritic processes can be identified
by special staining. Dispersion of groups of cells by the characteristic
fibrous stroma associated with solid carcinoma produces the organoid
neurogenic appearance.

Amyloid produced by the cells (Fig. 19) is eventually extruded and
may be found in the connective tissue septa (Albores-Saavedra *et al.*,

Fig. 17.—Solid carcinoma shown in whole-organ section of thyroid gland with deep
cervical lymph nodes attached. The right lobe is largely replaced with tumor which extends beyond the capsule to invade two deep cervical nodes. Two pericapsular lymph
nodes on the superior aspect of the isthmus are filled with tumor (arrows) (hematoxylin
and eosin, × 1.5).

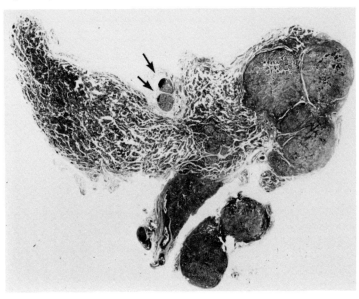

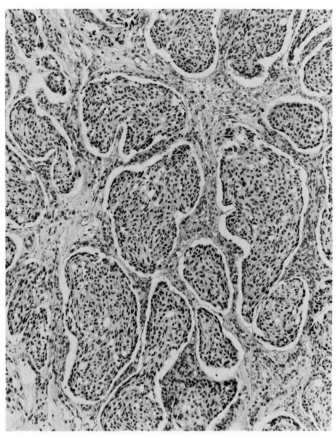

Fig. 18.—The organoid pattern of solid thyroid carcinoma is shown in this low power photomicrograph. Connective tissue septa divide groups of cells into compartments (hematoxylin and eosin, × 100).

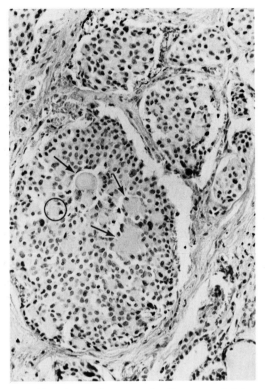

Fig. 19.—The organoid patterns of groups of cells surrounded by connective tissue shown at higher power. Irregular oval masses of hyalin material represent amyloid (arrows). A tumor cell with intracytoplasmic amyloid has a pyknotic nucleus pushed laterally (circle) (hematoxylin and eosin, × 180). (Courtesy of Ibanez, Cole, Russell, and Clark, 1967).

1964). Although occasionally the amyloid may be difficult to identify, with intensive study it has been found in every solid thyroid tumor in this series. Characteristic secretory granules have been demonstrated by electron microscopy (Meyer and Abdel-Bari, 1968; Braunstein, Stephens, and Gibson, 1968).

The phenomenon of anaplastic change has not been observed in patients with solid carcinoma of the thyroid gland seen at this institution.

Comment

Four aspects of primary thyroid carcinoma which merit further discussion are: (1) intraglandular spread of the tumors and metastases to regional lymph nodes, (2) incidence and significance of bilaterality, (3) therapeutic significance of anaplastic transformation in differentiated carcinoma, and (4) infrequent precursor changes.

Intraglandular spread and metastases to regional lymph nodes were clearly demonstrated in the study of 80 thyroid glands by whole-organ subserial sectioning (Russell, Ibanez, Clark, and White, 1963). It was determined that metastases occurred in all parts of the gland in both principal types of thyroid carcinoma through the plexus of intraglandular lymphatics around the clusters of follicles. The first barrier limiting extraglandular spread of a primary lesion was shown to be the thyroid capsule with its lymphatic network and small pericapsular lymph nodes illustrated in Figure 20.

The mechanism of spread and the significance of the capsular lymphatics and pericapsular lymph nodes were particularly well illustrated in one case (Russell, Ibanez, Clark, and White, 1963). The primary lesion observed in the superior pole of one lobe was disseminated within that lobe. With subserial whole-organ sectioning, no tumor was found in the opposite lobe but metastasis was detected in a pericapsular lymph node on the superior pole of the opposite lobe. The only routes of metastasis were through the intraglandular lymphatics across the isthmus or via the pericapsular lymphatics of the capsule. In any event, the clinical significance is obvious. Although the two lobes of the thyroid gland may be regarded as dual organs, the gland is, in fact, a single organ with a broad isthmus joining the two lobes. Metastases to either lobe may occur through the intraglandular lymphatic system, across the isthmus, or through the pericapsular lymphatics and lymph nodes (Clark, White, and Russell, 1959; Clark, Russell, and Ibanez, 1960; Rose et al., 1963; Clark, White, Russell, and Ibanez, 1965).

The incidence of bilateral involvement has direct bearing on decisions as to what constitutes adequate, successful surgical treatment for thyroid carcinoma. The problem of contralateral lobe or lymph node involvement has been carefully considered in the various studies of patients with primary thyroid carcinoma seen at this institution. The initial evaluation was based on observations in 50 thyroid glands studied by the whole-organ technique; bilateral involvement was found in 44 (88 per cent) of the glands (Clark, White, and Russell, 1959; Clark, Russell, and Ibanez, 1960).

These findings were further substantiated in a study of 138 patients treated by total thyroidectomy; 60 of the glands removed were examined by whole-organ techniques and routine pathologic procedures were performed in 78. Bilateral involvement was found in 53 (88 per cent) of the 60 glands studied by whole-organ subserial sectioning. Routine sectioning

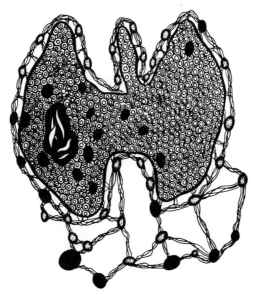

Fig. 20.—Diagram of intraglandular thyroid lymphatics. The lymph vessels are united in a network around the follicles, penetrate the capsule, and merge with the pericapsular lymph nodes, forming a plexus on the surface of the gland. The large black and white area on the left represents a primary carcinoma. From this site, the tumor spreads via the lymphatics to all parts of the gland and to the pericapsular and deep cervical lymph nodes, represented by the black areas. (Courtesy of Russell, Ibanez, Clark, and White, 1963.)

procedures demonstrated only 31 per cent bilateral involvement in the other 78 glands (Clark, 1961).

Another related study concerned 116 patients treated by total lobectomy on the affected side only, the majority of whom had undergone an operation elsewhere and subsequently were referred to this institution. In 34 of these patients, prophylactic removal of the remaining lobe of the thyroid gland was performed, and cancer was found in 61.7 per cent of the resected contralateral lobes. The other 82 patients were closely followed up, and in 27, masses subsequently developed necessitating resection of the remaining lobes. In other words, cancer was demonstrated in the contralateral lobes of 41 of the 116 patients, and the incidence of bilateral involvement was increased when resected lobes were examined by the whole-organ technique (Rose *et al.*, 1963).

In a review of 218 patients with primary thyroid carcinoma treated by total thyroidectomy, whole-organ studies showed bilateral involvement in 78.4 per cent of 102 glands, and routine pathologic procedures demonstrated bilateral involvement in 37.1 per cent of 116 glands (Clark, White, Russell, and Ibanez, 1965).

The general conclusion to be drawn from these studies is that bilateral involvement is sufficiently frequent to indicate total thyroidectomy as the treatment of choice for primary carcinoma of the gland. This is further supported by the known tendency of differentiated thyroid cancer of many years' duration to undergo malignant transformation.

Anaplastic change in differentiated thyroid carcinoma is a unique phenomenon in human neoplastic disease, representing the transformation of a relatively indolent tumor to what probably is the most rapidly growing human neoplasm. Moreover, with extremely rare exceptions, it is universally fatal and fails to respond to any of the available modalities of treatment, which means prevention is the only means of control.

As of January 1972, the M. D. Anderson Hospital series included 60 patients with anaplastic thyroid carcinoma (data in Tables 1 to 5 are based on the computer analysis of August 1971). In more than 80 per cent of these patients, the precursor differentiated thyroid tumor was identified. For 11 patients, the available histological materials were inadequate for detection of the antecedent lesion.

Some of the 60 patients were known to have thyroid carcinoma for as long as 20 years before anaplastic change occurred. The only way this fatal complication could have been prevented would have been total extirpation of the differentiated lesion.

The decision to remove immediately every thyroid nodule must be considered in the light of several factors—availability of appropriate medical facilities and surgical competence, age of the patient, and duration of the thyroid enlargement. Anaplastic carcinoma is a disease of older patients (Table 3), with 96 per cent of lesions being diagnosed in patients over 40 years of age and 59 per cent in the sixth to eighth decades. This appears to indicate the advisability of total removal of all thyroid masses detected in patients over age 40, giving the various temporizing factors less consideration with advancing age of the patients.

Precursor changes were rarely observed in this series of 777 patients with primary thyroid tumors. This factor distinguishes thyroid carcinoma from malignant lesions of many other anatomic sites where some antecedent phase of hyperplasia or atypical cellular changes usually are seen in the normal tissue elements before overt malignancy occurs. For example, adenomatous hyperplasia precedes carcinoma of the endometrium, and intraductal hyperplasia is associated with the development of breast cancer. Also, some benign tumors such as adenomatous polyps of the colon are known to precede the malignant state. In this context, thyroid adenomas might be expected to represent the precursor phase of differentiated carcinomas in this gland. However, in the cases of papillary and mixed thyroid lesions no precursor relationships with adenomas have been observed in this series. Even with whole-organ studies which provide three-dimensional observations from subserial sections, no association with previously existing adenomas could be detected for these two major subtypes of differentiated thyroid carcinoma (Russell, Ibanez, Clark, and White, 1963). Moreover, in studying primary tumors with foci as small as 2 mm. in diameter, no adenomatous precursor lesion or atypical cellular changes could be found in the tissue surrounding the tumor (Ibanez *et al.*, 1966). Therefore, based on present observations, papillary and mixed differentiated carcinomas apparently arise *de novo* in thyroid parenchyma.

Occasionally, an area of an encapsulated follicular carcinoma will closely resemble an adenoma, but a direct precursor relationship has not been clearly established. In Hürthle cell carcinoma, sequential developmental changes, with transitional phases from true adenomas to carcinoma and further malignant transformation to anaplastic carcinoma (Fig. 11) have been observed within a single gland (Russell, Ibanez, Clark, and White, 1963).

In solid carcinoma, the second major type of malignant thyroid tumor, no precursor changes have been observed in patients seen at this institution. Williams (1966) reported association with hyperplasia in his study of 24 spontaneously occurring rat thyroid tumors interpreted to be solid carcinoma; however, no similar observations have been described in man.

Association of solid carcinoma with follicular cell adenomas has not been seen in the M. D. Anderson Hospital series. Moreover, solid carcinoma has not been observed intermingled with a differentiated thyroid tumor, although two patients had both solid and differentiated carcinoma occurring as entirely separate and discrete primary lesions within the gland.

Thus, the distinctions between the differentiated thyroid lesions and solid carcinoma are further emphasized, reinforcing the concept that these two groups must be considered as histogenetically, biologically, and clinically separate neoplastic entities which apparently share no common factor beyond their origin in the parenchymal components of the thyroid gland.

Summary

Based on continuing clinicopathologic studies of 777 patients with primary thyroid carcinoma, including whole-organ subserial sectioning of 160 glands, a more workable classification of these tumors has been developed. Malignant neoplasms arising in the functional parenchymal components of the gland are divisible into two histogenetically, morphologically, and clinically distinct categories.

Differentiated carcinoma, with four subtypes, typifies the classical image of thyroid cancer, demonstrating all the varying degrees of differentiation of the follicular cells. All these tumors (follicular, papillary, mixed, and Hürthle cell) have the potential for transformation to anaplastic carcinoma.

Solid carcinoma, composed of pleomorphic, poorly differentiated cells, has no generally recognized, clinically significant subtypes. The tumors are characterized by amyloid formation, calcitonin production, and frequent association with genetically determined benign and malignant lesions. Anaplastic change has not been observed in solid carcinoma.

Anaplastic carcinoma of the thyroid gland, probably the most malignant tumor afflicting human beings, is not classified as a separate type because it represents highly malignant transformation of a precursor differentiated tumor. The anaplastic form is rapidly fatal and does not respond to any of the available modalities of therapy; prevention by early removal of the differentiated carcinoma is presently the only means of control.

In this series of 777 patients, 670 (89 per cent) had differentiated thyroid carcinoma; 47 of the tumors (6.8 per cent) developed anaplastic change. The 70 patients with solid carcinoma represented approximately 9 per cent of the series. Of the 777 patients, 556 are living. Thyroid cancer was cause of death in 53.8 per cent of deceased patients, representing 15 per cent of the total series.

Papillary and mixed differentiated carcinomas, as well as solid carcinoma, apparently arise *de novo* in the thyroid parenchyma. No adenomatous precursor lesions or atypical premalignant cellular changes have been observed with these tumors. However, with Hürthle cell carcinoma, sequential developmental changes from adenoma to carcinoma and anaplastic transformation have been observed within a single gland (Fig. 11). Occasionally, an area within an encapsulated follicular carcinoma will present the morphologic patterns of an adenoma but a definite precursor relationship has not yet been established.

Despite its anatomic structure formed of two lobes, the thyroid gland must be considered as a single organ with potential for metastasis to either lobe through the intraglandular lymphatic system or through the pericapsular lymphatics and lymph nodes.

Conclusions

Primary carcinomas arising from the follicular or the parafollicular cells of the thyroid parenchyma are divisible histogenetically, morphologically, and clinically into two separate types: (1) Differentiated thyroid carcinoma, which typifies the classical image of thyroid carcinoma, develops from follicular cells of thyroglossal duct derivation. The four subtypes of differentiated tumors, follicular, papillary, mixed, and Hürthle cell carcinoma, including those which develop anaplastic change, comprise approximately 90 per cent of all primary thyroid cancers seen in this series of 777 patients. Anaplastic carcinomas develop from precursor differentiated tumors and probably are the most malignant neoplasms afflicting human beings. Removal of the differentiated tumor before transformation appears to be the only means of controlling this highly malignant disease which fails to respond to any of the present therapies.

(2) Solid thyroid carcinoma is a functioning, calcitonin-producing tumor derived from parafollicular cells of neural crest origin incorporated in the gland from the ultimobranchial bodies. This tumor type was observed in approximately 10 per cent of the patients in this study. Solid carcinoma is frequently associated with various genetically determined benign and malignant conditions. Anaplastic transformation has not been observed in these tumors. In patients with solid carcinoma, the mortality rate from the disease is more than twice that observed for patients with differentiated carcinoma, including those with anaplastic transformation.

REFERENCES

Albores-Saavedra, J., Rose, G. G., Ibanez, M. L., Russell, W. O., Grey, C. E., and Dmochowski, L.: The amyloid in solid carcinoma of the thyroid gland. Staining characteristics, tissue culture, and electron microscopic observations. *Laboratory Investigation*, 13:77-93, January 1964.

Arey, L. B.: Developmental Anatomy: *A Textbook and Laboratory Manual of Embryology*. 7th edition. Philadelphia, Pennsylvania, W. B. Saunders Company, 1965, 695 pp.

Block, M. A., Horn, R. C., Jr., Miller, J. M., Barrett, J. L., and Brush, B. E.: Familial medullary carcinoma of the thyroid. *Annals of Surgery*, 166:403-412, September 1967.

Braunstein, H., Stephens, C. L., and Gibson, R. L.: Secretory granules in medullary carcinoma of the thyroid. Electron microscopic demonstration. *Archives of Pathology*, 85:306-313, March 1968.

Clark, R. L., Jr.: Intraglandular dissemination of thyroid cancer. In *Fourth National Cancer Conference Proceedings*. Philadelphia, Pennsylvania, J. B. Lippincott Company, 1961, pp. 665-668.

Clark, R. L., Jr., Russell, W. O., and Ibanez, M. L.: Cancer of the thyroid. Treatment by total thyroidectomy: Clinicopathologic considerations. *Acta Unio internationalis contra cancrum*, 16(6):1425-1433, 1960.

Clark, R. L., Jr., White, E. C., and Russell, W. O.: Total thyroidectomy for cancer of the thyroid. Significance of intraglandular dissemination. *Annals of Surgery*, 149:858-866, June 1959.

Clark, R. L., White, E. C., Russell, W. O., and Ibanez, M. L.: Clinicopathologic studies in 218 total thyroidectomies for thyroid cancer. In Cassano, C., and Andreoli, M., Eds.: *Current Topics in Thyroid Research*, New York, New York, and London, England, Academic Press, 1965, pp. 1045-1050.

Eisenberg, A. A., and Wallerstein, H.: Pheochromocytoma of the suprarenal medulla (paraganglioma): A clinicopathologic study. *Archives of Pathology*, 14: 818-836, June 1932.

Fries, J. G., Chamberlin, J. A., and Vandivier, T. G.: Primary fibrosarcoma of the thyroid. *Texas State Journal of Medicine*, 57:981-982, December 1961.

Gonzalez-Licea, A., Hartmann, W. H., and Yardley, J. H.: Medullary carcinoma. Ultrastructural evidence of its origin from the parafollicular cell and its possible relation to carcinoid tumors. *The American Journal of Clinical Pathology*, 49(4):512-520, April 1968.

Hazard, J. B., Hawk, W. A., and Crile, G., Jr.: Medullary (solid) carcinoma of the thyroid—a clinicopathologic entity. *The Journal of Clinical Endocrinology and Metabolism*, 19:152-161, January 1959.

Ibanez, M. L., Cole, V. W., Russell, W. O., and Clark, R. L.: Solid carcinoma of the thyroid gland: Analysis of 53 cases. *Cancer*, 20(5):706-723, May 1967.

Ibanez, M. L., Russell, W. O., Albores-Saavedra, J., Lampertico, P., White, E. C., and Clark, R. L.: Thyroid carcinoma—biologic behavior and mortality. Postmortem findings in 42 cases, including 27 in which the disease was fatal. *Cancer*, 19(8):1039-1052, August 1966.

Johnston, M. C.: A radioautographic study of the migration and fate of cranial neural crest cells in the chick embryo. *Anatomical Record*, 156:143-156, October 1966.

Le Douarin, N., and Le Lievre, C.: Demonstration of the neural origin of the cells producing calcitonin in the ultimobranchial body in the chick embryo. *Comptes Rendus Hebdomadaires des Séances de l'Académie des Sciences*, 270: 2857-2860, June 1970 (in French).

Ljungberg, O., Cederquist, E., and von Studnitz, W.: Medullary thyroid carcinoma and phaeochromocytoma: A familial chromaffinomatosis. *British Medical Journal*, 1:279-281, February 4, 1967.

Meyer, J. S., and Abdel-Bari, W.: Granules and thyrocalcitonin-like activity in medullary carcinoma of the thyroid gland. *The New England Journal of Medicine*, 278:523-529, March 7, 1968.

Prakash, A., Kukreti, S. C., and Sharma, M. P.: Primary squamous cell carcinoma of the thyroid gland. *International Surgery*, 50:538-541, December 1968.

Rose, R. G., Kelsey, M. P., Russell, W. O., Ibanez, M. L., White, E. C., and Clark, R. L.: Follow-up study of thyroid cancer treated by unilateral lobectomy. *The American Journal of Surgery*, 106:494-500, September 1963.

Russell, W. O., Ibanez, M. L., Clark, R. L., and White, E. C.: Thyroid carcinoma. Classification, intraglandular dissemination, and clinicopathological study based upon whole organ sections of 80 glands. *Cancer,* 16:1425-1460, November 1963.

Russell, W. O., Ibanez, M. L., Clark, R. L., Hill, C. S., Jr., and White, E. C.: Follicular (organoid) carcinoma of the thyroid gland. Report of 84 cases. In Hedinger, C. E., Ed.: *Thyroid Cancer,* UICC Monograph Series. Vol. 12, New York, New York, Springer-Verlag, 1969a, pp. 14-25.

Russell, W. O., Ibanez, M. L., Hill, C. S., Jr., Clark, R. L., and White, E. C.: Papillary and follicular thyroid carcinoma: Prognostic significance of type variation in 97 of 116 primary tumors studied by whole organ sections. In Young, S., and Inman, D. R.: *Thyroid Neoplasia.* London, England, and New York, New York, Academic Press, 1969b, pp. 109-133.

Schimke, R. N., Hartmann, W. H., Prout, T. E., and Rimoin, D. L.: Syndrome of bilateral pheochromocytoma, medullary thyroid carcinoma and multiple neuromas. A possible regulatory defect in the differentiation of chromaffin tissue. *The New England Journal of Medicine,* 279:1-7, July 4, 1968.

Sipple, J. H.: The association of pheochromocytoma with carcinoma of the thyroid gland. *The American Journal of Medicine,* 31:163-166, July 1961.

United States Department of Health, Education and Welfare: *Morbidity From Cancer In the United States,* Public Health Monograph No. 56, Washington, D. C., 1959, pp. 52-53.

Warren, S., and Meissner, W. A.: Tumors of the Thyroid Gland. In *Atlas of Tumor Pathology* Section IV-Fascicle 14, Washington, D. C., Armed Forces Institute of Pathology, 1953, 97 pp.

Williams, E. D.: Histogenesis of medullary carcinoma of the thyroid. *Journal of Clinical Pathology,* 19:114-118, March 1966.

Williams, E. D., Brown, C. L., and Doniach, I.: Familial syndromes associated with medullary carcinoma of the thyroid. In Cassano, C., and Andreoli, M., Eds.: *Current Topics in Thyroid Research, The Fifth International Thyroid Conference.* New York, New York, and London, England, Academic Press, 1965, pp. 1020-1022.

Williams, E. D., and Pollock, D. J.: Multiple mucosal neuromata with endocrine tumours: A syndrome allied to von Recklinghausen's disease. *The Journal of Pathology and Bacteriology,* 91(1):71-80, January 1966.

Trophoblastic Disease: Diagnosis and Management

JULIAN P. SMITH, M.D.

Department of Surgery, The University of Texas at Houston
M. D. Anderson Hospital and Tumor Institute,
Houston, Texas

TROPHOBLASTIC NEOPLASMS represent a complete spectrum of malignant diseases, beginning with the completely benign hydatidiform mole at one end, the occasionally malignant invasive mole in the middle, and choriocarcinoma, which is possibly the most malignant of all solid tumors, at the other end of the spectrum.

Because trophoblastic neoplasms are uncommon, few physicians have had the experience of treating more than an occasional patient with this disease. Patients with trophoblastic disease frequently are either undertreated since the attending physician may forget completely the potential for malignant transformation after the immediate problems of hemorrhage and passage of the hydatidiform mole have been managed, or the patient is overtreated with unnecessary surgical procedures and/or chemotherapy. Nevertheless, trophoblastic neoplasms hold special interest for physicians who treat women during their reproductive years. The anxiety that accompanies the severe vaginal bleeding that almost always occurs with the expulsion of a hydatidiform mole is followed by the specter of potential malignant disease.

Hydatidiform Mole

The incidence of hydatidiform mole varies throughout the world (Table 1). The incidence of hydatidiform moles is approximately 1 in every 1,700 deliveries in the United States or 1 of every 2,000 pregnancies. The incidence of choriocarcinoma is approximately 1 in every 50,000 pregnancies. Approximately one half of all choriocarcinomas occur after hydatidiform moles, one-fourth after incomplete abortions, and one-fourth after term

TABLE 1.—INCIDENCE OF HYDATIDIFORM MOLE

COUNTRY	INCIDENCE	AUTHOR
U.S.A.	1:1,500 pregnancies	Goldstein and Reid (1967)
	1:1,699 deliveries	Brewer and Gerbie (1967)
	1:2,093 pregnancies	
Great Britain	1:835 pregnancies	Das (1938)
Australia	1:695 pregnancies	Beischer and Fortune (1968)
France	1:500 pregnancies	Brindeau *et al.* (1952)
Mexico	1:200 pregnancies	Marquez-Monter *et al.* (1963)
Philippines	1:173 pregnancies	Acosta-Sison (1959)
Taiwan	1:120 pregnancies	Wei-Ouyang (1963)

pregnancies. Since choriocarcinoma may evolve from a benign mole, prevention of this malignant change by early diagnosis, adequate treatment, and careful follow-up of all hydatidiform moles is important.

DIAGNOSIS

The diagnosis of hydatidiform mole can usually be made by a combination of clinical signs, laboratory tests, and roentgenographic examinations (Table 2).

The most important clinical sign is vaginal bleeding. This almost always is associated with lower abdominal pain or discomfort. Approximately 50 per cent of the patients with hydatidiform moles have a uterus that is larger than would be expected for the length of pregnancy, and 25 per

TABLE 2.—DIAGNOSIS OF MOLAR PREGNANCY

Clinical
  Vaginal bleeding
  Lower abdominal pain
  Uterine size larger than gestational dates
  Absent fetal heart tones
  Early toxemia
  Uterus probes easily

Laboratory
  HCG greater than 500,000 I.U./L.
  Absent fetal heart by ECG
  Absent fetal heart by electrical amplification
  Ultrasound sonogram of uterus

Radiographic
  Pelvic roentgenogram
  Pelvic arteriography
  Amniography

cent have a uterus that is smaller than expected. The absence of fetal heart tones in a patient with a uterus that is larger than 20 weeks' gestational size or the presence of hypertension or albuminuria in a previously normal pregnant woman before the third trimester is suggestive of a mole. The passage of vesicular placenta tissue is pathognomonic of a mole.

The several laboratory tests that may be helpful in diagnosing a hydatidiform mole include urinary or serum assays of chorionic gonadotropin (HCG), fetal electrocardiograms, and ultrasound sonograms of the uterus. A pelvic roentgenogram may demonstrate the presence or absence of fetal skeleton after 16 to 18 weeks of gestation. A pelvic arteriogram may demonstrate the multiple vesicles present in the uterus or the characteristic vascular pattern of the hydatidiform or invasive mole. Pelvic arteriograms, however, are seldom used to diagnose a suspected mole because of the high dose of radiation that might be given to a normal fetus with the multiple exposures. The injection of 15 to 20 cc. of water-soluble radiopaque material into the uterine cavity through the lower abdominal wall, followed by a roentgenogram of the pelvis, frequently will show the typical moth-eaten or vesicular pattern of a hydatidiform mole. This is a safe, easy, and highly reliable examination in patients with suspected moles.

Another simple but often forgotten test for diagnosing a hydatidiform mole consists of gently probing the cervix. The amniotic sac in an intact pregnancy will provide resistance to the probe; however, the small vesicles of a hydatidiform mole will allow the probe to easily pass through the uterus to the top of the fundus.

TREATMENT

When the diagnosis of hydatidiform mole is established, preparation should be made for immediate evacuation of the uterus. If the uterus is under 12 to 14 weeks' gestational size, the mole can be evacuated by dilatation of the cervix and curettage of the uterus with an oxytocin infusion during curettage. A suction evacuation is equally effective with early moles and can be performed when the uterus is at the level of the umbilicus or larger, if adequate facilities are available for rapid transfusion of blood and if the uterus is stimulated by a continuous infusion of dilute intravenous oxytocin.

If facilities for suction curettage are not available, or if distant metastases are present and the uterus is too large to be safely evacuated by curettage, a hysterotomy should be performed. The possibility of perforation of the uterus in an area of choriocarcinoma in the myometrium may, on occasion, outweigh the ease of evacuation of the uterus from below.

The role of prophylactic chemotherapy both before and after evacuation of a hydatidiform mole is unsettled. If facilities are available for accurate determination of HCG in either the serum or urine, it is difficult to justify treating all patients with moles with prophylactic chemotherapy. Eight of 10 patients with hydatidiform mole will have a fall of their HCG titer to normal values within eight weeks after expelling a mole, leaving only 20 per cent of the patients with an abnormal HCG assay (Delfs, 1959). Only 10 per cent of the total number of patients with hydatidiform moles will develop malignant changes to either an invasive mole or choriocarcinoma. Since these patients can be detected by frequent HCG assays, it is not reasonable to give potentially toxic medications, such as methotrexate or actinomycin D, to all patients with hydatidiform moles when only 20 per cent of the patients will have abnormal HCG titers eight weeks after expelling a mole and only 50 per cent of these patients will have an invasive mole or choriocarcinoma.

Following evacuation of the mole, the patient should have HCG assays performed each week until the titers begin to fall. Titration then should be performed again in two weeks and if levels continue to fall, should be repeated every month for at least one year. The patient should be instructed to avoid pregnancy during this time. Combination birth control pills are an excellent way of preventing pregnancy while the patient is being observed after hydatidiform mole. These pills suppress the pituitary gonadotropins so that the assays performed will measure only gonadotropins from the trophoblast and the gonadotropin assay will not show the cyclic variation of the normally menstruating woman.

In every patient who has passed a mole, the uterus should be curetted with a sharp curette. The mole and the curettage specimen should be examined by the pathologist. The uterine contents may contain fragments of myometrium and may allow the pathologist to make a diagnosis of invasive mole or, rarely, choriocarcinoma.

Invasive Mole and Choriocarcinoma

Chorionic Gonadotropin in Trophoblastic Disease

The availability of an accurate quantitative assay of HCG either in the serum or urine is necessary for the diagnosis and management of invasive moles and choriocarcinoma. HCG has been called a "tumor specific index" (Bagshawe and Wilde, 1965). It accurately reflects the number of growing and proliferating trophoblasts and serves as a guide to the duration and effectiveness of treatment.

The quantitative methods of HCG assay that are available include pregnancy tests such as the biological tests using the frog or toad and the immunological test utilizing HCG-coated tanned red cells. The pregnancy tests using the female frog or male toad are not satisfactory for following up patients with trophoblastic disease. The semiquantitative immunological pregnancy test can be utilized when the patient is receiving chemotherapy. This test, however, is not accurate enough for patients with low titers of gonadotropin to follow minimal disease or to follow patients who are in remission of their disease as a result of chemotherapy.

The quantitative bioassays on 24-hour urine collections have been the standard HCG assays in the United States for managing patients with metastatic trophoblastic disease or persistent trophoblastic disease after hydatidiform mole. The quantitative bioassay is performed on a concentrated 24-hour urine specimen or a serum sample and requires approximately 4 to 5 days.

The radioimmune assay of HCG has been used in the Southwestern Trophoblastic Disease Center at The University of Texas at Houston M. D. Anderson Hospital and Tumor Institute. It is a very sensitive assay and has been entirely satisfactory. During the first year that the radioimmunoassay was performed in this laboratory, all patients were studied simultaneously with both bioassays and radioimmunoassays for HCG. The results were identical, so the slower and more cumbersome bioassay has been abandoned.

The radioimmunoassay for HCG as currently used at M. D. Anderson Hospital is capable of detecting 0.07 I.U./ml. of serum or urine and can be performed in eight hours. The results of the assay are expressed in international units of HCG per liter of serum, since this figure represents the approximate value that would be found in 1 L. of urine, a value which closely approximates the 24-hour urine excretion.

DIAGNOSIS

Although there is considerable disagreement among pathologists about the histological diagnosis of trophoblastic tumors, the only differentiation that need be made for the clinician who treats patients with these tumors is the distinction between metastatic and nonmetastatic tumors. This does not mean that the prognosis for the invasive mole is as bleak as the prognosis for choriocarcinoma, but rather that the treatment depends on whether the patient has metastatic or nonmetastatic disease and not on the histologic diagnosis.

TREATMENT

Of all the malignant diseases that are treated with chemotherapy, possibly none requires more expertise than metastatic trophoblastic disease. Metastatic trophoblastic disease is extremely rare and few physicians outside of cancer treatment centers have had the occasion to treat more than one or two patients with this disease. Unfortunately, the high reported success rate, the apparent good health, and the young age of patients tempt the physician to treat these patients despite his meager experience.

NONMETASTATIC TUMORS.—Patients with nonmetastatic trophoblastic tumors are curable by hysterectomy, and practically all are curable by chemotherapy. Patients who are more than 35 years of age, those who have completed their family and have persistent nonmetastatic trophoblastic disease eight weeks or more after expelling a mole, or those who have a histological diagnosis of choriocarcinoma after a mole, abortion, or pregnancy should undergo a hysterectomy. Patients who are under 35 or who desire more children can be satisfactorily treated with chemotherapy.

METASTATIC TUMORS.—Patients with metastatic trophoblastic tumors should be treated by chemotherapy and should have a hysterectomy only when the metastatic lesions have disappeared after chemotherapy and when there is reason to believe that there is persistent unresponsive tumor in the uterus. An occasional patient with metastatic trophoblastic neoplasms will require a hysterectomy because of severe bleeding or infection.

There is some evidence that trophoblastic neoplasms can progress from a less malignant to a more malignant state. In six patients treated at the National Institutes of Health who had a histological diagnosis of invasive mole and died of their disease, four had only choriocarcinoma in their metastases at autopsy (Hertz, Lewis, Lipsett, 1961).

The chemotherapeutic drugs which are useful in the treatment for trophoblastic tumors include methotrexate, actinomycin D, and a combination of actinomycin D, methotrexate, and chlorambucil. In England and in China, 6-mercaptopurine has been used to manage this disease. Vinblastine was used at the National Institutes of Health in the early 1960's, but it is seldom effective in tumors that are resistant to methotrexate; 6-diazo-5-oxo-L-norleucine has also been used, but it is ineffective in patients with metastatic trophoblastic disease.

Methotrexate has been the drug of choice in treating patients with trophoblastic tumors in the United States. It is usually given in doses of 20 to 30 mg. intramuscularly daily for 5 days, and these five-day courses of treatment are repeated as soon as the toxicity from the previous course of chemotherapy has subsided. Methotrexate produces complete remissions in approximately 50 per cent of patients with metastatic tumors. It should not be given to patients with decreased renal function or hepatic disease.

Actinomycin D is the second drug of choice in patients with trophoblastic disease; it is useful in treating patients with liver or renal disease and is effective in treating patients who are not responding to methotrexate or who have growing disease despite treatment with methotrexate. The usual dose of actinomycin D is 7 to 12 μg./kg. body weight intravenously daily for 5 days. These 5-day courses of chemotherapy are repeated as soon as all evidence of toxicity from the previous course of chemotherapy has subsided. Actinomycin D will produce a complete remission in approximately 40 to 50 per cent of patients with metastatic trophoblastic disease. It is effective in treating patients who are resistant to methotrexate, and when used following methotrexate, the two drugs produced a complete remission in 74 per cent of patients treated at the National Institutes of Health (Hertz, 1967).

Patients who do not respond to either methotrexate or actinomycin D may respond to a combination of methotrexate, actinomycin D, and chlorambucil. The methotrexate is given in doses of 5 mg./day orally for 25 days; chlorambucil is given in doses of 10 mg./day orally for 25 days; actinomycin D is given at the dosage of 0.5 mg./day intravenously for five days starting on day 3, 12, and 21 (Li, 1961). This is an extremely toxic combination and must be used with great care in patients who have received previous chemotherapy.

ALTERNATE SEQUENTIAL CHEMOTHERAPY WITH METHOTREXATE AND ACTINOMYCIN D

Since 1965, at M. D. Anderson Hospital, patients with trophoblastic tumors who receive chemotherapy have been treated with alternate sequential methotrexate and actinomycin D (Table 3). All patients receive methotrexate as the first drug at a dosage of 15 to 30 mg./day intravenously for five days. All patients receive 25 mg./day with the first course of chemotherapy. Approximately three to five days after completing the methotrexate the patient is given actinomycin D 0.5 mg./day intravenously for five days, if there is no evidence of stomatitis or gastrointestinal ulceration, the white blood cell count is above 3,000, and the platelet count is above 150,000. As soon as all evidence of toxicity from the actinomycin D has subsided, the methotrexate is started again. All patients are given one course of either methotrexate or actinomycin D after the gonadotropin

TABLE 3.—ALTERNATE SEQUENTIAL THERAPY FOR
TROPHOBLASTIC TUMORS

DRUG[*]	DOSAGE
Methotrexate	15 to 30 mg. intravenously daily for five days
Actinomycin D	0.5 mg. intravenously daily for five days

[*]The drugs are given sequentially and alternately as soon as the oral and hematological toxicity from the preceding drug has subsided.

titer has returned to normal. The HCG titers are followed weekly for three weeks, then every two weeks, and finally every month for 12 months if the titers remain normal.

The methotrexate is given intravenously because there is some evidence that in other neoplasms intravenous methotrexate is more effective than oral or intramuscular medication. The intravenous medication is better tolerated than oral or intramuscular methotrexate, causing fewer severe toxic reactions. This combination of drugs given alternately and sequentially is well tolerated and allows a maximum amount of medication to be given in the minimum amount of time, thereby utilizing the sensitivity of the tumor to both of these medications before it can develop resistance. This treatment plan takes advantage of the slightly different mode of action and different toxicity of these two drugs and allows a larger number of courses of medication to be given in a shorter period of time than if the two medications were given separately.

Results of Chemotherapy of Trophoblastic Tumors

METASTATIC TUMORS

Since 1961, 37 patients with metastatic trophoblastic tumors have been seen at M. D. Anderson Hospital. Five of these patients will be excluded from the discussion of results. Three of the five were treated before referral to this hospital and had growing tumors; another died in a coma on the day of admission and the fifth, who was admitted in pulmonary failure from extensive pulmonary metastases, died on her fifth hospital day. These five patients all died of their disease or their treatment.

Thirty-two patients with metastatic trophoblastic disease received all their treatment at M. D. Anderson Hospital. Of these patients, 19 had a histological diagnosis of choriocarcinoma and 13 had a diagnosis of invasive mole or were presumed to have an invasive mole since tissue was not available to make the diagnosis of choriocarcinoma. Of these 32 patients,

24 had pulmonary metastases, six had vaginal metastases, five had an elevated HCG titer after abdominal hysterectomy, one had tumor in the bladder, and one had brain metastases.

Hertz (1967) has reported that the two most important prognostic factors in determining the results of chemotherapy for patients with metastatic trophoblastic disease were the time interval from the antecedent pregnancy to the onset of treatment for metastatic trophoblastic disease and the chorionic gonadotropin titer at the time treatment was instituted. Patients who were treated less than four months after a prior pregnancy had an 85 per cent complete remission rate with chemotherapy, and patients who were treated more than four months afterwards had 61 per cent survival. Bagshawe (1971) reported 95 per cent survival in patients who were treated less than six months after their prior pregnancy, 70 per cent survival in patients treated six to 12 months after pregnancy, and only 30 per cent survival in patients treated more than 24 months after their antecedent pregnancy.

The results of treatment of the 32 patients are detailed in Table 4 by interval from pregnancy to treatment. The pregnancy-treatment interval varied from one week to 30 months, with the average interval being five months. Eight patients were treated more than five months after their preceding pregnancy. Only one patient of the 32 failed to achieve a complete remission with chemotherapy; this patient was treated two months after a term delivery.

The chorionic gonadotropin titers varied from 1,000 to 3,100,000 I.U./L. of serum, 14 of the 32 patients having titers greater than 100,000 I.U./L. of serum. The only patient who did not achieve a complete remission with chemotherapy had a titer of less than 100,000 I.U./L. of serum when her treatment was started (Table 5). This patient was the only patient in this series who died. She was referred to M. D. Anderson Hospital several weeks after a normal vaginal delivery. A choriocarcinoma of the cervix was thought to be an undifferentiated squamous carcinoma. After four weeks of X-ray therapy, she developed multiple large pulmonary metasta-

TABLE 4.—RESULTS OF TREATMENT FOR METASTATIC
TROPHOBLASTIC NEOPLASMS

START OF THERAPY	NUMBER OF PATIENTS	COMPLETE REMISSIONS
Less than four months from gestation to treatment	21	95%
Greater than four months from gestation to treatment	11	100%
Totals	32	97%

TABLE 5.—HCG TITERS AS RELATED TO TREATMENT FOR
METASTATIC TROPHOBLASTIC NEOPLASMS

TITER LEVEL	NUMBER OF PATIENTS	COMPLETE REMISSIONS
HCG greater than 100,000 I.U./L. serum	14	100%
HCG less than 100,000 I.U./L. serum	18	95%
Totals	32	97%

ses. Her failure to respond to chemotherapy is possibly related to her prior radiation treatment.

The patients treated before 1965 received single-agent chemotherapy, always starting with methotrexate. They required two to 18 courses of chemotherapy with a mean of 5.2 courses before the HCG titers were normal. Their HCG titers returned to normal after two to 19 weeks of treatment, with the mean treatment time of nine weeks.

Since 1965, all patients have been treated with alternate sequential methotrexate and actinomycin D. These patients have required one to seven courses of chemotherapy, with the average patient requiring 3.3 courses before her HCG titers were normal. The treatment was given over one to nine weeks, with a mean treatment of 5.6 weeks.

NONMETASTATIC TUMORS

The results of chemotherapy in patients with nonmetastatic trophoblastic disease are seen in Table 6. The histological diagnoses of these 18 patients were: choriocarcinoma (1), invasive mole (4), and hydatidiform moles with persistently elevated HCG titers more than eight weeks after termination of a molar pregnancy (13). The HCG titers in these patients varied from 200 to 220,000 I.U./L. of serum, and they were seen from two weeks to eight months after expelling a hydatidiform mole.

All were treated with alternative sequential methotrexate and actinomy-

TABLE 6.—RESULTS OF TREATMENT FOR NONMETASTATIC
TROPHOBLASTIC NEOPLASMS

HISTOLOGICAL DIAGNOSIS	NUMBER OF PATIENTS	COMPLETE REMISSIONS
Hydatidiform mole	12	100%
Invasive mole	5	100%
Choriocarcinoma	1	100%
Totals	18	100%

TABLE 7.—Triple Therapy for Trophoblastic Tumors

Drug	Dosage
Actinomycin D	0.5 mg. intravenously daily for five days*
Methotrexate	10 to 15 mg. orally daily for five days
Cytoxan	150 to 250 mg. orally daily for five days

*The five-day courses of treatment are repeated as soon as the oral and hematological toxicity from the preceding treatment has subsided.

cin D. They required from one to seven courses of chemotherapy before their titers returned to normal, with the average patient receiving 2.2 courses. The treatment time varied from two to eight weeks, with a mean treatment time of 3.4 weeks.

Only one patient among the 32 patients with metastatic disease and none of the patients with nonmetastatic disease has had recurrence of tumor after completing treatment. This one patient had normal titers for three months before her recurrence was discovered. She had complete remission of her disease after three courses of triple therapy with five-day courses of actinomycin D, methotrexate, and cyclophosphamide (Table 7).

Thirty-eight patients with metastatic trophoblastic disease who were treated by outside physicians have been followed with HCG titers at the Southwestern Trophoblastic Disease Center at M. D. Anderson Hospital. Many of these patients were treated under the direction of the Center, but other patients were treated by an outside physician without advice or recommendations. Of these patients, 29 per cent have died of their disease, and a similar percentage have not attained a complete remission.

It is tragic that any physician with limited experience in chemotherapy for metastatic trophoblastic tumors would undertake to treat these young, potentially curable patients when facilities are easily available in the several centers throughout the country. The 29 per cent death rate in these patients is inexcusable. Doctor Brewer, in a similar study at Northwestern Trophoblastic Disease Center in Chicago, Illinois, has reported that 14 of 65 patients with metastatic trophoblastic disease treated by inexperienced physicians outside the Trophoblastic Disease Center at Passavant Memorial Hospital died of their disease, and 22 failed to achieve a complete remission of their disease and were referred to the Center for treatment.

Ovarian Choriocarcinoma

Ovarian choriocarcinoma is a very rare tumor of the ovary. Only three patients with ovarian choriocarcinoma have been found in more than 1,800

TABLE 8.—Nongestational Trophoblastic Neoplasms

Pathology	Metastases	Remarks	Results
Pure choriocarcinoma	Rapidly rising HCG titer after operation	Complete response	Living and well
Embryonal carcinoma, dysgerminoma teratoma, choriocarcinoma	Pulmonary metastases hepatic metastases	Complete response followed by rising HCG titers	Dead
Gonadoblastoma, choriocarcinoma	Brain, omentum	Intestinal obstruction	Dead

patients with ovarian cancer at M. D. Anderson Hospital. One of these patients had choriocarcinoma in association with a gonadoblastoma; one had choriocarcinoma in combination with embryonal carcinoma, dysgerminoma, and other elements of a malignant teratoma; the third patient had a pure choriocarcinoma. Choriocarcinoma of the ovary has been reported to be unresponsive to chemotherapy; however, three of four patients treated at the National Institutes of Health had complete remission of their cancer after treatment with actinomycin D, methotrexate, and chlorambucil (Wider *et al.*, 1969). All three of the patients at the M. D. Anderson Hospital have received similar treatment. Two of the three patients are dead of their disease; however, the third patient has had a complete remission (Table 8).

Summary

1. Hydatidiform moles occur in approximately 1 of 1,500 pregnancies in the United States, and approximately 10 per cent of the patients with moles will have malignant changes in their tumors.

2. Metastatic trophoblastic disease is highly curable by experienced physicians who have adequate laboratory facilities available for performing HCG assays and who are experienced in the chemotherapy and have knowledge of the natural history of this disease.

3. Nonmetastatic trophoblastic disease is 100 per cent curable. Most patients can be cured with chemotherapy without loss of their childbearing potential.

4. An accurate, readily available HCG assay is essential to adequately manage patients with trophoblastic disease.

5. Alternate sequential chemotherapy of metastatic trophoblastic dis-

ease with methotrexate and actinomycin D is more effective than use of single drugs.

6. Ovarian choriocarcinoma can be effectively treated with triple chemotherapy utilizing methotrexate, actinomycin D, and chlorambucil.

Acknowledgments

This investigation was supported by United States Public Health Services Research Grants No. 73965, 06-H-000 and 004-03-0.

REFERENCES

Acosta-Sison, H.: The chance of malignancy in a repeated hydatidiform mole. *American Journal of Obstetrics and Gynecology*, 78:876-877, October 1959.

Bagshawe, K. D.: The treatment of trophoblastic tumors. In Dealey, T. J., Ed.: *Modern Radiotherapy of Gynecological Cancer*. London, England, Butterworths, 1971, pp. 228-242.

Bagshawe, K. D., and Wilde, C. E.: Some aspects of the excretion of gonadotrophic hormones by patients with trophoblastic tumors. *Journal of Obstetrics and Gynecology of the British Commonwealth*, 72:59-64, February 1965.

Beischer, N. A., and Fortune, D. W.: Significance of chromatin patterns in cases of hydatidiform mole with an associated fetus. *American Journal of Obstetrics and Gynecology*, 100:276-282, January 15, 1968.

Brewer, J. I., and Gerbie, A. B.: Early development of choriocarcinoma. In Holland, J. F., and Hreshchyshyn, M. M., Eds.: *Choriocarcinoma, Transactions of a Conference of the International Union Against Cancer*. Berlin, Germany, Springer-Verlag, 1967, pp. 45-53.

Brindeau, A., Hinglais, A., and Hinglais, M.: La mole hydatiforme. *Bulletin de la Fédération des Sociétés de Gynécologie et d'Obstétrique de Langue Française*, 4:3-36, 1952.

Das, P. C.: Hydatidiform mole: A statistical and clinical study. *Journal of Obstetrics and Gynecology of the British Empire*, 45:265-280, April 1938.

Delfs, E.: Chorionic gonadotropin determinations in patients with hydatidiform mole. *Annals of the New York Academy of Sciences*, 80:125-135, 1959.

Goldstein, D. P., and Reid, D. E.: Recent developments in the management of molar pregnancy. *Clinical Obstetrics and Gynecology*, 10:313-322, June 1967.

Hertz, R.: Eight years experience with the chemotherapy of metastatic choriocarcinoma and related trophoblastic tumors in women. In Holland, J. F., and Hreshchyshyn, M. M., Eds.: *Choriocarcinoma*. U.I.C.C. Monograph Series III, Berlin, Germany, Springer-Verlag, 1967, pp. 66-71.

Hertz, R., Lewis, J. L., and Lipsett, M. B.: Five years experience with the chemotherapy of metastatic choriocarcinoma and related trophoblastic tumors in women. *American Journal of Obstetrics and Gynecology*, 82:631-640, September 1961.

Li, M. C.: Management of choriocarcinoma and related tumors of uterus and testis. *Medical Clinics of North America*, 45:661-676, May 1961.

Marquez-Monter, H., Alfara de la Vegga, G., Robles, M., and Bolio-Cicero, A.: Epidemiology and pathology of hydatidiform mole in the General Hospital of Mexico: study of 104 cases. *American Journal of Obstetrics and Gynecology,* 85:856-864, April 1, 1963.

Wei, P.-Y., and Ouyang, P.-C.: Trophoblastic disease in Taiwan: A review of 157 cases in a 10 year period. *American Journal of Obstetrics and Gynecology,* 85:844-849, April 1, 1963.

Wider, J. A., Marshall, J. R., Bardin, C. W., Lipsett, M. B., and Ross, C. T.: Sustained remissions after chemotherapy for primary ovarian cancers containing choriocarcinoma. *The New England Journal of Medicine,* 280:1439-1442, June 26, 1969.

Hormone Production by Testicular Tumors

EMIL STEINBERGER, M.D., AND
KEITH D. SMITH, M.D.

*Program in Reproductive Biology and Reproductive Endocrinology,
The University of Texas Medical School at Houston,
Houston, Texas*

THE TESTICLE has the capacity to give rise to a bewildering array of neoplasms. This is not surprising since it is composed of a number of different tissues. This heterogeneity has seriously hampered attempts to arrive at unanimity concerning classification of testicular tumors. The most widely accepted classifications are those used by the Testicular Tumor Registry of The Armed Forces Institute of Pathology (Dixon and Moore, 1952) and by the Testicular Tumor Panel and Registry of Great Britain and Ireland (Collins and Pugh, 1964). The former system will be followed in the subsequent discussion.

TABLE 1.—INCIDENCE OF TESTICULAR TUMORS

TYPE OF TUMOR	INCIDENCE PER CENT
Germinal tumors	
1. Seminoma	40
a. Typical	
b. Anaplastic	
c. Spermatocytic	
2. Embryonal carcinoma	15 to 20
3. Teratoma	1 to 5
4. Teratocarcinoma	20 to 25
5. Choriocarcinoma	1
6. Mixed tumor	15 to 20
Nongerminal tumors	1 to 2
1. Gonadal stromal tumors (mixtures of Sertoli, Leydig, and stromal cells)	
2. Interstitial cell tumors	

413

Tumors originating from the germinal cells of the testis comprise 97 per cent of this organ's neoplasms. The remaining 3 per cent originate from the nongerminal elements. The incidence of various types of testicular tumors is listed in Table 1. Testicular tumors of children differ from the adult neoplasms in their behavior and characteristics. They are usually divided into three groups: (1) teratoma, (2) embryonal carcinoma, and (3) gonadal stromal tumors. The embryonal carcinomas are highly malignant, while teratomas and gonadal stromal tumors are usually benign. Interstitial cell tumors are the most common of the latter group.

Hormone Production by Testicular Tumors

It is generally accepted that choriocarcinoma, a tumor originating from the germinal elements, and interstitial cell tumor, a neoplasm developing from the stromal tissue, are clearly hormone-producing neoplasms of the testis. The production of gonadotropins by other types of testicular tumors has been alluded to sporadically (Moormann and König, 1967). Except for rare cases of gynecomastia associated with these tumors, no systemic hormonal effects have been noted (Hobson, 1965). Consequently, little attention has been directed toward the possible significance of hormone production by these tumors.

Newer, more sensitive and more specific techniques have prompted re-evaluation of the question of hormone production by testicular tumors. Elevation of urinary gonadotropins in patients with seminoma and teratoma has been described (Symington and Wallace, 1964; Hobson, 1965). The gonadotropin elevation has been attributed to interference with the pituitary-gonadal axis secondary to testicular damage caused by the tumor (Symington and Wallace, 1964).

Recently, Wieland *et al.* (1969) described a patient with teratoma and embryonal carcinoma of the testis whose circulating levels of gonadotropin were only modestly elevated but whose testicular vein levels were extremely high. This finding provides direct evidence of gonadotropin secretion by a testicular tumor other than choriocarcinoma.

If it could be shown that most testicular tumors secrete significant amounts of gonadotropin, this would assume diagnostic importance and offer a sensitive laboratory parameter for follow-up of such patients.

CHORIOCARCINOMA

This testicular tumor is a highly malignant, hormone-producing neoplasm of germinal cell origin. Its capacity to produce massive quantities of human chorionic gonadotropin (HCG) has been utilized for years as both a diagnostic tool and a means of follow-up. The biologic parameters of the tumor HCG do not differ from those of placental HCG. Since HCG is capable of stimulating Leydig cell activity (Kirschner, Lipsett, and Collins, 1965), a notable increase of testosterone production would be expected in patients with this neoplasm. However, measurements of plasma testosterone in the peripheral and spermatic veins of patients with HCG-producing testicular tumors failed to reveal elevated levels of this hormone (Kirschner, Wider, and Ross, 1970). Furthermore, administration of HCG of placental origin, as well as purified tumor HCG, failed to increase plasma testosterone levels in these patients, while suppression of endogenous luteinizing hormone (LH) induced a significant drop in plasma testosterone levels. This drop could be reversed by HCG administration, but the presuppression levels of testosterone could not be exceeded (Kirschner, Wider, and Ross, 1970).

Despite normal testosterone levels in these patients, estrogen production and excretion were markedly elevated. This elevated level of estrogens may explain the gynecomastia frequently present in these patients. The estrogens probably do not originate in the testis, but most likely result from aromatization of dehydroepiandrosterone (DHEA) sulfate. The aromatization seems to occur in trophoblastic tissues, since in normal women and men, circulating DHEA sulfate is not readily converted to estrogens; however, during pregnancy rapid conversion does occur (MacDonald and Siiteri, 1965; Kirschner, Wiqvist, and Diczfalusy, 1966). Furthermore, tissue cultures of choriocarcinoma vigorously aromatize DHEA (Kohler, Bridson, Vanha-Parttula, and Hammond, 1969; Pattillo, Gey, Delfs, and Mattingly, 1969). The ability of the trophoblastic tumor to aromatize DHEA may become a sensitive tool for detection of small remnants of trophoblastic tissue after therapy.

Interstitial Cell Tumors

These rare tumors often present with gynecomastia in adult males and sexual precocity in prepubertal males. They are usually benign, invariably hormone producing, and difficult to differentiate from adrenal rest tumors on the basis of morphologic criteria. This is not surprising since both Leydig and adrenal cortical cells are closely related embryologically (Langman, 1969). Even the presence of crystalloids of Reinke (Reinke, 1896), characteristically Leydig cell inclusions, is not diagnostic since the crystalloids were also observed in a tumor with steroid biogenetic pathways characteristic of adrenal cortical tissue (Savard *et al.*, 1960). Conversely, in some classic Leydig cell tumors, crystalloids of Reinke could not be detected (Smith, Breuer, and Schriefers, 1964; Wegienka and Kolb, 1967; Gittes, Smith, Conn, and Smith, 1970).

Benign interstitial cell tumors produce testosterone and androstenedione as their major steroids and thus fit the classic biochemical parameters of Leydig cells. The malignant interstitial cell tumors more closely resemble adrenocortical carcinoma in their steroid biogenetic behavior (Engel *et al.*, 1964; Lipsett *et al.*, 1966). It has to be stressed that some benign interstitial cell tumors may also produce considerable amounts of C_{21} steroids of the adrenocortical series (Glenn and Boyce, 1962; Wegienka and Kolb, 1967). These tumors most likely have their origin in adrenal rests. Consequently, the pattern of steroid biogenesis of the interstitial cell tumors is not a reliable index to either their classification or their malignant behavior.

The occurrence of androgen-producing tumors in testes of prepubertal males provides a natural experiment to evaluate the local effects of androgens on the initiation of spermatogenesis in the human. The respective roles of androgens and gonadotropins in this process is unclear (Steinberger, 1971). For example, administration of testosterone to adult men results in atrophy of the seminiferous epithelium (Hotchkiss, 1944; Heller *et al.*, 1950). Its administration to hypogonadotropic eunuchs or to hypophysectomized men fails to induce or support the spermatogenic process. However, in certain lower species, after hypophysectomy, spermatogenesis may be maintained by systemic administration of high doses of testosterone or by implantation of testosterone-containing pellets into the testis (Ludwig, 1950; Dvoskin, 1944).

Initiation of spermatogenesis has been demonstrated recently in testes of prepubertal boys harboring Leydig cell tumors (Gittes, 1970; Steinberger, 1970) or Leydig cell hyperplasia (Bergada, 1970). In each instance, the unaffected testicle revealed immature seminiferous tubules. In one case (Steinberger, 1970), evaluation of the hormonal parameters revealed low levels of plasma gonadotropins and testosterone. The androstenedione was well above adult range. The spermatic vein draining the tumor-bearing testicle contained high concentrations of both testosterone and androstenedione. Incubation of the tumor tissue with appropriate radiolabeled precursors revealed an active androgen-biogenetic pathway (Steinberger *et al.*, submitted for publication).

These observations provide direct evidence for the role of testosterone in initiation of spermatogenesis in human testes. The apparent incongruity of the observations on the effects of systemic administration of testosterone in lower species and man could possibly be explained by the fact that in man, even the highest dose of systemically administered testosterone was not sufficient to create adequate local concentrations of this steroid in the seminiferous epithelium. If one calculates the equivalent dose for man compared to the rat in milligrams per kilogram of body weight, a 60-kg. man would require a daily dose of 300 to 1,000 mg. of testosterone propionate. To our knowledge, no attempt has ever been made to administer testosterone at this level to man.

Summary

1. A brief discussion of the classification of testicular tumors is presented.

2. Evidence of hormonal production by testicular tumors other than choriocarcinoma or interstitial cell tumor is reviewed.

3. It is pointed out that recently developed, highly sensitive techniques for determination of plasma gonadotropin levels have been instrumental in demonstrating gonadotropin production by a variety of testicular tumors. The application of this knowledge to routine follow-up of patients with testicular tumors is suggested.

4. Recent information on steroid metabolism by trophoblastic neoplasms has been summarized. The extraordinary capacity of trophoblastic tissue to aromatize DHEA may provide a much more sensitive technique for follow-up of patients with choriocarcinoma than does the presently utilized determination of HCG levels.

5. Androgen production by interstitial cell tumors and its effect on spermatogenesis is discussed.

Acknowledgments

Supported in part by a grant from the Ford Foundation and N.I.H. Grant H.D. 06316.

REFERENCES

Bergada, C.: Personal communication, 1970.

Collins, D. H., and Pugh, R. C. B.: Classification and frequency of testicular tumours. *British Journal of Urology*, (Supplement) 36:1-11, 1964.

Dixon, F. J., and Moore, R. A.: Tumors of the male sex organs. In *Armed Forces Institute of Pathology Atlas of Tumor Pathology*, Section 8, Part 31b and 32. Washington, D. C., Armed Forces Institute of Pathology, 1952, pp. 48-127.

Dvoskin, S.: Local maintenance of spermatogenesis by intratesticularly implanted pellets of testosterone in hypophysectomized rats. *American Journal of Anatomy*, 75:289-327, November 1944.

Engel, F. L., McPherson, H. T., Fetter, B. F., Baggett, B., Engel, L. L., Carter, P., Fielding, L. L., Savard, K., and Dorfman, R. I.: Clinical, morphological and biochemical studies on a malignant testicular tumor. *The Journal of Clinical Endocrinology and Metabolism*, 24:528-542, June 1964.

Gittes, R. F., Smith, G., Conn, C. A., and Smith, F.: Local androgenic effect of interstitial cell tumor of the testis. *Journal of Urology*, 104:774-777, November 1970.

Glenn, J. F., and Boyce, W. H.: Adrenogenitalism with testicular adrenal rests simulating interstitial cell tumor. *Transactions of American Association of Genito-Urinary Surgeons*, 54:59-66, 1962.

Heller, C. G., Nelson, W. O., Hill, I. B., Henderson, E., Maddock, W. O., Jungck, E. C., Paulsen, C. A., and Mortimore, G. E.: Improvement in spermatogenesis following depression of human testis with testosterone. *Fertility Sterility*, 1:415-422, September 1950.

Hobson, B. M.: The excretion of chorionic gonadotropin by men with testicular tumours. *Acta endocrinologica*, 49:337-348, July 1965.

Hotchkiss, R. S.: Effects of massive doses of testosterone propionate upon spermatogenesis. *The Journal of Clinical Endocrinology and Metabolism*, 4:117-120, March 1944.

Kirschner, M. A., Lipsett, M. B., and Collins, D. R.: Plasma ketosteroids and testosterone in man: A study of the pituitary-testicular axis. *The Journal of Clinical Investigation*, 44:657-665, April 1965.

Kirschner, M. A., Wiqvist, N., and Diczfalusy, E.: Studies on oestriol synthesis from dehydroepiandrosterone sulphate in human pregnancy. *Acta endocrinologica*, 53:584-597, December, 1966.

Kirschner, M. A., Wider, J. A., and Ross, G. T.: Leydig cell function in men with gonadotropin-producing testicular tumors. *The Journal of Clinical Endocrinology and Metabolism*, 30:504-511, April 1970.

Kohler, P. O., Bridson, W. E., Vanha-Perttula, T., and Hammond, J. M.: Isolation of hormone-producing clonal strains of human choriocarcinoma (Abstract). *Program of the Fifty-First Meeting of the Endocrine Society*, Abstract 44, 1969, p. 52.

Langman, J.: Special embryology. In *Medical Embryology*. 2nd edition. Baltimore, Maryland, The Williams and Wilkins Company, 1969, pp. 163-166, 329-332.

Lipsett, M. B., Sarfaty, G. A., Wilson, H., Bardin, C. W., and Fishman, L. M.: Metabolism of testosterone and related steroids in metastatic interstitial cell carcinoma of the testis. *The Journal of Clinical Investigation*, 45:1700-1709, November 1966.

Ludwig, D. J.: The effect of androgen on spermatogenesis. *Endocrinology*, 46: 453-481, May 1950.

MacDonald, P. C., and Siiteri, P. K.: Origin of estrogen in women pregnant with an anencephalic fetus. *The Journal of Clinical Investigation*, 44:465-474, March 1965.

Moormann, J. G., and König, K.: Diagnose und Klassifikation der malignen Hodentumoren. *Deutsche medizinische Wochenschrift*, 92:1502-1505, August 1967.

Pattillo, R. A., Gey, G. O., Delfs, E., and Mattingly, R. F.: Gonadotropin hormone specificity of the new trophoblast cell line (Abstract). *Program of the Fifty-First Meeting of the Endocrine Society*, Abstract 43, 1969, p. 52.

Reinke, F.: Beiträge zur Histologie des Menschen. I. Ueber Krystalloidbildungen in den interstitiellen Zellen des menschlichen Hodens. *Archiv für mikroskopische Anatomie*, 47:34-44, 1896.

Savard, K., Dorfman, R. I., Baggett, B., Fielding, L. L., Engel, L. L., McPherson, H. T., Lister, L. M., Johnson, D. S., Hamblen, E. C., and Engel, F. L.: Clinical, morphological and biochemical studies of a virilizing tumor in the testis. *The Journal of Clinical Investigation*, 39:534-553, March 1960.

Smith, E. R., Breuer, H., and Schriefers, H.: A study of the steroid metabolism of an interstitial cell tumour of the testis. *Biochemical Journal*, 93:583-587, December 1964.

Steinberger, E.: Discussion of Vilar, O.: Histology of the human testis from neonatal period to adolescence. In Rosenberg, E., and Paulsen, C. A., Eds.: *The Human Testes*. New York, New York, London, England, Plenum Press, 1970, p. 110.

————: Hormonal control of mammalian spermatogenesis. *Physiological Reviews*, 51:1-22, January 1971.

Steinberger, E., Ficher, M., Root, A. W., and Smith, K. D.: The role of androgens in the initiation of spermatogenesis in man. (Submitted for publication.)

Symington, T., and Wallace, N.: Hormone investigations in cases of testicular tumour. *British Journal of Urology*, (Supplement) 36:103-106, June 1964.

Tamm, J., Apostolakis, M., and Voigt, K. D.: The effects of ACTH and HCG on the urinary excretion of testosterone in male patients with various endocrine disorders. *Acta endocrinologica*, 53:61-72, September 1966.

Wegienka, L. C., and Kolb, F. O.: Hormonal studies of a benign interstitial cell tumour of the testis producing androstenedione and testosterone. *Acta endocrinologica*, 56:481-489, September 1967.

Wieland, R. G., Guevara, A., Hallberg, M. C., Zorn, E. M., and Pohlman, C.: Spermatic and peripheral venous levels of gonadotropin and testosterone in a teratoma with embryonal cell carcinoma. *The Journal of Clinical Endocrinology and Metabolism*, 29:398-400, March 1969.

Index

421